2025

ADVANCES IN
CLINICAL RADIOLOGY

AF903337

EDITOR-IN-CHIEF

Frank H. Miller, MD, FACR, FSAR, FSABI

SECTION EDITORS

Amichai J. Erdfarb, MD

Ankur Garg, MD, MBA

Edward Y. Lee, MD, MPH

Robert J. Lewandowski, MD, FSIR

ELSEVIER

Director, Continuity Publishing: Dolores Meloni
Editor: Stacy Eastman
Developmental Editor: Nitesh Barthwal

Publishing Office:
Elsevier Inc.
1600 John F. Kennedy Boulevard,
Suite 1600
Philadelphia, PA 19103
United States

International Standard Serial Number: 2589-8701
International Standard Book Number: 13: 978-0-443-41343-8

ADVANCES IN CLINICAL RADIOLOGY

EDITOR-IN-CHIEF

FRANK H. MILLER, MD, FACR, FSAR, FSABI
Lee F. Rogers MD Professor of Medical Education Chief, Body Imaging Section Medical Director, MRI Department of Radiology, Northwestern Memorial Hospital, Northwestern University Feinberg School of Medicine, Chicago, Illinois, USA

SECTION EDITORS

AMICHAI J. ERDFARB, MD
Chief of Radiology, NewYork-Presbyterian Hudson Valley Hospital Assistant Professor of Radiology, Division of Neuroradiology, Columbia University Irving Medical Center, New York, New York, USA

ANKUR GARG, MD, MBA
Vice Chair, Health Network Radiology Program Director, Diagnostic Radiology Residency Associate Program Director, Integrated Interventional Radiology Residency Associate Professor, Department of Radiology, Musculoskeletal Imaging Section, Northwestern University Feinberg School of Medicine, Chicago, Illinois, USA

EDWARD Y. LEE, MD, MPH
Director, Advanced Imaging Professor of Radiology, Departments of Radiology, Boston Children's Hospital and Harvard Medical School, Boston, Massachusetts, USA

ROBERT J. LEWANDOWSKI, MD, FSIR
Professor of Radiology, Medicine, and Surgery Director of Interventional Oncology, Northwestern University Feinberg School of Medicine, Chicago, Illinois, USA

CONTRIBUTORS

EDITOR

FRANK H. MILLER, MD, FACR, FSAR, FSABI
Lee F. Rogers MD Professor of Medical Education, Chief, Body Imaging Section, Medical Director, MRI, Department of Radiology, Northwestern Memorial Hospital, Northwestern University Feinberg School of Medicine, Chicago, Illinois, USA

AUTHORS

IAN S. ACKERS, DO, PhD
Resident, Adjunct Instructor, Department of Physical Medicine and Rehabilitation, Michigan State University, University of Michigan Health - Sparrow, Lansing, Michigan, USA

ULAS BAGCI, PhD
Professor, Department of Radiology, Northwestern Memorial Hospital, Northwestern University Feinberg School of Medicine, Chicago, Illinois, USA

KAREN BUCH, MD
Associate Professor, Department of Radiology, Massachusetts General Hospital, Boston, Massachusetts, USA

LUCAS BUCHLER, MD
Assistant Professor, Department of Orthopaedic Surgery, Northwestern University Feinberg School of Medicine, Chicago, Illinois, USA

JULIE C. BULMAN, MD, RPVI
Assistant Professor, Section of Interventional Radiology, Department of Radiology, Beth Israel Deaconess Medical Center, Harvard Medical School, Boston, Massachusetts, USA

GABRIEL ORTIZ CELEMIN, BA
Medical Student, Diagnostic Radiology Department, Northwestern University Feinberg School of Medicine, Chicago, Illinois, USA

PATRICK CHEUNG, MD, FRCPC
Professor, Department of Radiation Oncology, Sunnybrook Odette Cancer Centre, University of Toronto, Toronto, Ontario, Canada

NATHAN DAVID P. CONCEPCION, MD
Head and Assistant Head, Section of Pediatric Radiology, Institute of Radiology, St. Luke's Medical Center - Quezon City, Philippines; Global City, Taguig, Philippines; Immediate Past President, Philippine Society for Pediatric Radiology, Fellow, Philippine College of Radiology, Metro Manila, Philippines

ANIL K. DASYAM, MD
Professor, Department of Radiology, University of Pittsburgh Medical Center, Pittsburgh, Pennsylvania, USA

ADAM DELORA, MD
Neuro-Critical Care Fellow, Cerebrovascular Center, Neurological Institute, Cleveland Clinic, Cleveland, Ohio, USA

ALEXANDER DOUBEK, DO
Spine Medicine Fellow, Center for Spine Health, Neurological Institute, Cleveland Clinic, Cleveland, Ohio, USA

CHRISTOPHER G. FILIPPI, MD
Professor, Department of Radiology, Hospital for Sick Children, Toronto, Ontario, USA

JEREMY FORD, MD, MBA
Instructor, Department of Radiology, Massachusetts General Hospital, Boston, Massachusetts, USA

ANKUR GARG, MD
Associate Professor, Diagnostic Radiology Department, Northwestern University Feinberg School of Medicine, Chicago, Illinois, USA

RACHEL GLICKSMAN, MD, MSc, FRCPC
Assistant Professor, Radiation Medicine Program, Department of Radiation Oncology, Princess Margaret Cancer Centre, University Health Network, Toronto, Canada

KUSH K. GOYAL, MD
Assistant Professor, Department of Physical Medicine and Rehabilitation, Cleveland Clinic Lerner College of Medicine, Case Western Reserve University, Center for Spine Health, Neurological Institute, Cleveland Clinic, Cleveland, Ohio, USA

TING GUO, PhD
Senior Research Associate, Department of Neurosciences and Mental Health, The Hospital for Sick Children Research Institute, Toronto, Canada

NANCY HAMMOND, MD
Radiologist, Department of Radiology, Northwestern Memorial Hospital, Northwestern University Feinberg School of Medicine, Chicago, Illinois, USA

JOHN HUDSON, MD, PhD, FRCPC
Assistant Professor, Department of Radiation Oncology, Sunnybrook Odette Cancer Centre, University of Toronto, Toronto, Ontario, Canada

NATHAN C. HULL, MD
Associate Professor, Division of Pediatric Radiology, Department of Radiology, Mayo Clinic, Rochester, Minnesota, USA

EMILIO J. INAREJOS CLEMENTE, MD
Pediatric Radiologist, Department of Radiology, Sant Joan de Deu Barcelona Hospital, Esplugues de Llobregat, Barcelona Spain

SRIRAM JAGANATHAN, MD
Assistant Professor, Department of Radiology, University of Texas Health (UT Health), San Antonio, Texas, USA

VENKAT S. KATABATHINA, MD
Professor, Department of Radiology, University of Texas Health (UT Health), San Antonio, Texas, USA

VISHAL KATHARDEKAR, BBA
Medical Student, Northeast Ohio Medical University, Rootstown, Ohio, USA

RAJESH N. KESWANI, MD
Associate Professor of Medicine, Department of Gastroenterology, Northwestern Memorial Hospital, Northwestern University Feinberg School of Medicine, Chicago, Illinois, USA

TARUNJEET KLAIR, MD
Associate Professor, Department of Hepatobiliary Surgery, University of Texas Health (UT Health), San Antonio, Texas, USA

ETHAN KLEPITSCH, MD
Radiology Resident, Diagnostic Radiology Department, Northwestern University Feinberg School of Medicine, Chicago, Illinois, USA

JILLIAN KRAUSS, MD
Section Head, Emergency Radiology, Instructor of Radiology, Ann and Robert H. Lurie Children's Hospital of Chicago, Northwestern University Feinberg School of Medicine, Chicago, Illinois, USA

SATHEESH KRISHNA, MD
Associate Professor, Department of Medical Imaging, University of Toronto, University Medical Imaging Toronto, University Health Network, Sinai Health System, Women's College Hospital, Toronto, Ontario, Canada

JESSICA KURIAN, MD
Professor, Department of Radiology, Westchester Medical Center, New York Medical College, Valhalla, New York, USA

RITA MARIA LAHOUD, MD
Resident, Department of Radiology, Tufts Medical Center, Boston, Massachusetts, USA

ANGEL M. LANCHARRO-ZAPATA, MD
Radiologist, Department of Radiology, Hospital Materno-Infantil Gregorio Marañon, Madrid, Spain

BERNARD F. LAYA, MD, MHM, DO
Professor of Radiology and Associate Dean for Research and Scholarly Work, St. Luke's Medical Center College of Medicine - William H. Quasha Memorial, Head, Section of Pediatric Radiology, Institute of Radiology, St. Luke's Medical Center - Quezon City, Philippines; Academic and Research Officer, Institute of Radiology St. Luke's Medical

Center - Global City, Philippines; Founding President, Philippine Society for Pediatric Radiology, Fellow, Philippine College of Radiology, Metro Manila, Philippines

EDWARD Y. LEE, MD, MPH
President, International Society of Pediatric Thoracic Imaging, Past President, NERRS and MSO at BCH, Director, Advanced Imaging, Professor, Department of Radiology, Boston Children's Hospital, Harvard Medical School, Boston, Massachusetts, USA

CHRISTOPHER S. LIM, MD, FRCPC
Assistant Professor, Department of Medical Imaging, Sunnybrook Health Sciences Centre, University of Toronto, Toronto, Ontario, Canada

CAMILA LOPES VENDRAMI, MD
Clinical Research Associate, Department of Radiology, Northwestern Memorial Hospital, Northwestern University Feinberg School of Medicine, Chicago, Illinois, USA

NEEL MADAN, MD
Faculty Member, Department of Radiology, Tufts Medical Center, Boston, Massachusetts, USA

JORDI CATALÀ MARCH, MD
Director, Department of Radiology, Instituts Guirado, Barcelona Spain

OUSSAMA METROUH, MD
Research Assistant, Section of Interventional Radiology, Department of Radiology, Beth Israel Deaconess Medical Center, Harvard Medical School, Boston, Massachusetts, USA

FRANK H. MILLER, MD, FACR, FSAR, FSABI
Lee F. Rogers MD Professor of Medical Education, Chief, Body Imaging Section, Medical Director, MRI, Department of Radiology, Northwestern Memorial Hospital, Northwestern University Feinberg School of Medicine, Chicago, Illinois, USA

PARDEEP MITTAL, MD
Radiologist, Department of Radiology and Imaging, Medical College of Georgia, Augusta, Georgia, USA

MARIA NAVALLAS, MD
Radiologist, Department of Radiology, Sant Joan de Deu Barcelona Hospital, Esplugues de Llobregat, Barcelona, Spain

VIVEK PAI, MD
Staff Neuroradiologist, Division of Neuroradiology, Department of Diagnostic and Interventional Radiology, The Hospital for Sick Children, Department of Medical Imaging, University of Toronto, Toronto, Ontario, Canada

DOMEN PLUT, MD, PhD
Assistant Professor, Department of Radiology, Faculty of Medicine, University of Ljubljana, Director, Division of Pediatric Radiology, Institute of Radiology, University Medical Centre Ljubljana, Ljubljana, Slovenia

ALISON ESTEVA SANDERS, MD
Assistant Professor, Diagnostic Radiology Department, Northwestern University Feinberg School of Medicine, Chicago, Illinois, USA

IRENE DIXE DE OLIVEIRA SANTO, MD, CIIP
PGY5 Radiology Resident, Department of Radiology, Yale University, New Haven, Connecticut, USA

JONATHAN D. SAMET, MD
Head, Body Imaging Division, Associate Professor of Radiology and Orthopaedic Surgery, Ann and Robert H. Lurie Children's Hospital of Chicago, Northwestern University Feinberg School of Medicine, Chicago, Illinois, USA

NICOLA SCHIEDA, MD, FRCPC
Professor of Radiology, Radiation Oncology and Medical Physics, Department of Medical Imaging, The Ottawa Hospital, University of Ottawa, Ottawa, Ontario, Canada

BINDU N. SETTY, MD
Clinical Associate Professor, Department of Radiology, Boston University, Boston, Massachusetts, USA

MANOHAR SHROFF, MD, FRCPC
Professor, Division of Neuroradiology, Department of Diagnostic and Interventional Radiology, The Hospital for Sick Children, Department of Medical

Imaging, University of Toronto, Toronto, Ontario, Canada

PETER SLAK, MD
Research Assistant, Department of Radiology, Faculty of Medicine, University of Ljubljana, Division of Pediatric Radiology, Institute of Radiology, University Medical Centre Ljubljana, Ljubljana, Slovenia

CONSTANTINOS T. SOFOCLEOUS, MD, PhD
Interventional Oncologist, Radiologist, Department of Radiology, Interventional Radiology Service, Memorial Sloan Kettering Cancer Center, New York, New York, USA

VLASIOS S. SOTIRCHOS, MD
Interventional Radiologist, Department of Radiology, Interventional Radiology Service, Memorial Sloan Kettering Cancer Center, New York, New York, USA

ABHIJIT SUNNAPWAR, MD
Professor, Department of Radiology, University of Texas Health (UT Health), San Antonio, Texas, USA

MAUDE S. TABIGUE, MD
Fellow, Philippine College of Radiology, Fellow, CT-MRI Society of the Philippines, Fellow, Philippine Society for Pediatric Radiology; Section of Pediatric Radiology, Institute of Radiology, St. Luke's Medical Center - Quezon City, Philippines

JOSHUA TUBLIN, MD
Integrated Interventional Radiology Resident, Section of Interventional Radiology, Department of Radiology, Beth Israel Deaconess Medical Center, Harvard Medical School, Boston, Massachusetts, USA

JEFFREY L. WEINSTEIN, MD, FSIR
Assistant Professor, Section of Interventional Radiology, Department of Radiology, Beth Israel Deaconess Medical Center, Harvard Medical School, Boston, Massachusetts, USA

ABBEY J. WINANT, MD
Attending Radiologist, Department of Radiology, Boston Children's Hospital, Harvard Medical School, Boston, Massachusetts, USA

DIMITRIOS XENOS, MD
Thoracic Surgeon, Department of Radiology, Interventional Radiology Service, Memorial Sloan Kettering Cancer Center, New York, New York, USA

CONTENTS

VOLUME 7 • 2025

Current Status of Pulmonary Embolism Intervention, *57*

By Joshua Tublin, Oussama Metrouh, Julie C. Bulman, and Jeffrey L. Weinstein

Pulmonary embolism (PE) represents a major cause of morbidity and mortality. The overall severity, presentation, and morbidity of each patient with a PE vary. The optimum treatment strategy for patients that are not in frank hemodynamic collapse is evolving. This article reviews the current state of the classification of PE, risk stratification strategies, endovascular catheter-based intervention options, and studies that shaped the current landscape along with upcoming trials that will shape the future. At the present time, pulmonary embolism response teams are a sound strategy for making treatment decisions on a case-by-case basis in this rapidly evolving space.

Rapid MRI for Acute Pediatric Emergencies: Increasing Efficiency with Noninvasive Imaging, *71*

By Jillian Krauss and Jonathan D. Samet

Rapid, noncontrast, nonsedated MRI techniques are being utilized in pediatric body, brain, and musculoskeletal imaging and have proven to be both effective and efficient in assessing commonly encountered pathologies in the emergency department, often negating the need for other imaging workup.

A Scoping Review of Current Techniques in Posterior Cruciate Ligament Injury Management and Reconstruction, *83*

By Gabriel Ortiz Celemin, Ethan Klepitsch, Lucas Buchler, Ankur Garg, and Alison Esteva Sanders

This article discusses the consensus on the postoperative functional superiority of single-bundle versus double-bundle posterior cruciate ligament (PCL); there is evidence to support that double-bundle PCL reconstruction is superior at returning posterior tibial translation to near-normal. Work remains to be done directly comparing PCL remnant-preserving approaches to traditional techniques, but there is a theoretic benefit to preserving this tissue for proprioceptive function. The posterior tibial slope affects graft failure rates following posterior cruciate ligament reconstruction (PCLr). Several techniques reduce or eliminate

Ultrasound (US) is a first-line imaging tool in neonates due to its non-invasive nature, safety, mobility, and effectiveness in visualizing soft tissues. It is especially valuable for assessing detailed organ structure and blood flow. Recent advancements, such as contrast-enhanced US (CEUS), microvascular flow (MV-flow) imaging, and elastography, have expanded its clinical utility. CEUS aids in assessing vascularity and organ perfusion, while MV-flow imaging enhances the detection of small blood vessels without the use of contrast. Elastography measures tissue stiffness, which can be an important sign of a disease. These methods offer non-invasive alternatives to more invasive imaging techniques in neonates.

Disease processes affecting the intrinsic muscles of the head and neck region can result in great functional impairment and psychological distress. Additionally, in certain cases, this may be a manifestation of an occult systemic disease and its recognition is important for timely therapy. We review a plethora of muscle-related entities with illustrative cases and offer clues to diagnosis to the interpreting radiologist. These include named muscular entities like fibromatosis colli, true and pseudohypertrophy, denervation atrophy, trauma-related complications, thyroid and non–thyroid-related orbital myositis, infection, and neoplasms.

This article provides practical information regarding the advantages of dual-energy computed tomography (CT) over single-energy CT and its commonly used and emerging clinical applications in the imaging of the pediatric chest and abdomen.

Advances in Clinical Radiology 7 (2025) xvii–xviii
ADVANCES IN CLINICAL RADIOLOGY

Preface

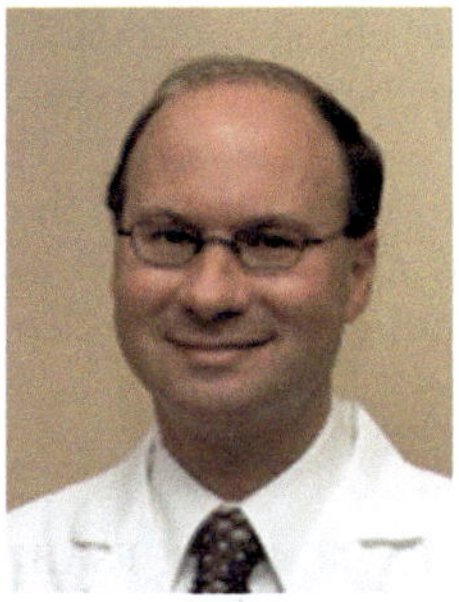

Frank H. Miller, MD, FACR, FSAR, FSABI
Editor

It is with great pleasure that we present our seventh annual issue of *Advances in Clinical Radiology* with a comprehensive issue of cutting-edge review articles and expert perspectives in the field of radiology. We are deeply grateful to our readers and authors for their tremendous support, which enables us to maintain the high quality and relevance of this series.

We are privileged to work with a talented team of co-editors, Drs Amichai Erdfarb, Ankur Garg, Edward Lee, and Robert Lewandowski, who have been integral in planning this issue. Their efforts include inviting outstanding authors, coauthoring several articles, and thoroughly reviewing the submissions. We would like to express our deepest appreciation to them for their invaluable contributions, which have been integral to the success of this series.

The articles featured in this issue of *Advances in Clinical Radiology* span a wide range of recent developments across multiple radiology subspecialities. Abdominal topics include "Advances in MR Imaging in the Evaluation of Chronic Pancreatitis and the Less Common Forms of Pancreatitis" (by Drs Camila Lopes Vendrami, Nancy Hammond, Pardeep Mittal, Rajesh N. Keswani, Ulas Bagci, and Frank H. Miller), as well as "Imaging of Hepatic Segment 4: Management and Surgical Implications" (by Drs Sriram Jaganathan, Abhijith Sunnapwar, Anil K. Dasyam, Tarunjeet Klair, and Venkat S. Katabathina), and "Radiotherapy of Primary Renal Cell Carcinoma: Imaging Considerations Before and After Therapy" (by Drs Christopher S. Lim, Patrick Cheung, John Hudson, Rachel Glicksman, Satheesh Krishna, and Nicola Schieda). Related to interventional radiology, we discuss "Curative Intent Percutaneous Thermal Ablation for Colorectal Liver Metastases: 2025 Update" (by Drs Dimitrios Xenos, Vlasios S. Sotirchos, and Constantinos T. Sofocleous), "Current Status of Pulmonary Embolism Intervention" (by Drs Joshua Tublin, Oussama Metrouh, Julie C. Bulman, and Jeffrey L. Weinstein), and the Musculoskeletal Imaging articles, featuring "A Scoping Review of Current Techniques in Posterior Cruciate Ligament Injury Management and Reconstruction" (by Drs Gabriel Ortiz Celemin, Ethan Klepitsch, Lucas Buchler, Ankur Garg, and Alison Esteva Sanders) and "Therapeutic Effectiveness of Lumbar Medial Branch Block and Lumbar Intra-Articular Facet Injections: A Review of Current Concepts" (by Drs Adam Delora, Alexander Doubek, Vishal Kathardekar, Ian S. Ackers, and Kush K. Goyal).

https://doi.org/10.1016/j.yacr.2025.06.006
2589-8701/25/

Neuroradiology advances include "Updates and Advances in Neuroimaging of Neonatal Encephalopathy" (by Drs Vivek Pai, Ting Guo, and Manohar Shroff), "Advances in Imaging the Glymphatic System" (by Drs Jeremy Ford, Neel Madan, Christopher G. Filippi, and Karen Buch), and "An Overview of the Different Intrinsic Muscular Abnormalities of the Head and Neck" (by Drs Irene Dixe de Oliveira Santo and Bindu N. Setty).

Pediatric radiology is well represented with "Advances in Neonatal Ultrasound Imaging: Beyond Grayscale and Color Doppler Assessment" (by Drs Domen Plut, Peter Slak, Abbey J. Winant, and Edward Y. Lee), "Rapid MRI for Acute Pediatric Emergencies: Increasing Efficiency with Noninvasive Imaging" (by Drs Jillian Krauss and Jonathan D. Samet), "Technical Advances in Pediatric Musculoskeletal Imaging: Theory to Daily Clinical Practice" (by Drs Emilio J. Inarejos Clemente, Maria Navallas, Angel M. Lancharro-Zapata, Jordi Català March, Abbey J. Winant, and Edward Y. Lee), "Up-to-Date Imaging Evaluation of Pediatric Syndromes Associated with Neoplasms: What Radiologists Need to Know" (by Drs Jessica Kurian, Rita M. Lahoud, Nathan C. Hull, and Edward Y. Lee), and "Dual-Energy Computed Tomographic Applications of Pediatric Disorders: Practical Imaging Approach to Diagnosis" (by Drs Maude S. Tabigue, Nathan David P. Concepcion, Bernard F. Laya, and Edward Y. Lee).

We would like to express our deep appreciation to the Elsevier team for their exceptional support throughout the publication process. Special thanks go to Nitesh Barthwal, the developmental editor, and Stacy Eastman, the associate publisher, along with their colleagues, Shyamala Kavikumaran and Samuel Gnanakumar. Without their dedication and expertise, this series would not have been possible.

We want to express our sincere appreciation to our readers. Your continued interest and engagement motivate us to ensure that we provide the best available content for this series.

Last, we extend our gratitude to the authors of the outstanding state-of-the art review articles featured in this issue. We hope you enjoy reading them as much as we did preparing them.

Sincerely,

Frank H. Miller, MD, FACR, FSAR, FSABI
Body Imaging Section
Department of Radiology
Northwestern Memorial Hospital
Northwestern University
Feinberg School of Medicine
676 North Saint Clair, Suite 800
Chicago, IL 60611, USA

E-mail address: Frank.Miller@nm.org

Advances in Clinical Radiology 7 (2025) 1–14
ADVANCES IN CLINICAL RADIOLOGY

Advances in MRI in the Evaluation of Chronic Pancreatitis and the Less Common Forms of Pancreatitis

Camila Lopes Vendrami, MD[a], Nancy Hammond, MD[a], Pardeep Mittal, MD[b], Rajesh N. Keswani, MD[c], Ulas Bagci, PhD[a], Frank H. Miller, MD[a,*]

[a]Department of Radiology, Northwestern Memorial Hospital, Northwestern University Feinberg School of Medicine, Chicago, IL 60611, USA; [b]Department of Radiology and Imaging, Medical College of Georgia, Augusta, GA 30912, USA; [c]Department of Gastroenterology; Northwestern Memorial Hospital, Northwestern University Feinberg School of Medicine, Chicago, IL 60611, USA

KEYWORDS

• Pancreatitis • MRCP • Magnetic resonance imaging (MRI) • Pancreas • Autoimmune • Annular • Paraduodenal

KEY POINTS

- Understanding MRI features of the less common pancreatitis.
- Understanding MRI features that can differentiate the less common pancreatitis from mimickers.
- Use and interpretation of T1-mapping and secretin-magnetic resonance magnetic resonance cholangiopancreatography.

INTRODUCTION

Pancreatic MRI is a robust modality that is commonly used to detect, characterize, and diagnose a wide range of pancreatic abnormalities including inflammatory conditions, neoplasms, variant ductal anatomy, and ductal injuries. Ongoing technical innovations have enabled most sequences to be performed in a single or few breath-holds resulting in decreased motion artifact and allowing for better evaluation of the pancreas. Diagnosing pancreatic conditions can be challenging, especially in the early stages as the functional reserve of the pancreas is high. MR (magnetic resonance) with MR cholangiopancreatography (MRCP) is a noninvasive technique with equivalent or better diagnostic capability than endoscopic retrograde pancreatography (ERCP) regarding pancreatitis, with the added benefit of avoiding potential complications that can occur from the ERCP [1]. The diagnostic accuracy of MRCP for ductal assessment can be further improved by the administration of secretin for the exocrine evaluation of pancreatic function. More recently, T1 mapping of the pancreas has shown promising results in distinguishing between mild chronic pancreatitis and the disease-free pancreas.

Pancreatitis, the most common pancreatic disease in children and adults, is an example of pancreatic pathology where MRI has potential advantages when compared to computed tomography (CT). Pancreatitis can be an acute or chronic inflammatory process and may result in progressive, permanent structural changes that involve the parenchyma and ductal system. Less common forms of pancreatitis include autoimmune pancreatitis, paraduodenal (groove) pancreatitis, heterotopic pancreatitis, and annular pancreatitis. In this

*Corresponding author. *E-mail address:* Frank.Miller@nm.org

https://doi.org/10.1016/j.yacr.2025.05.001
www.advancesinclinicalradiology.com
2589-8701/25/

ABBREVIATIONS

AI	artificial intelligence
AIP	autoimmune pancreatitis
CBD	common bile duct
ECV	extracellular volume fraction
ERCP	endoscopic retrograde cholangiopancreatography
MPD	main pancreatic duct
MR	magnetic resonance
MRCP	magnetic resonance cholangiopancreatography
ms	milliseconds
PDP	paraduodenal pancreatitis
SI	signal intensity
SIR	signal intensity ratio
SVM	support vector machine
WI	weighted image

article, we aim to review the key MRI features to help diagnose the less common types of pancreatitis and how to differentiate them from mimickers, including a brief review of the use of secretin-MRCP.

Autoimmune Pancreatitis

Autoimmune pancreatitis (AIP) is a rare type of chronic pancreatitis that occurs more frequently in males than females [2–4]. The exact cause is unknown, but a multifactorial process related to autoimmunity, genetic susceptibility, and exposure to environmental factors probably explains the etiology and pathogenesis of AIP. AIP is classified in 2 subtypes (type 1 and type 2). Type 1 is the more common subtype and is an immunoglobulin G4 (IgG4)-related systemic disease that may have extrapancreatic involvement. Unlike type 1, type 2 only involves the pancreas and histologically demonstrates idiopathic duct-centric pancreatitis with the hallmark granulocytic epithelial lesions [5] and normal or only mildly elevated serum IgG4 levels [6]. Serum IgG4 levels higher than 300 mg/dL (or >2-fold higher than the normal range) are highly suggestive of type 1 AIP. The ratio of serum IgG4/IgG greater than 10% is typical in type 1 AIP, thus this calculation is helpful with mild IgG4 elevations [6]. Although there are no specific serologic markers for type 2 AIP, antineutrophil cytoplasmic antibodies can be detected in some cases [6]. Type 2 AIP is associated with inflammatory bowel disease, more commonly ulcerative colitis [7].

Diffuse enlargement of the pancreas with loss of the lobular structure and straightening of the pancreatic margin is the most typical imaging feature of AIP, creating a *sausage-like* enlargement appearance of the pancreas (Fig. 1). Peripancreatic fat stranding and a low-density capsule on CT or low T2 signal intensity (SI) rim on MRI with delayed parenchymal enhancement may be seen in up to 80% of cases [8]. Morphologic findings of AIP can be diffuse, focal or multifocal, depending on the pattern resulting in enlargement of the involved portion of the pancreas. On T1-weighted image (WI), the involved area is hypointense, while on T2WI image it shows mild hyperintensity.

Approximately, 28% to 41% of cases of AIP present as a focal mass-forming pancreatitis, which can be challenging to distinguish from pancreatic adenocarcinoma since imaging and clinical characteristics often overlap [4,9–11]. Differentiation between these entities is essential as the prognosis and management are vastly different, with AIP responding favorably to corticosteroids, while pancreatic adenocarcinoma's only curative therapy is radical surgical resection [12]. A response to corticosteroid therapy can be helpful in the diagnosis of AIP and may result in pancreatic atrophy. Focal AIP has been described to more likely show a *speckled* enhancement pattern on the pancreatic phase of imaging than cancer [13]. Careful evaluation of the pancreatic ductal system is also crucial in the diagnosis of AIP. The *duct-penetrating* sign has been described in cases of focal AIP and is characterized as the main pancreatic duct (MPD) penetrating the lesion without occluding the duct [9,13,14]. This finding is best demonstrated with secretin-enhanced MRCP and is in distinction to pancreatic cancer where the underlying lesion typically results in ductal occlusion [4,15]. Upstream pancreatic ductal dilatation occurring from focal AIP typically shows less dilatation (<4 mm) compared with pancreatic cancer (>4 mm) [9,14,16]. Irregular narrowing of the MPD is also seen in focal AIP with a longer length of narrowing (≥3 cm) than from pancreatic duct adenocarcinoma [16–20]. The *icicle sign* has also been described with focal AIP and is characterized as smooth tapered narrowing of the upstream pancreatic duct resulting in the appearance of an icicle [21]. Even if the parenchymal changes are segmental, a reported prevalence of 61.5% of multifocal strictures along the whole extent of the MPD, at MRCP, can be identified in focal AIPs [22].

Additional features of AIP include delayed homogeneous enhancement of the lesion and a hypointense capsule-like rim. In contrast, pancreatic cancer demonstrates a hypoenhancing mass with associated peripancreatic infiltration and vascular encasement (Fig. 2), upstream pancreatic atrophy, and peripancreatic lymphadenopathy. Diffusion-weighted imaging (DWI) can be helpful in the diagnosis of AIP and to assess therapy.

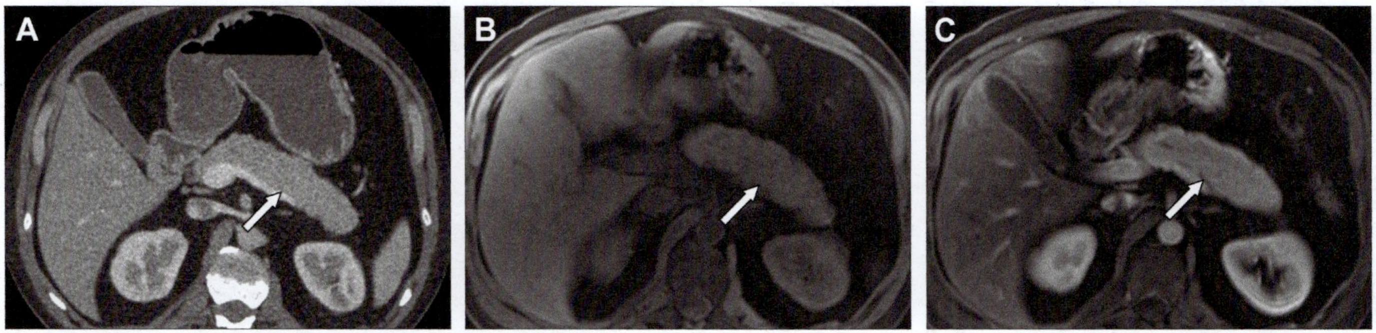

FIG. 1 58-year-old man with history of eosinophilic esophagitis. (**A**) Axial contrast-enhanced CT image, axial T1 fat-suppressed (FS) unenhanced (**B**) and contrast-enhanced (**C**) MR images show enlargement of the body and tail of the pancreas with loss of normal lobulation resulting in the characteristic sausage-shaped appearance of AIP (*arrows*)

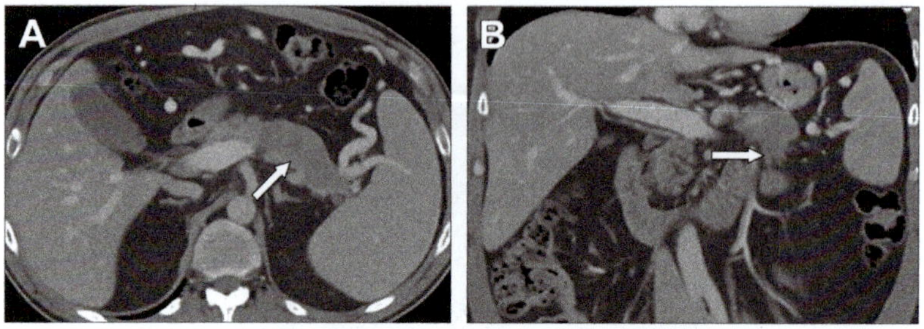

FIG. 2 56-year-old man presenting with new onset diabetes and weight loss. (**A**) Axial CT image shows enlargement and hypoenhancement of the pancreatic tail (*arrow*). While findings can be seen with pancreatitis including AIP, closer inspection of the (**B**) coronal CT image shows irregular soft tissue extension from the pancreatic tail (*arrow*) raising concern for an invasive ductal adenocarcinoma over AIP or pancreatitis, which was confirmed on biopsy.

AIP tends to have more restricted diffusion than pancreatic cancer with the apparent diffusion coefficient (ADC) shown to be significantly lower in AIP than pancreatic cancer or normal pancreatic parenchyma [4,14,23].

Type 2 AIP mostly involves the pancreas making the diagnosis more difficult (Fig. 3). Radiologists can be the first to suggest the diagnosis of AIP based on the evaluation for the presence of extrapancreatic features of AIP. MRI can be especially helpful to show the extrapancreatic disease and typically demonstrates the findings more clearly than CT (Fig. 4). Extrapancreatic lesions include sclerosing cholangitis, retroperitoneal fibrosis, and interstitial nephritis. These findings are in distinction to the usual sites and appearance of metastatic pancreatic cancer and can assist in the differentiation between the 2 entities [4]. Extrapancreatic manifestations of AIP can also occur in the salivary/lacrimal glands. Pancreatic metastases, on the other hand, usually involve primarily the liver, lungs, peritoneum, omentum, and lymph nodes [4,17].

Biliary involvement associated with AIP usually manifests as a long segment stricture with prestenotic

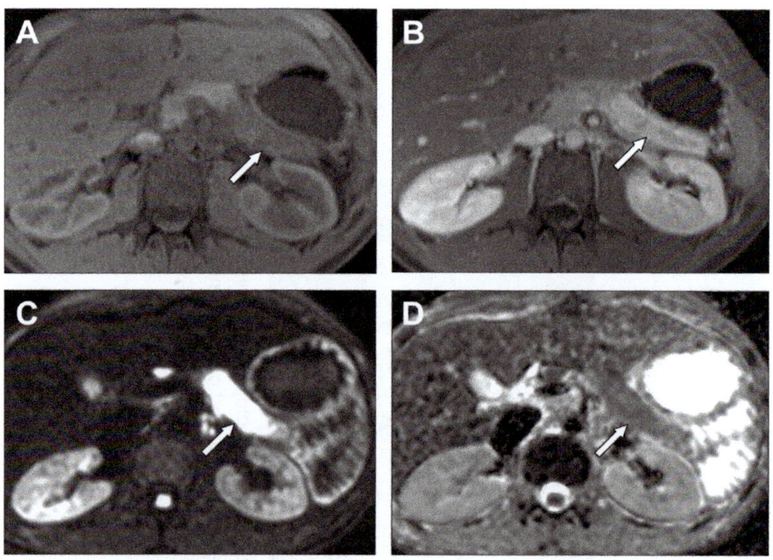

FIG. 3 25-year-old woman with type II AIP. (**A, B**) Axial T1 FS unenhanced MRI shows abnormal hypointense signal of the pancreatic tail (*arrow*) relative to the uninvolved pancreas (*arrow*). (**B**) Axial T1 FS contrast-enhanced MR image shows delayed enhancement to the involved pancreatic tail (*arrow*). (**C, D**) DWI (b800 s/mm^2) and ADC map images show restricted diffusion of the involved portion of the pancreas (*arrow*)

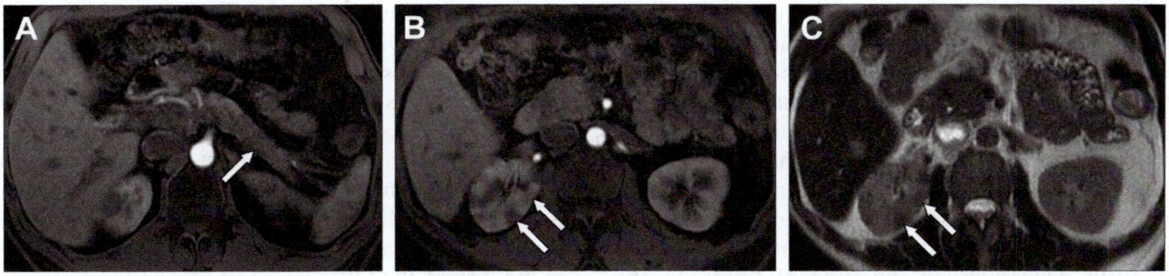

FIG. 4 56-year-old man with history of AIP. (**A**) Axial T1 FS contrast-enhanced MR image shows hypoenhancing pancreas from AIP (*arrow*). (**B**, **C**) Axial T1 FS contrast-enhanced (**B**) and T2-weighted (**C**) MR images show multiple hypoenhancing (**B**; *arrows*) and T2 hypointense (**C**; *arrows*) renal lesions, compatible with tubulointerstitial nephritis associated with AIP.

dilatation of the distal common bile duct [17]. Multifocal strictures or thickening of the intrahepatic or extrahepatic bile ducts, similar to primary sclerosing cholangitis, may also be seen. Gallbladder involvement appears as decreased signal intensity on T2WI, diffuse mural thickening and delayed contrast enhancement [17]. Renal involvement, which primarily occurs in the renal cortex, is seen as isointense or hypointense lesions on T1-and hypointense lesions on T2-weighted MR images [8], gradual enhancement on contrast-enhanced images and restricted diffusion [17]. At CT imaging, renal lesions are hypodense on early-phase contrast-enhanced imaging and have gradual enhancement on delayed phases [24]. Gallium-67 scintigraphy demonstrates increased uptake in the involved renal lesions [25]. Retroperitoneal fibrosis appears as a fibrotic mass around the aorta or inferior vena cava. Entrapment of the ureters leading to hydronephrosis may also be seen [8,17]. At MRI, a low or intermediate signal intensity lesion on T1-weighted images, with variable signal intensity on T2WI, and variable contrast-enhancement are observed [24]. Mikulicz disease consists of bilateral swelling of the lacrimal and major salivary glands with homogeneous T1 and T2 hypointensity, and enhancement on contrast-enhanced sequences. Kuttner disease is a chronic sclerosing sialadenitis of the submandibular gland that appears isointense on T1WI, hypointense on T2WI, and enhances homogeneously [8]. IgG4-related prostatitis appears as a diffusely enlarged prostate gland with low signal intensity lesions and surrounding inflammatory stranding [26], with high signal intensity on diffusion weighted image (DWI), mimicking prostatitis and prostate cancer [25].

At PET imaging, both AIP and pancreatic cancer demonstrate extrapancreatic fluorodeoxyglucose (FDG) uptake; however, increased uptake in the kidneys and salivary glands should lead to the diagnosis of AIP. In addition, AIP usually shows increased FDG activity of the extrapancreatic portion of the bile duct, slower liver clearance of FDG activity, and higher standardized uptake volume (SUV) max for the prostate gland [27].

Paraduodenal Pancreatitis

Paraduodenal pancreatitis (PDP), also known as groove pancreatitis, is a type of focal chronic pancreatitis involving the pancreaticoduodenal groove (PDG). The groove is normally a thin anatomic space in the anterosuperior pararenal space bordered medially by the pancreatic head, superiorly by the duodenal bulb, laterally by the descending duodenum, inferiorly by the transverse duodenum, and posteriorly by the inferior vena cava [28]. The incidence of PDP is not completely established; however, in a surgical series of patients undergoing pancreaticoduodenectomies for chronic pancreatitis, a variable incidence of 2.7% to 24.4% has been reported [29]. PDP is found mostly in middle-aged men (40–50 years of age). A history of alcohol overconsumption occurs in most cases, suggesting it is a precipitating factor and is a helpful clinical information to suspect the diagnosis. The pathogenesis of PDP is unclear, but various factors may be related to this condition, such as true duodenal wall cyst, pancreatic heterotopia in the duodenum, peptic ulcer, gastric hypersecretion, gastric resection, or disturbance of the flow of pancreatic juice through the Santorini duct [29,30]. There are 2 described patterns of PDP [1]: pure pattern that affects only the groove, and [2] segmental pattern that extends medially to involve the pancreatic head [28,29]. Both forms may show attenuated and narrowed MPD, which is best appreciated on the coronal multiplanar reformatted images. This narrowing is often relatively smooth, tapered, and regular, without evidence of *shouldering*, irregularity, or abrupt margins. The pancreatic duct can also be narrowed toward the downstream pancreatic head, usually in a smooth gradual fashion [31]. In some cases of pure PDP, progressive narrowing of the pancreatic duct occurs, which eventually results in diffuse changes of chronic pancreatitis in the entirety of the pancreas [29].

MRI shows a sheet-like mass between the head of the pancreas and the duodenal C loop, which is hypointense on T1WI and hypointense to slightly hyperintense on T2WI depending on the time of onset. In the subacute phase of PDP, the area involved is hyperintense on T2WI because of edema, while in the chronic phase, it demonstrates hypointensity because of fibrosis. Dynamic contrast-enhanced images show delayed enhancement because of the fibrous nature of the tissue. T2 hyperintense cysts in the duodenal wall and in the PDG (Fig. 5) can occur with similar appearance to pancreatic pseudocysts, duplication cysts, and/or cystic tumors. Both the pure and segmental patterns of PDP demonstrate medial duodenal wall thickening. In the segmental PDP, mass-like enlargement of the pancreatic head obscures the groove and shows T1 hypointensity and delayed enhancement, which can mimic pancreatic adenocarcinoma (Fig. 6). The common bile duct (CBD) can appear attenuated or narrowed in both patterns of PDP and smoothly tapers to the ampulla without shouldering or irregular/abrupt margins, which is best depicted on the coronal plane or on MRCP images. The pancreatic duct may also narrow in a gradual and smooth fashion toward the pancreatic head. An ancillary finding in PDP is the widened distance between the ampulla and duodenal lumen that is associated with a dilated banana-shaped gallbladder because of the narrowing at the ampulla and strictures of the distal CBD [29].

Imaging features that are suggestive of paraduodenal pancreatic adenocarcinoma that can help in the differentiation from PDP, include invasion and obstruction of the MPD by tumor resulting in upstream ductal dilatation and atrophy of the pancreas and abrupt cutoff and irregular dilatation of the duct [32]. Though both have similar features on T1WI and T2WI, the enhancement pattern is more homogeneously hypointense in adenocarcinomas. Pancreatic adenocarcinoma infiltrates the retroperitoneal space and usually encases major vessels, including the gastroduodenal artery. Thickening of the duodenal wall or luminal stenosis can also occur in adenocarcinomas but cystic changes in the groove or medial wall of the duodenum are more suggestive of PDP.

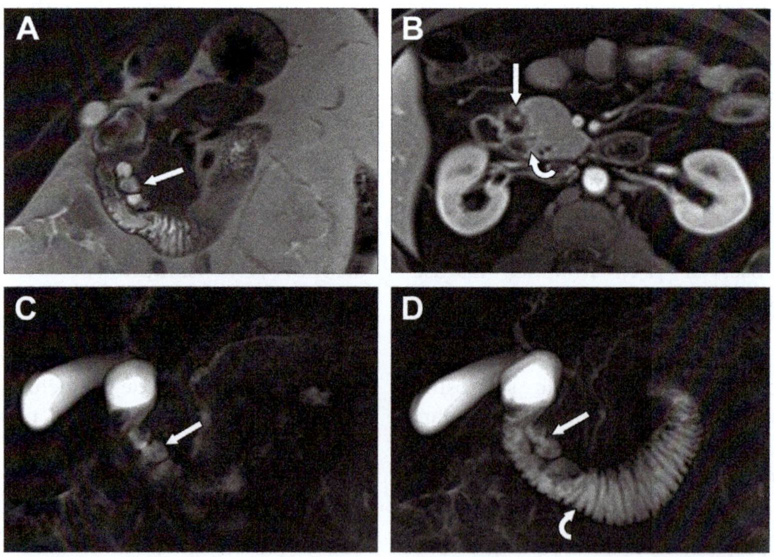

FIG. 5 56-year-old man with alcohol overuse and abdominal pain. (**A**) Coronal T2-weighted MR image shows cystic changes in the paraduodenal groove (*arrow*). (**B**) Axial T1 FS contrast-enhanced MR image shows cystic changes (*straight arrow*) and abnormal tissue with delayed enhancement in the paraduodenal groove (*curved arrow*). (**C**, **D**) MRCP pre (**C**) and 5 minutes (**D**) post-secretin administration images show cysts (*straight arrow*) and increasing fluid in the duodenum and proximal jejunum consistent with intact exocrine pancreatic function (*curved arrow*).

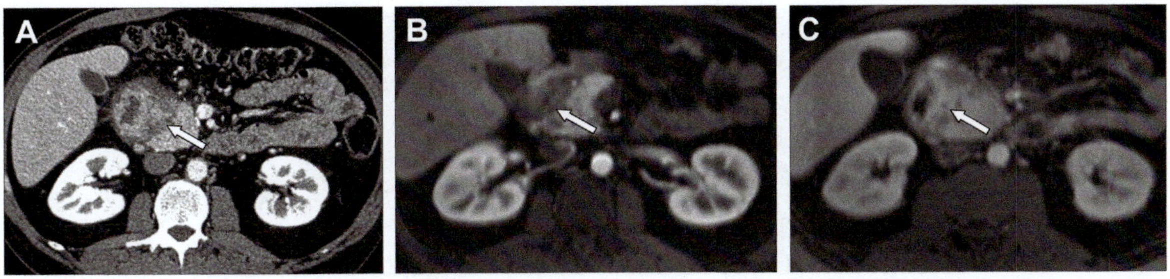

FIG. 6 Fig. 6: 39-year-old man with abdominal pain and history of alcohol overuse. (**A**) Axial contrast-enhanced CT image shows heterogeneous inflammatory changes involving the paraduodenal groove (*arrow*). (**B, C**) Axial T1 FS contrast-enhanced MR images show mass-like area between the pancreatic head and duodenum (*arrow*) that is hypoenhancing on pancreatic phase (**B**) and shows delayed enhancement on the later phase (**C**), compatible with PDP

Jaundice and elevated tumor markers cancer antigen 19-9 (CA 19–9) are more likely to occur with pancreatic adenocarcinoma [29].

Heterotopic Pancreatitis

Heterotopic pancreas is a congenital abnormality of aberrantly located pancreatic tissue without anatomic or vascular continuity with the orthotopic pancreas. It is typically found during the fourth to sixth decades of life and is seen more frequently in males. Patients are often asymptomatic, and heterotopic pancreas is generally identified incidentally during imaging, surgery, or autopsy [33]. Heterotopic pancreas is mostly found in the stomach (26%–38%), duodenum (28%–36%), and jejunum (16%) [34,35]. It is typically found in the submucosa or muscularis propria, especially along the great curvature of the gastric antrum or proximal duodenum. Other potential locations include Meckel's diverticulum, ileum, gallbladder, colon, bile ducts, umbilicus, liver, spleen, mesentery, mediastinum, esophagus, and fallopian tubes [33,35].

MRI has advantages over CT in the diagnosis of heterotopic pancreas. The characteristic high signal intensity of pancreatic tissue on T1 fat-suppressed images that is also seen in heterotopic pancreatic parenchyma is readily identifiable [33]. When not inflamed, heterotopic pancreas is isointense to the orthotopic pancreas on unenhanced imaging including T1WI, T2WI, and DWI sequences and shows a similar enhancement pattern to the orthotopic pancreas following contrast-enhanced imaging. When inflamed, heterotopic pancreas shows similar findings of pancreatitis as seen in the orthotopic pancreas [33,36,37]. The visualization of a central high signal area representing the pancreatic duct on T2WI and MRCP is an important confirmatory finding for diagnosing this condition [38,39]. When pancreatitis occurs in the heterotopic pancreas, nonspecific imaging features may appear as a soft-tissue mass at the center of inflammatory changes and bowel wall thickening. The inflamed heterotopic pancreas may show decreased enhancement [40] (Fig. 7). A high index of suspicion is required to make the diagnosis of heterotopic pancreas and should be based on the enhancement pattern of the heterotopic pancreas, at both CT and MRI, being similar to the orthotopic pancreas, with avid enhancement during the arterial/pancreatic phase (see Fig. 7), With chronic pancreatitis, the heterotopic pancreas may show low signal intensity on T1 fat-suppressed images with decreased enhancement [33] and may be associated with pseudocysts or dilated ducts similar to chronic pancreatitis in the orthotopic pancreas [41].

Annular Pancreatitis

Annular pancreas is a congenital anomaly that occurs during organogenesis because of failure of the ventral pancreatic bud to rotate properly resulting in pancreatic tissue encircling the duodenum, most commonly involving the second duodenal segment [33]. Two types of annular pancreas, extramural and intramural, have been described. The intramural type is characterized by pancreatic tissue that is incorporated into the duodenal wall with multiple small ducts draining directly into the duodenum, while the extramural type shows a well-defined duct encircling the duodenum and joining the main pancreatic duct [35,42]. Approximately one-third of annular pancreas cases coexist with pancreas divisum, and although congenital, it may not be diagnosed until adulthood [43]. Symptoms are associated with peptic ulcer disease or acute pancreatitis. Repeated episodes of inflammation of the annulus may worsen obstructive symptoms [33].

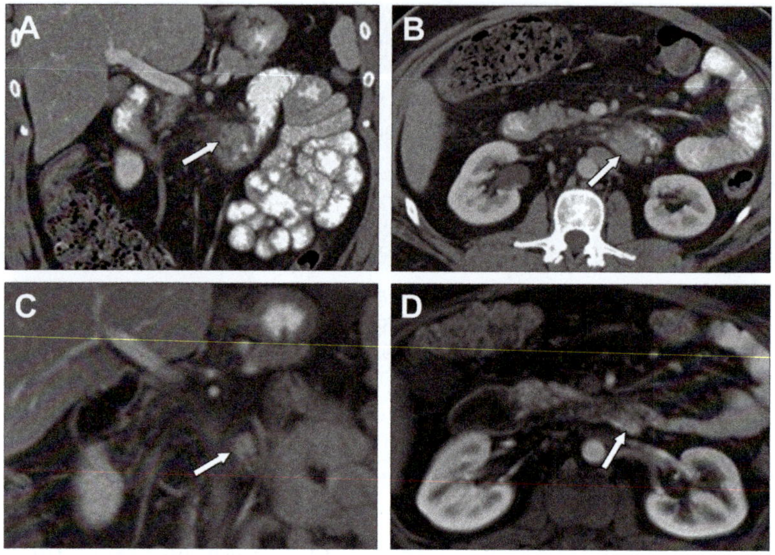

FIG. 7 43-year-old woman presenting with abdominal pain and elevated serum lipase consistent with pancreatitis. (**A**, **B**) Coronal and axial CT images show enhancing soft tissue lesion with mild adjacent fat stranding (*arrow*) at the duodenal/jejunal junction, which has a similar appearance to the pancreatic head consistent with heterotopic pancreatitis. (**C**, **D**) Coronal and axial T1 FS contrast-enhanced MR images (obtained 1 year-later) show that the area at the duodenal-jejunal junction follows pancreatic signal and enhancement consistent with heterotopic pancreas without inflammation (*arrow*)

On cross-sectional imaging, annular pancreas appears as pancreatic tissue partially or fully (two-thirds of cases) surrounding the duodenum [40,44]. In cases of complete annular pancreas, cross-sectional imaging shows the bowel to be encircled by pancreatic parenchyma. The annular pancreas is better assessed and diagnosed with MRI than CT imaging as it shows characteristic high signal intensity on T1 fat-suppressed imaging from pancreatic tissue that surrounds the duodenum. On T2WI including MRCP images, the annular pancreatic duct can be visualized surrounding the duodenum in extramural annular pancreas. This is also seen during ERCP or surgery. The pancreatic head may have a rounded or triangular appearance in incomplete annular pancreas, resulting in a *crocodile-jaw* appearance. The most sensitive and specific feature for diagnosing annular pancreas is the presence of pancreatic tissue along the posterolateral aspect of the duodenum [33,40].

Acute pancreatitis from annular pancreatitis usually affects the annulus and pancreatic head, sparing the body and tail (Fig. 8). An increased risk of pancreatitis is possibly related to poor drainage in the annular duct. Imaging features include the enlargement of the annulus and head with duodenal wall thickening that may result in upstream bowel dilatation [45,46], which can mimic pancreatic neoplasm. In cases with significant symptoms that are attributed to annular pancreas, surgery remains the therapy of choice to relieve duodenal or gastric outlet obstruction by bypassing the annulus. Resection of the annulus should be avoided because it is correlated with pancreatic fistula formation, incomplete relief of obstruction, and pancreatitis [33,47,48].

T1 MAPPING USE FOR CHRONIC PANCREATITIS

Chronic pancreatitis is characterized by fibrosis, loss of acinar and islet cells as well as ductal changes [49] leading to permanent impairment of exocrine and endocrine pancreatic functions [50]. Cross-sectional imaging studies are recommended by the American College of Gastroenterology as the first diagnostic modality as biopsy is generally not performed [49,51]. The imaging findings of chronic pancreatitis can be grouped into early and late findings. Early findings include low-signal-intensity of the pancreas on T1-weighted fat-suppressed images, dilated side branches, and decreased and delayed enhancement after contrast administration (Fig. 9) [50]. Late findings include pseudocysts, parenchymal atrophy or enlargement,

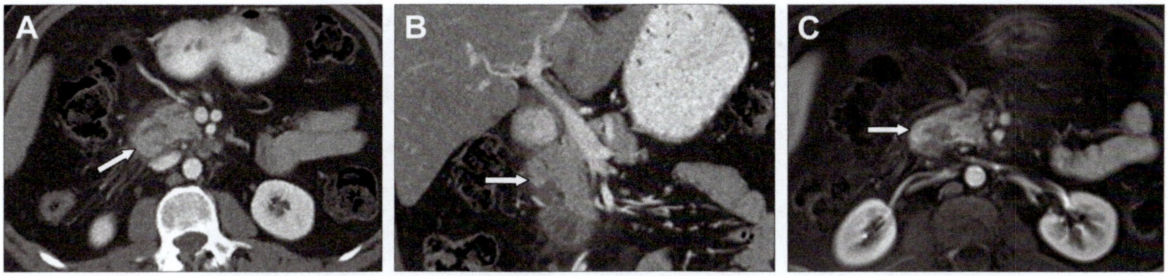

FIG. 8 27-year-old man with history of abdominal pain and elevated serum lipase. (**A**, **B**) Axial and coronal contrast-enhanced CT images show an annular pancreas with adjacent fat stranding consistent with pancreatitis. (**C**) Contrast-enhanced axial T1FS MR confirms the annular pancreas surrounding the duodenum (*arrow*) to be of the same signal intensity as the adjacent pancreatic head

and dilatation and beading of the pancreatic duct usually with intraductal calcifications [50]. Particularly in patients with milder forms of pancreatitis that demonstrate less severe ductal abnormalities on MRCP or lack calcifications on CT, the diagnosis of chronic pancreatitis can be challenging [49]. Using MRI, T1 mapping may play a role in the early detection and staging of chronic pancreatitis. Typically, the normal pancreas has higher signal intensity than other organs based on the presence of acinar proteins (Fig. 10). In chronic pancreatitis, there is a loss of acinar cells with replacement by fibrosis that increases the T1 relaxation time and decreases the signal intensity of the pancreas. The acquisition time for T1 mapping takes about 20 seconds making it a potentially useful tool in the clinical setting to diagnose chronic pancreatitis, with no additional cost to the scan time [52]. T1 signal intensity ratio (SIR) can be used to assess chronic pancreatitis by comparing the pancreas to a reference organ such as spleen or muscle [53]. The region of interest for SIR is obtained on axial precontrast, T1-weighted, fat-suppressed, 3D gradient echo sequences. SIR is calculated by dividing the average pancreas signal intensity (SI) by the SI of the reference organ (spleen or muscle); SIR = SI Pancreas/SI Reference [53]. A decreased pancreatic T1-SIR reflects the degree of fibrosis and loss of normal acinar tissue [54]. Tirkes T et al reported a statistically significant increase of T1 relaxation time in mild chronic pancreatitis cases [52]. A T1 relaxation cutoff time of 900 milliseconds (ms) was shown to yield 80% sensitivity and 69% specificity in the diagnosis of mild chronic pancreatitis (see Fig. 10) [52,55].

Cheng and colleagues evaluated T1 mapping for the diagnosis of early chronic pancreatitis, correlating it with Cambridge classification system of chronic pancreatitis based on morphologic changes in the pancreatic ducts using ERCP. A significant difference in the mean T1 relaxation time was found between the combined Cambridge 0 (normal) and 1 (equivocal) group and the Cambridge 2 (mild chronic pancreatitis) group [56].

A higher extracellular volume fraction (ECV) has also been described in individuals with chronic pancreatitis [49]. The extracellular matrix is increased because

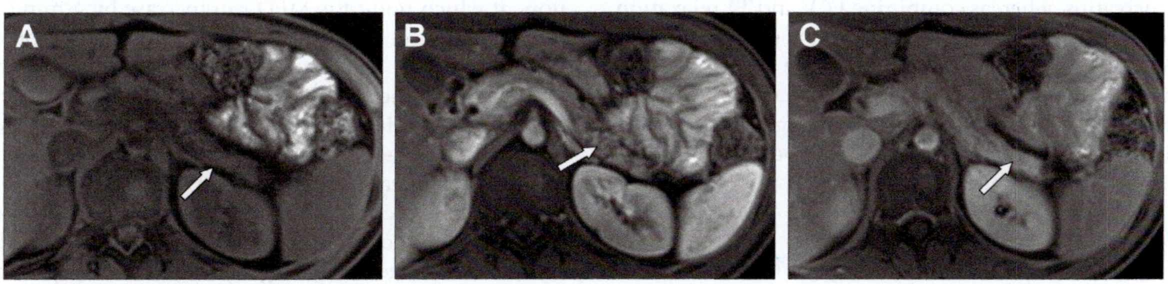

FIG. 9 21-year-old woman with history of chronic pancreatitis. (**A**, **B**, **C**) Axial T1FS MR images show pancreatic atrophy and relatively low signal intensity of the pancreatic tail on the unenhanced T1FS image (**A**) with decreased enhancement on early phase (**B**) and delayed enhancement on later phase (**C**) of the pancreatic body and tail (*arrow*)

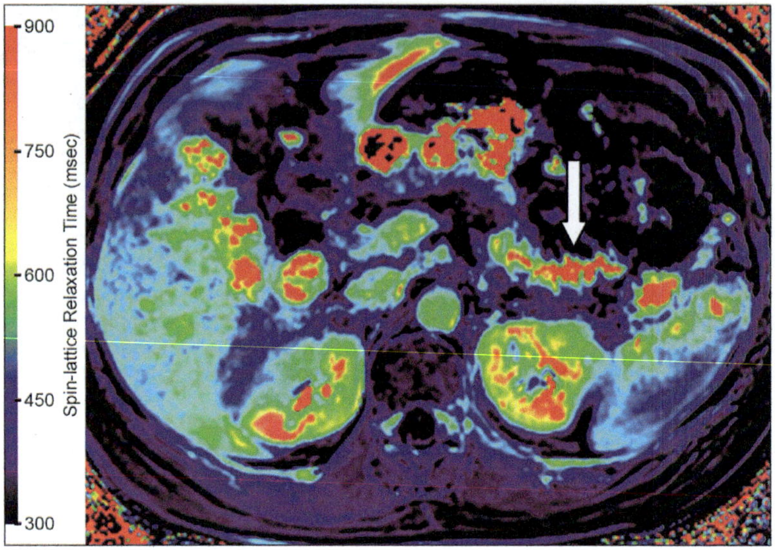

FIG. 10 36-year-old woman with severe chronic pancreatitis. Axial color T1 map (scaled from 300 to 900 ms) shows the average T1 relaxation time was 710 milliseconds, suggestive of chronic pancreatitis. (*Image Courtesy of* Temel Tirkes, MD, Department of Radiology, Indiana University School of Medicine.)

of detrimental tissue remodeling resulting in fibrosis. ECV imaging allows dichotomization of tissues into their intracellular and extracellular elements by using T1 relaxation times obtained before and after MR contrast enhancement administration. Most of current gadolinium-based contrast agents are extracellular during the late enhancement phase, thus T1 shortening of the tissues shows their concentration in the extracellular space. Extracellular volume imaging can divide tissues into their intracellular and extracellular components by employing T1 relaxation times acquired before and after contrast administration [49]. Extracellular volume imaging has been shown to yield 92% sensitivity and 77% specificity for diagnosing chronic pancreatitis, whereas combining ECV and T1 relaxation time yielded sensitivity of 85% and specificity of 92% [54,57]. Another study by the same group showed that T1 higher than 950 ms yielded 64% sensitivity and 88% specificity, while ECV higher than 0.27 yielded 92% sensitivity and 77% specificity for the diagnosis of chronic pancreatitis [57].

SECRETIN-MRCP USE FOR CHRONIC PANCREATITIS

Secretin MRCP has potential advantages over conventional MRCP in some patients with chronic pancreatitis. Secretin can assess pancreatic function by inducing fluid production from the pancreas to fill the duodenum and detect impaired function associated with chronic pancreatitis. It is used less commonly than standard MRCP because it requires an additional 15 minutes of scanner time including the imaging and slow intravenous (IV) infusion required of secretin and due to additional expenses and nursing involvement [52]. Also, secretin is relatively contraindicated in cases of severe acute pancreatitis [58].

Secretin is a gastrointestinal hormone that stimulates the pancreas to secrete pancreatic fluid (bicarbonate-rich) while temporarily increasing the tone of the sphincter of Oddi [52,59,60]. The optimum effect of secretin typically occurs 3 to 5 minutes after administration, at which point the MPD can increase by 1 mm or more from onset and side branch radicals may become identifiable and excretion is seen in the duodenum [58]. The exocrine response to secretin can be enhanced by fasting for at least 4 hours before MRI [59], and the infusion of a negative contrast agent (diluted gadolinium in water or pineapple juice at 100% concentration or other fluids) to conceal the high-intensity fluid in the stomach and duodenum on MRCP is advised [58,59]. Antiperistaltic agents (glucagon) may be employed to avoid motion artifact from bowel peristalsis [58].

An indirect estimate of exocrine function has been shown to be provided by measuring the volume of fluid filling the duodenum after secretin administration during MRCP. Thick slab two-dimensional (2D) MRCP images are acquired every 30 seconds over 10 minutes. The qualitative description of duodenal fluid uses a grading scale [1]: grade 0 with no increased fluid in duodenum (Fig. 11) [2], grade 1 with increased fluid in the duodenal bulb only [3], grade 2 with increased fluid to the proximal third duodenal segment), and [4] grade 3 with increased fluid in the distal third duodenal segment or beyond [61,62]. Secretin-MRCP has been shown to have a strong correlation with histopathologic fibrosis (having 2 or more secretin-MRCP features, such as MPD irregularity, MPD stenosis, MPD dilatation, and/or dilated side branches, yields sensitivity of 65% and specificity of 89% for detecting fibrotic glands, and sensitivity of 88% and specificity of 78% for identifying severe fibrosis) [62]. Secretin MRCP may be useful in early chronic pancreatitis; however, normal duodenal filling after secretin administration does not preclude mild exocrine dysfunction [60,62].

NEW IMAGING TECHNIQUES AND ARTIFICIAL INTELLIGENCE

Several software and hardware technologies are under development, including artificial intelligence (AI) and radiomics, that will improve diagnostic accuracy, differential diagnosis, and manage treatment response [63]. Shiraishi M and colleagues reported that when using a conventional machine learning approach (ie, support vector machine (SVM), the mean 2D-ADC and three-dimensional (3D)-ADC values are lower in focal-AIP cases when compared to PDAC with good inter-reader reliability. Their study also revealed that the nonlinear SVM using a combination of mean 2D-ADC object volume, and exponential-energy (the texture parameter with the highest area under the curve [AUC]) may help in differentiating focal AIP from PDAC [64]. Other studies based on CT radiomics, and other newer techniques also show promising results; however, most of the published studies have limitations of single-center, retrospective, limited sample size, and low radiomics quality score, which make further studies required [63].

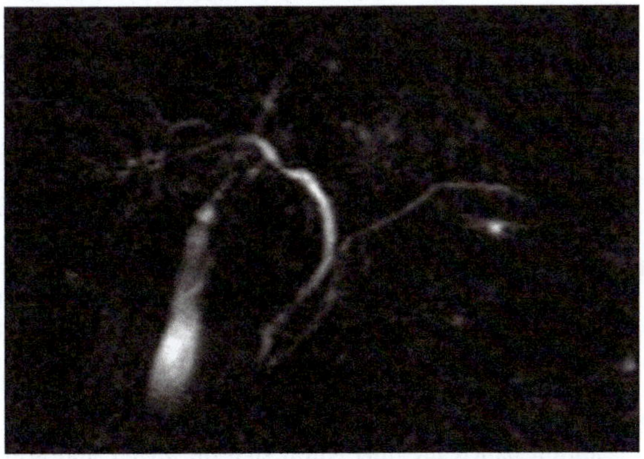

FIG. 11 28-year-old man with history of alcohol overuse and suspected chronic pancreatitis. MRCP post-secretin administration image shows no increased fluid in the duodenum on dynamic imaging 10 minutes post injection of secretin, suggestive of pancreatic exocrine dysfunction. There was no caliber change of the pancreatic duct also suggestive of chronic pancreatitis

It is important to note that AI algorithms, particularly those using deep learning, have shown exceptional promise in automating the detection and characterization of many diseases. More specifically, pancreatitis and its subtypes are starting to be evaluated by AI but it is still in its infancy [65–67]. AI algorithms are usually trained on large datasets of medical images with expert-derived labels or ground truths, enabling them to recognize complex patterns and subtle features that may be missed by human radiologists. For instance, convolutional neural networks, or more recently Transformers and Foundational Models [68], can differentiate between acute and chronic pancreatitis with high accuracy by analyzing CT and MRI scans [65–67]. Additionally, AI models have great potential to assist in identifying less common forms of pancreatitis, such as AIP and PDP (groove), by highlighting specific imaging biomarkers associated with these conditions. By integrating clinical data with imaging findings, AI systems, called multimodal AI now, can potentially provide a comprehensive assessment of patient status, offering predictions about disease progression, risk of complications, and likely outcomes [69,70]. The application of AI in pancreatitis extends to therapeutic decision-making and treatment monitoring [71]. AI algorithms can also evaluate the effectiveness of therapeutic interventions by analyzing follow-up imaging studies, thereby aiding in the optimization of treatment protocols [72]. In the context of chronic pancreatitis, AI can help monitor disease progression and response to therapies such as enzyme replacement or pain management strategies [73]. These insights can guide clinicians in selecting the most effective treatments and adjusting them based on real-time feedback from AI analyses, ultimately improving patient outcomes.

SUMMARY

MRI is a robust modality in the assessment of a wide spectrum of pancreatic abnormalities such as neoplasms, inflammatory conditions, variant ductal anatomy, and ductal injuries. Advances in MRI have allowed for improved evaluation of the pancreas and less artifacts that could impair its proper assessment. Pancreatitis can be acute or chronic, with less common forms including AIP, PDP, heterotopic pancreatitis, and annular pancreatitis. Techniques such as T1-mapping and secretin-MRCP are being used with greater frequency in evaluating chronic pancreatitis and thus, understanding of their use and interpretation is helpful in the clinical setting. Radiologists should be aware of the imaging features of these less common forms of pancreatitis as they can play a vital role in their diagnosis.

CLINICS CARE POINTS

- Pancreatic MRI is a powerful modality often used to detect, characterize, and diagnose a wide spectrum of pancreatic disorders including inflammatory conditions, neoplasms, variant ductal anatomy, and ductal injuries.
- Pancreatitis, the most common pancreatic disease in children and adults, and the less common forms of pancreatitis include autoimmune pancreatitis, paraduodenal (groove) pancreatitis, heterotopic pancreatitis, and annular pancreatitis are discussed. These conditions can be detected with MRI based on certain characteristic features, which may also help differentiate them from mimickers.
- Novel techniques such as T1-mapping, and secretin-magnetic resonance cholangiopancreatography are being used with greater frequency in evaluating chronic pancreatitis. Software and hardware technologies are being developed, including AI and radiomics, which may assist in improving diagnostic accuracy, differential diagnosis, and management of treatment response.

FUNDING

NIH, United States/NIDDK #U01 DK127384-02S1; NIH/NCI #R01 CA246704-01.

DISCLOSURES

None.

REFERENCES

[1] Sica GT, Braver J, Cooney MJ, et al. Comparison of endoscopic retrograde cholangiopancreatography with MR cholangiopancreatography in patients with pancreatitis. Radiology 1999;210(3):605–10.

[2] Cao Z, Tian R, Zhang T, et al. Localized autoimmune pancreatitis: report of a case clinically mimicking pancreatic cancer and a literature review. Medicine (Baltim) 2015;94(42):e1656. https://doi.org/10.1097/MD.0000000000001656.

[3] Kim KP, Kim MH, Song MH, et al. Autoimmune chronic pancreatitis. Am J Gastroenterol 2004;99(8):1605–16.

[4] Lopes Vendrami C, Shin JS, Hammond NA, et al. Differentiation of focal autoimmune pancreatitis from pancreatic ductal adenocarcinoma. Abdom Radiol (NY) 2020;45(5):1371–86.

[5] Madhani K, Farrell JJ. Autoimmune pancreatitis: an update on diagnosis and management. Gastroenterol Clin N Am 2016;45(1):29–43.

[6] Zen Y. Type 2 autoimmune pancreatitis: consensus and controversies. Gut Liver 2022;16(3):357–65.

[7] Kamisawa T, Chari ST, Lerch MM, et al. Recent advances in autoimmune pancreatitis: type 1 and type 2. Gut 2013;62(9):1373–80.

[8] Hafezi-Nejad N, Singh VK, Fung C, et al. MR imaging of autoimmune pancreatitis. Magn Reson Imag Clin N Am 2018;26(3):463–78.

[9] Muhi A, Ichikawa T, Motosugi U, et al. Mass-forming autoimmune pancreatitis and pancreatic carcinoma: differential diagnosis on the basis of computed tomography and magnetic resonance cholangiopancreatography, and diffusion-weighted imaging findings. J Magn Reson Imag 2012;35(4):827–36.

[10] Al-Hawary MM, Kaza RK, Azar SF, et al. Mimics of pancreatic ductal adenocarcinoma. Cancer Imaging 2013;13(3):342–9.

[11] Kothari K, Lopes Vendrami C, Kelahan LC, et al. Inflammatory mimickers of pancreatic adenocarcinoma. Abdom Radiol (NY) 2020;45(5):1387–96.

[12] Slodkowski M, Wronski M, Karkocha D, et al. Current approaches for the curative-intent surgical treatment of pancreatic ductal adenocarcinoma. Cancers (Basel) 2023;15(9). https://doi.org/10.3390/cancers15092584.

[13] Sugiyama Y, Fujinaga Y, Kadoya M, et al. Characteristic magnetic resonance features of focal autoimmune pancreatitis useful for differentiation from pancreatic cancer. Jpn J Radiol 2012;30(4):296–309.

[14] Choi SY, Kim SH, Kang TW, et al. Differentiating mass-forming autoimmune pancreatitis from pancreatic ductal adenocarcinoma on the basis of contrast-enhanced MRI and DWI findings. AJR Am J Roentgenol 2016;206(2):291–300.

[15] Johnston A, Serhal A, Lopes Vendrami C, et al. The abrupt pancreatic duct cutoff sign on MDCT and MRI. Abdom Radiol (NY) 2020;45(8):2476–84.

[16] Wakabayashi T, Kawaura Y, Satomura Y, et al. Clinical and imaging features of autoimmune pancreatitis with focal pancreatic swelling or mass formation: comparison with so-called tumor-forming pancreatitis and pancreatic carcinoma. Am J Gastroenterol 2003;98(12):2679–87.

[17] Agrawal S, Daruwala C, Khurana J. Distinguishing autoimmune pancreatitis from pancreaticobiliary cancers: current strategy. Ann Surg 2012;255(2):248–58.

[18] Kamisawa T, Tu Y, Egawa N, et al. Can MRCP replace ERCP for the diagnosis of autoimmune pancreatitis? Abdom Imaging 2009;34(3):381–4.

[19] Naitoh I, Nakazawa T, Hayashi K, et al. Clinical differences between mass-forming autoimmune pancreatitis and pancreatic cancer. Scand J Gastroenterol 2012; 47(5):607–13.

[20] Nishino T, Oyama H, Toki F, et al. Differentiation between autoimmune pancreatitis and pancreatic carcinoma based on endoscopic retrograde cholangiopancreatography findings. J Gastroenterol 2010;45(9):988–96.

[21] Chang WI, Kim BJ, Lee JK, et al. The clinical and radiological characteristics of focal mass-forming autoimmune pancreatitis: comparison with chronic pancreatitis and pancreatic cancer. Pancreas 2009;38(4):401–8.

[22] Negrelli R, Manfredi R, Pedrinolla B, et al. Pancreatic duct abnormalities in focal autoimmune pancreatitis: MR/MRCP imaging findings. Eur Radiol 2015;25(2):359–67.

[23] Hur BY, Lee JM, Lee JE, et al. Magnetic resonance imaging findings of the mass-forming type of autoimmune pancreatitis: comparison with pancreatic adenocarcinoma. J Magn Reson Imag 2012;36(1):188–97.

[24] Vlachou PA, Khalili K, Jang HJ, et al. IgG4-related sclerosing disease: autoimmune pancreatitis and extrapancreatic manifestations. Radiographics 2011;31(5):1379–402.

[25] Fujinaga Y, Kadoya M, Kawa S, et al. Characteristic findings in images of extra-pancreatic lesions associated with autoimmune pancreatitis. Eur J Radiol 2010;76(2): 228–38.

[26] Kozoriz MG, Chandler TM, Patel R, et al. Pancreatic and extrapancreatic features in autoimmune pancreatitis. Can Assoc Radiol J 2015;66(3):252–8.

[27] Zhang J, Jia G, Zuo C, et al. (18)F- FDG PET/CT helps differentiate autoimmune pancreatitis from pancreatic cancer. BMC Cancer 2017;17(1):695.

[28] Bello HR, Sekhar A, Filice RW, et al. Pancreaticoduodenal groove: spectrum of disease and imaging features. Radiographics 2022;42(4):1062–80.

[29] Mittal PK, Harri P, Nandwana S, et al. Paraduodenal pancreatitis: benign and malignant mimics at MRI. Abdom Radiol (NY) 2017;42(11):2652–74.

[30] Triantopoulou C, Dervenis C, Giannakou N, et al. Groove pancreatitis: a diagnostic challenge. Eur Radiol 2009;19(7):1736–43.

[31] Raman SP, Salaria SN, Hruban RH, et al. Groove pancreatitis: spectrum of imaging findings and radiology-pathology correlation. AJR Am J Roentgenol 2013; 201(1):W29–39.

[32] Miller FH, Lopes Vendrami C, Hammond NA, et al. Pancreatic cancer and its mimics. Radiographics 2023; 43(11):e230054. https://doi.org/10.1148/rg.230054.

[33] Wood CG, Lopes Vendrami C, Craig E, et al. Pancreatitis in the developmentally anomalous pancreas. Abdom Radiol (NY) 2020;45(5):1316–23.

[34] Rezvani M, Menias C, Sandrasegaran K, et al. Heterotopic pancreas: histopathologic features, imaging findings, and complications. Radiographics 2017;37(2):484–99.

[35] Mortele KJ, Rocha TC, Streeter JL, et al. Multimodality imaging of pancreatic and biliary congenital anomalies. Radiographics 2006;26(3):715–31.

[36] Thangasamy SJ, Zheng L, McIntosh L, et al. Dynamic contrast-enhanced MRI findings of acute pancreatitis in ectopic pancreatic tissue: case report and review of the literature. JOP 2014;15(4):407–10.

[37] Bhasin DK, Rana SS, Nanda M, et al. Ansa pancreatica type of ductal anatomy in a patient with idiopathic acute pancreatitis. JOP 2006;7(3):315–20.

[38] Silva AC, Charles JC, Kimery BD, et al. MR cholangiopancreatography in the detection of symptomatic ectopic pancreatitis in the small-bowel mesentery. AJR Am J Roentgenol 2006;187(2):W195–7.

[39] Ginsburg M, Ahmed O, Rana KA, et al. Ectopic pancreas presenting with pancreatitis and a mesenteric mass. J Pediatr Surg 2013;48(1):e29–32.

[40] Sandrasegaran K, Patel A, Fogel EL, et al. Annular pancreas in adults. AJR Am J Roentgenol 2009;193(2): 455–60.

[41] Kung JW, Brown A, Kruskal JB, et al. Heterotopic pancreas: typical and atypical imaging findings. Clin Radiol 2010;65(5):403–7.

[42] Johnston DW. Annular pancreas: a new classification and clinical observations. Can J Surg 1978;21(3):241–4.

[43] Zyromski NJ, Sandoval JA, Pitt HA, et al. Annular pancreas: dramatic differences between children and adults. J Am Coll Surg 2008;206(5):1019–25, ; discussion 1025-1017.

[44] Jadvar H, Mindelzun RE. Annular pancreas in adults: imaging features in seven patients. Abdom Imaging 1999;24(2):174–7.

[45] Rondelli F, Bugiantella W, Stella P, et al. Symptomatic annular pancreas in adult: report of two different presentations and treatments and review of the literature. Int J Surg Case Rep 2016;20S(Suppl):21–4.

[46] Huddleston VS, Lippuner V, Dyer AW. Annular pancreas in an adult presenting with acute pancreatitis. J Radiol Case Rep 2018;12(10):11–6.

[47] Hidaka T, Hirohashi S, Uchida H, et al. Annular pancreas diagnosed by single-shot MR cholangiopancreatography. Magn Reson Imaging 1998;16(4):441–4.

[48] Sencan A, Mir E, Gunsar C, et al. Symptomatic annular pancreas in newborns. Med Sci Monit 2002;8(6): CR434–7.

[49] Tirkes T, Yadav D, Conwell DL, et al. Consortium for the Study of Chronic Pancreatitis, Diabetes, Pancreatic Cancer. Quantitative MRI of chronic pancreatitis: results from a multi-institutional prospective study, magnetic resonance imaging as a non-invasive method for assessment of pancreatic fibrosis (MINIMAP). Abdom Radiol (NY) 2022;47(11):3792–805.

[50] Miller FH, Keppke AL, Wadhwa A, et al. MRI of pancreatitis and its complications: part 2, chronic pancreatitis. AJR Am J Roentgenol 2004;183(6):1645–52.

[51] Conwell DL, Lee LS, Yadav D, et al. American Pancreatic Association practice guidelines in chronic pancreatitis: evidence-based report on diagnostic guidelines. Pancreas 2014;43(8):1143–62.

[52] Tirkes T, Lin C, Fogel EL, et al. T(1) mapping for diagnosis of mild chronic pancreatitis. J Magn Reson Imag 2017;45(4):1171–6.

[53] Tirkes T, Fogel EL, Sherman S, et al. Detection of exocrine dysfunction by MRI in patients with early chronic pancreatitis. Abdom Radiol (NY) 2017;42(2):544–51.

[54] Tirkes T, Yadav D, Conwell DL, et al. Consortium for the Study of Chronic Pancreatitis, Diabetes, Pancreatic Cancer. Magnetic resonance imaging as a non-invasive method for the assessment of pancreatic fibrosis (MINI-MAP): a comprehensive study design from the consortium for the study of chronic pancreatitis, diabetes, and pancreatic cancer. Abdom Radiol (NY) 2019;44(8): 2809–21.

[55] Serai SD, Robson MD, Tirkes T, et al. T(1) mapping of the abdomen, from the AJR "how we do it" special series. AJR Am J Roentgenol 2024. https://doi.org/10.2214/AJR.24.31643.

[56] Cheng M, Gromski MA, Fogel EL, et al. T1 mapping for the diagnosis of early chronic pancreatitis: correlation with Cambridge classification system. Br J Radiol 2021; 94(1121):20200685. https://doi.org/10.1259/bjr.20200685.

[57] Tirkes T, Lin C, Cui E, et al. Quantitative MR evaluation of chronic pancreatitis: extracellular volume fraction and MR relaxometry. AJR Am J Roentgenol 2018;210(3): 533–42.

[58] Siddiqui N, Vendrami CL, Chatterjee A, et al. Advanced MR imaging techniques for pancreas imaging. Magn Reson Imag Clin N Am 2018;26(3):323–44.

[59] Tirkes T, Sandrasegaran K, Sanyal R, et al. Secretin-enhanced MR cholangiopancreatography: spectrum of findings. Radiographics 2013;33(7):1889–906.

[60] Chamokova B, Bastati N, Poetter-Lang S, et al. The clinical value of secretin-enhanced MRCP in the functional and morphological assessment of pancreatic diseases. Br J Radiol 2018;91(1084):20170677. https://doi.org/10.1259/bjr.20170677.

[61] Matos C, Metens T, Deviere J, et al. Pancreatic duct: morphologic and functional evaluation with dynamic MR pancreatography after secretin stimulation. Radiology 1997;203(2):435–41.

[62] Swensson J, Zaheer A, Conwell D, et al. Secretin-enhanced MRCP: how and why-AJR expert panel narrative review. AJR Am J Roentgenol 2021;216(5):1139–49.

[63] Yan G, Yan G, Li H, et al. Radiomics and its applications and progress in pancreatitis: a current state of the art review. Front Med 2022;9:922299. https://doi.org/10.3389/fmed.2022.922299.

[64] Shiraishi M, Igarashi T, Hiroaki F, et al. Radiomics based on diffusion-weighted imaging for differentiation between focal-type autoimmune pancreatitis and pancreatic carcinoma. Br J Radiol 2022;95(1140):20210456. https://doi.org/10.1259/bjr.20210456.

[65] Liang H, Wang M, Wen Y, et al. Predicting acute pancreatitis severity with enhanced computed tomography scans using convolutional neural networks. Sci Rep 2023;13(1): 17514. https://doi.org/10.1038/s41598-023-44828-7.

[66] Gorris M, Hoogenboom SA, Wallace MB, et al. Artificial intelligence for the management of pancreatic diseases. Dig Endosc 2021;33(2):231–41.

[67] Tirkes T, Shah ZK, Takahashi N, et al. Consortium for the Study of Chronic Pancreatitis, Diabetes, Pancreatic Cancer. Reporting standards for chronic pancreatitis by using CT, MRI, and MR cholangiopancreatography: the consortium for the study of chronic pancreatitis, diabetes, and pancreatic cancer. Radiology 2019;290(1): 207–15.

[68] Medetalibeyoglu A, Velichko YS, Hart EM, Bagci U. Foundational artificial intelligence models and modern medical practice. BJR Artif Intell 2024;2(1):ubae018.

[69] Jha D, Rauniyar A, Hagos D, et al. Practical and ethical considerations for generative AI in medical imaging. In: MICCAI workshop on fairness of AI medical imaging. 2024. 2024. p. 176–87. https://doi.org/10.13140/RG.2.2.34105.99681.

[70] Acosta JN, Falcone GJ, Rajpurkar P, et al. Multimodal biomedical AI. Nat Med 2022;28(9):1773–84.

[71] Hameed BS, Krishnan UM. Artificial intelligence-driven diagnosis of pancreatic cancer. Cancers (Basel) 2022; 14(21). https://doi.org/10.3390/cancers14215382.

[72] Bi WL, Hosny A, Schabath MB, et al. Artificial intelligence in cancer imaging: clinical challenges and applications. CA Cancer J Clin 2019;69(2):127–57.

[73] Hu JX, Zhao CF, Wang SL, et al. Acute pancreatitis: a review of diagnosis, severity prediction and prognosis assessment from imaging technology, scoring system and artificial intelligence. World J Gastroenterol 2023; 29(37):5268–91.

Advances in Clinical Radiology 7 (2025) 15–30
ADVANCES IN CLINICAL RADIOLOGY

Imaging of Hepatic Segment 4

Management and Surgical Implications

Sriram Jaganathan, MD[a], Abhijit Sunnapwar, MD[a], Anil K. Dasyam, MD[b], Tarunjeet Klair, MD[c], Venkat S. Katabathina, MD[a,*]

[a]Department of Radiology, University of Texas Health (UT Health), San Antonio, TX, USA; [b]Department of Radiology, University of Pittsburgh Medical Center, Pittsburgh, PA, USA; [c]Department of Hepatobiliary Surgery, University of Texas Health (UT Health), San Antonio, TX, USA

KEYWORDS

• Hepatic segment 4 • Bile leak • Pseudotumors • And mucinous cystic neoplasm

KEY POINTS

- Due to its unique embryologic development, hepatic segment 4 (S4) possesses distinct anatomic characteristics with varied vascular and biliary configurations.
- Understanding the functional segmental anatomy forms the basis of various hepatic resections and can help mitigate potential post-operative complications, especially in living donor liver transplantation.
- Because of its developmental nature, S4 is a unique location for select pathologies, including ciliated-hepatic foregut cysts and mucinous cystic neoplasms. S4 is a common location for pseudotumors, including focal fatty infiltration, fatty sparing areas, and perfusion abnormalities.

INTRODUCTION

Hepatic segment 4 (S4), also known as the left medial segment, possesses distinct anatomic, physiologic, and surgical characteristics and exhibits unique vascular and biliary configurations due to factors of embryologic development [1,2]. Understanding these anatomic configurations and segmental anatomy of the S4 is essential for surgical planning, including various hepatic resections described by the International Hepato-Pancreatico-Biliary Association Brisbane committee and the recent "New World" terminology [3–5]. S4 anatomy and vascular/biliary variations also play a crucial role in transplant surgeries, especially in living donor liver transplantation (LDLT), where the resection planes involve S4, potentially impacting both the donor and recipient. Additionally, S4 is prone to specific pathologies and pseudotumor formations due to its unique blood supply, anatomic position, and embryologic origins (Table 1).

This article describes embryology, essential surgical anatomy, arterial and portal venous supply, and hepatic venous and biliary drainage of the S4. This article also discusses various surgical resections involving the S4, associated post-operative complications, and potential anatomic details that may help mitigate these complications. It reviews imaging findings of unique conditions affecting the S4, including pseudotumors, inflammatory conditions, and neoplasms, to help radiologists better understand the conditions that can impact patient-care.

IMAGING TECHNIQUES

Ultrasound (US) is the initial imaging modality to assess the liver echotexture and focal hepatic lesions. Doppler US plays a crucial role, especially in post-liver donor transplant (LDLT), in evaluating the arterial and

*Corresponding author. Department of Radiology, 7703 Floyd Curl Drive, San Antonio, TX 78229. *E-mail address:* Katabathina@uthscsa.edu

https://doi.org/10.1016/j.yacr.2025.05.002
www.advancesinclinicalradiology.com
2589-8701/25/

ABBREVIATIONS

CHA	common hepatic artery
CHFC	ciliated hepatic foregut cyst
CT	computed tomography
CT	Computed tomography
FFD	focal fatty deposition
FFS	focal fatty sparing
GI	gastrointestinal
HS	hepatic segment
IPNB	intraductal papillary neoplasm of the bile duct
LDLT	living donor liver transplantation
LGA	left gastric artery
LHD	left hepatic duct
LPV	left portal vein
MCN	mucinous cystic neoplasm
MHA	middle hepatic artery
MHV	middle hepatic vein
S4	hepatic segment 4
SLT	split liver transplant
SMA	superior mesenteric artery
SVC	superior vena cava
THED	transient hepatic enhancement difference
US	ultrasound

venous blood flow, including the vascular evaluation of the S4 in the donor. US also helps identify post-surgical collections and guides therapeutic aspiration/drainage catheter placement. Computed tomography (CT) is the commonest modality utilized to evaluate the focal lesions further when identified on the US. Multiphasic CT helps assess the vascular anatomy, particularly in LDLT/hepatic resections, based on segmental distribution, and precisely delineates any anatomic variation in arterial or venous structures. In addition, post-operative complications can be better evaluated on CT scans, including fluid collections, hematomas, and vascular complications. MRI is a problem-solving modality in focal liver lesions indeterminate on CT and accurately differentiates focal fat deposition or sparing from other lesions. Magnetic resonance cholangio pancreatography (MRCP) is the modality of choice for assessing biliary anatomy, which plays a crucial role in various hepatic resections and LDLT. Hepatobiliary phase images obtained 20 to 30 min after contrast administration on Gadoxetic acid-enhanced (Eovist) MRI liver are especially useful in the evaluation of biliary anatomy and post-operative bile leaks.

LIVER SEGMENTAL ANATOMY

The Couinaud segmentation and International Hepato-Pancreatico-Biliary Association Brisbane committee segmentation are the commonly used classification systems to describe segmental liver anatomy and help in hepatic segmental resections [3–5]. The arrangement of the hepatic vasculature and the biliary drainage forms the basis of the functional anatomic classification systems. Cantlie's line (from the middle of the gallbladder fossa anteriorly to the inferior vena cava posteriorly) along the middle hepatic vein (MHV) divides the liver into functional right and left lobes [6]. The right and left hepatic veins, the falciform ligament, and the right and left portal veins (LPVs) divide the liver into 8 functionally independent hepatic segments (HSs), each with its own vascular inflow, outflow, and biliary drainage, although with some variant overlap [1,3,5] (Fig. 1). This arrangement enables the surgical resection of individual HSs without compromising the remaining segments [3]. The "New World" terminology simplifies the current classification systems, adding specifications for non-anatomical resections, multiple resections, and combined bilio-vascular resections [4].

TABLE 1
List of the Unique Pathologies of Hepatic Segment 4

	Unique S4 Pathologies
Post-surgical Complications	Bile leak & hepatic infarction
Related to the distinct vascular supply	Pseudotumors include abnormal vascular enhancement, focal fat deposition & focal fat sparing.
Embryologic/developmental origin	Ciliated hepatic foregut cyst
Neoplasms	Mucinous cystic neoplasm
Anatomic location related	Ingested-gastric foreign bodies perforating S4. Extension of pathologies from the gall bladder, stomach, and peritoneum.

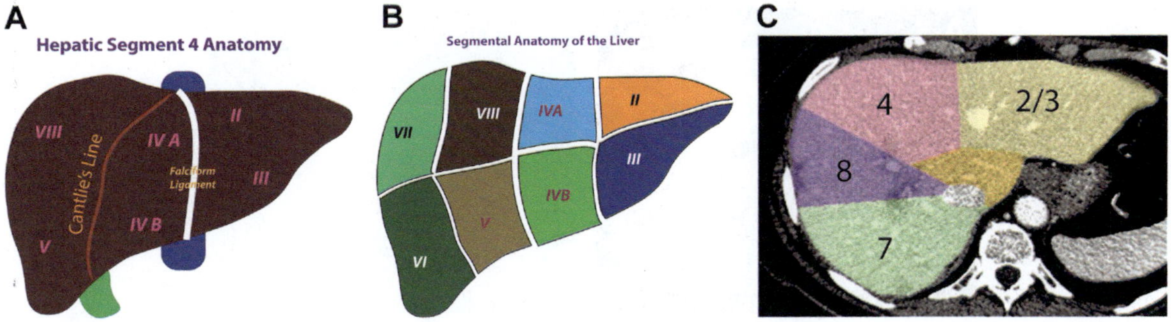

FIG. 1 (**A, B**) Illustrations demonstrate segmental anatomy of the liver based on Cantlie's line, falciform ligament, gallbladder fossa, portal venous supply, and hepatic venous drainage (**C**). Axial CT image utilizing the CT volumetry software superior to the portal venous bifurcation depicts various hepatic segments in different colors.

SEGMENT 4 EMBRYOLOGY

The primordial liver appears as an outgrowth from the endoderm of the ventral foregut during the third week of gestation [2]. The epithelium of this primordial liver proliferates to form future liver and intrahepatic biliary system. The persistent communication between the primordial liver and foregut forms the extrahepatic bile ducts. The umbilical vein lies within the left portion of the primitive middle hepatic lobe, marking the future plane that divides S3 from S4. As the liver increases in mass, the middle lobe rapidly enlarges, forming a larger S4 and a smaller S3, while the primitive left lobe regresses to become S2.

There are 3 principal arteries during the developmental stages of life, beginning at 8 w of gestation: 1. The left gastric artery (LGA) supplies the left lateral segment (S2). 2. An artery from the celiac axis supplies the paramedian sectors (S5, S8, S4, and S3). 3. The superior mesenteric artery (SMA) supplies the right lateral segments (S6 and S7). The 3 arteries later fuse to form a single artery—originating from the celiac axis, known as the common hepatic artery (CHA). If the right or left embryonic hepatic artery does not regress, it remains an aberrant hepatic artery (Fig. 2) [2,4,6,7]. Thus, S4 develops from the embryologic middle lobe, with arterial supply from the middle hepatic artery (MHA) and drainage by the MHV [2]. The S4 biliary ductules variably drain into the S2 and S3, forming the left hepatic duct (LHD).

This aspect of embryologic development makes S4 unique in its vascular and biliary configurations. Knowledge of standard anatomy and variations is essential for surgical planning, particularly in the context of transplant surgery, where the resection planes for split liver transplant (SLT) and living donor transplant (LDLT) involve S4, with potential consequences for both the recipient and the donor. It also becomes essential when planning interventions, such as targeted embolization or complex and segmental hepatic mass resections.

SEGMENT 4 ANATOMY

S4 is a part of the left hepatic lobe that lies between the left and MHVs and is subdivided into S4A and S4B subsegments by the transverse plane of the main portal vein [1,3,5]. S4B, often called the 'quadrate lobe' by

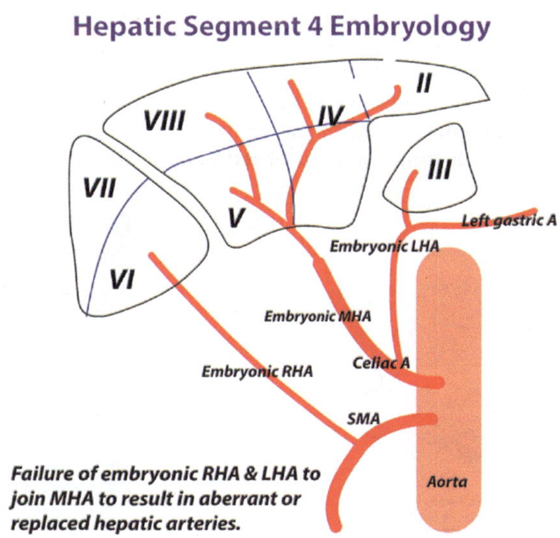

FIG. 2 Illustration demonstrates hepatic segment 4 embryology, and the evolution of segment 4 arteries based on the development.

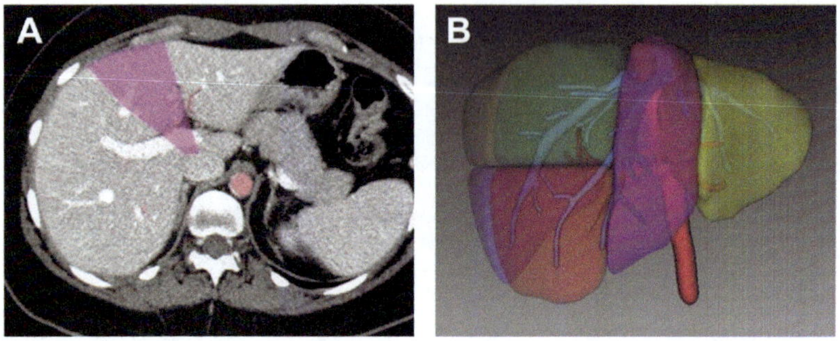

FIG. 3 Post processed images using CT liver volumetry software identifying segment 4. Axial post contrast CT image (**A**) and post processed volume rendered image (**B**) that demonstrate the different functional hepatic segments. Segment 4 is shown in purple color.

anatomists, is clinically recognized for its reliability as a landmark for bile duct anatomy, particularly during laparoscopic cholecystectomy. The quadrate lobe is bounded externally by the gallbladder fossa on the right, the umbilical fossa on the left, the anterior border of the liver below, and the porta hepatis above [2]. On CT/MRI, S4 is located between the MHV and the origin of the left hepatic vein superiorly (S4A) or the umbilical fissure inferiorly (S4B) (Fig. 3) [1,3,5].

SEGMENT 4 ARTERIAL ANATOMY

The proper hepatic artery supplies the liver, which gives rise to the right and left hepatic arteries. However, there are considerable variations in the arterial supply, with the more common being the replaced left hepatic artery from LGA and the replaced right hepatic artery from SMA. The main arterial supply to S4 originates from the MHA, also known as the medial segmental artery, the left medial artery, or the segment 4 artery (A4). A4 arises either from the right or left hepatic arteries, with variations in the portion of parenchyma being supplied [8–13]. Based on origin as either extrahepatic or intrahepatic branches of right HA, left HA, or proper HA, A4 is classified into 4 different types (Fig. 4) [7]. 1. Left HA Type: An extrahepatic or intrahepatic branch of the proximal left hepatic artery. 2. Right HA Type: A4 arises either from the right hepatic artery or the right anterior hepatic artery. Most right hepatic artery (RHA)-type A4s are extrahepatic branches of the proximal RHA. 3. Proper HA Type: It arises directly from the proper HA, forming a trifurcation. 4. Dual Type: Defined as 2 principal arteries stemming from 2 different origins [7].

SEGMENT 4 PORTAL VENOUS ANATOMY

The LPV is divided into transverse and vertical segments. The transverse segment lies at the base of S4, and the vertical segment runs in the umbilical fissure. The vertical segment gives rise to the branches that supply S4, with branches to S4A at right angles and branches to S4B to arise posteriorly (Fig. 5) [2].

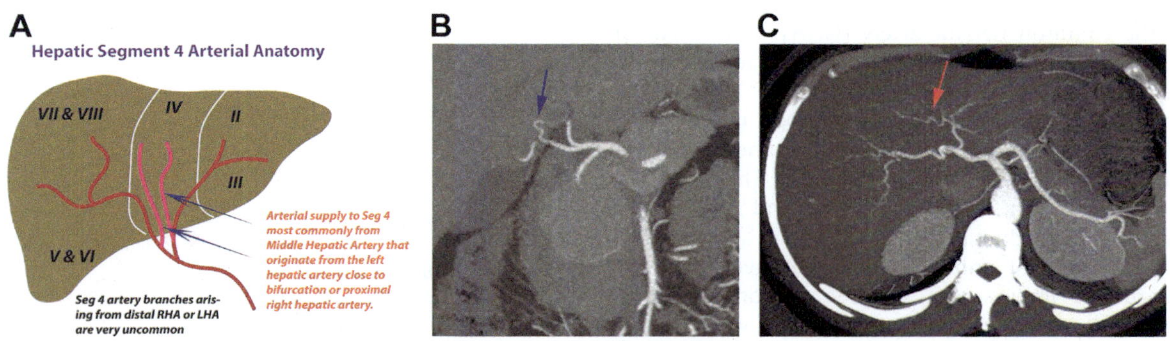

FIG. 4 Illustration demonstrates hepatic segment 4 arterial anatomy (**A**). Coronal MIP image (**B**) that demonstrates origin of S4 artery from the right hepatic artery (*blue arrow*). An axial MIP image (**C**) that demonstrates the origin of the S4 artery from the left hepatic artery (*red arrow*).

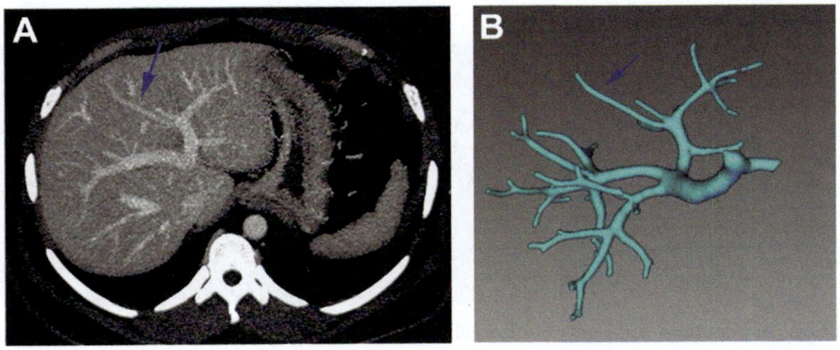

FIG. 5 Axial post contrast CT MIP image (**A**) that demonstrates segment 4A (*blue arrow*) portal venous branch from left portal vein. Volume rendered image (**B**) that shows segment 4 portal vein from the left portal vein (*blue arrow*).

SEGMENT 4 HEPATIC VENOUS ANATOMY

A precise understanding of the hepatic veins and their anatomic relationship with the inferior vena cava (IVC) is essential for safe liver surgeries, including partial hepatectomy, liver transplantation, and managing hepatic trauma. The major venous drainage of S4 is the MHV, with S4B and S5 hepatic veins joining to form the main trunk of MHV (Fig. 6). Additionally, MHV receives tributaries from S4A (superiorly) and S8. MHV ultimately drains into the IVC, along with the LHV, as a common trunk. The intersegmental zone between S4 and S2/S3 is a watershed between the drainage of MHV and LHV [2]. Occasionally, small hepatic veins draining S4A can directly join the suprahepatic IVC close to the MHV-LHV trunk.

SEGMENT 4 BILIARY ANATOMY

Biliary drainage of S4 closely follows the portal veins. S4 duct joins ducts from S2 and S3 in several configurations to form the LHD. Reichert and colleagues described 4 different anatomic variations of the LHD, and Cho and colleagues described 3 variations [14,15]. The most common (~55 – 78%) configuration involves the S4 duct joining the left lateral segment duct, formed by the union of the S3 and S2 ducts, to create the LHD (Fig. 7) [14–16]. Because S4 in this arrangement does not cross segment boundaries/surgical resection planes, it is least at risk of injury. The following is the most common variant: the S2 duct joins the common trunk formed by S4 and S3. The less common variations include 2 S4 ducts joining the LHD; all 3 left HS ducts converge simultaneously to form the LHD; and S4 drains into the right hepatic duct [2,14–16].

HEPATIC SURGICAL RESECTIONS INVOLVING SEGMENT 4: SURGICAL SIGNIFICANCE OF S4 ANATOMY AND POST-OPERATIVE COMPLICATIONS

Surgical resections involving S4 include S4 hepatectomy, left hepatectomy, extended left hepatectomy,

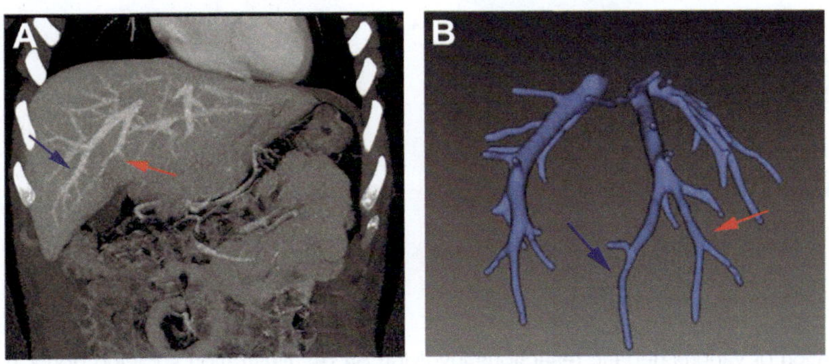

FIG. 6 Coronal MIP image (**A**) and volume rendered reformatted hepatic venous image (**B**) demonstrate segment 4B *(red arrows)* and segment 5 (*red arrows*) join to form the middle hepatic vein.

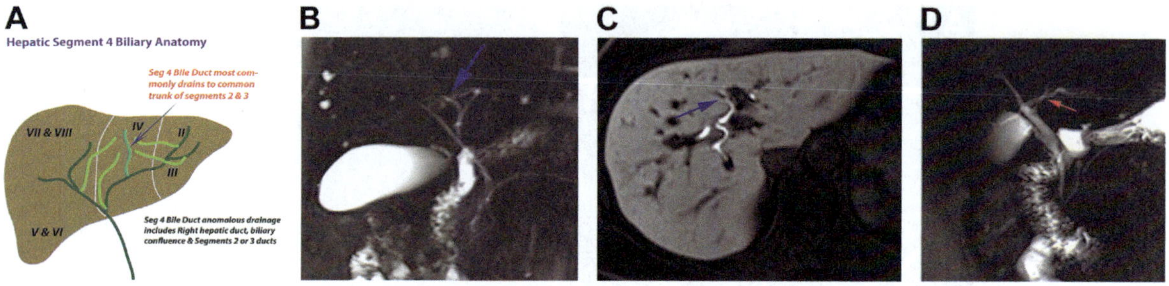

FIG. 7 Illustration (**A**) demonstrates segment 4 bile duct anatomy including the common pattern and variations. 2D MRCP image (**B**) and axial post Eovist hepatobiliary phase MR image (**C**) demonstrates segment 4 bile duct (*blue arrows*) draining into the common trunk of segment 2/3 ducts forming left hepatic duct. Variant anatomy: 2D MRCP image (**D**) demonstrates segment 4 duct (*red arrow*) draining into the common hepatic duct.

and extended right hepatectomy. S4 is also involved in right hepatectomy and left lateral segmentectomy for adult LDLT and pediatric LDLT, respectively (Fig. 8) [2]. In these hepatectomies, the surgical transection plane passes through or involves S4; hence, understanding S4 vascular, biliary, and parenchymal anatomy is crucial for minimizing post-operative complications, such as bile leaks, vascular injuries, and impaired graft function [2].

Pre-operative identification of variant arterial/portal venous/hepatic venous anatomy of S4 is very important before LDLT and other hepatic resections and has significant clinical implications. In LDLT surgeries, preserving donor A4 is crucial, whether it involves a right hepatic lobe graft or an S2/3 graft, as ischemia of S4 can compromise the functional liver remnant. For right lobe donors, a complete segment II-IV blood supply needs to be maintained to the left lobe remnant [2]. Thrombosis of the A4 was one of the common complications of LDLT before the advent of advanced microsurgical techniques. However, the incidence of A4 thrombosis has decreased due to the improvement in surgical techniques used for its reconstruction and dissection away from the hepatectomy plane in the setting of variant anatomy [8–13]. On CT, the S4 infarct appears as a well-defined hypodensity in the lateral aspect of the S4, abutting the cut surface of the liver (Fig. 9).

In the right lobe transplant, the LPV is preserved so that S4 is unaffected. However, in the left lateral segment

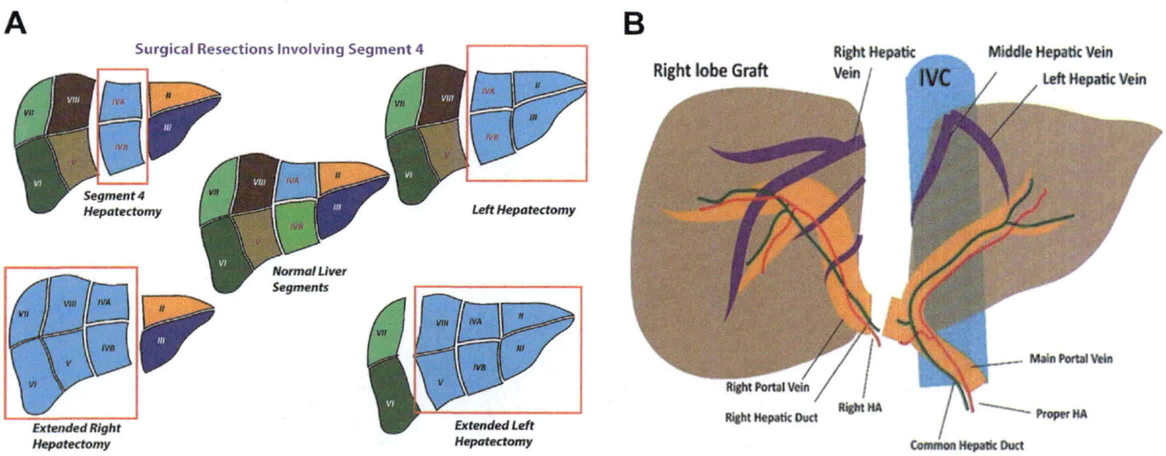

FIG. 8 Illustration of various hepatic resections involving S4 (**A**). Illustration showing donor hepatectomy resection plane on living donor right hepatic lobe liver transplant (**B**). Note that the transection plane in LDLT traverses along the middle hepatic vein involving S4.

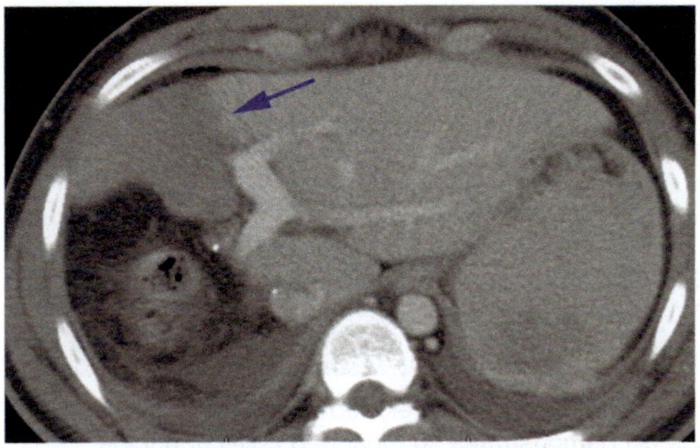

FIG. 9 A 20-year-old healthy donor who presented with abdominal pain nearly a week after the right hepatic lobe liver donation. Axial contrast enhanced CT image demonstrates infarct in segment 4 (*blue arrow*), likely due to S4 hepatic arterial injury.

transplant, though the S4 arterial supply is maintained, S4 portal venous branches are ligated at the umbilical fissure, resulting in relative S4 ischemia [2]. Additionally, preserving the hepatic venous drainage of S4 is crucial to prevent congestion and impact the future regeneration of S4 in the right lobe LDLT. Hence, retaining the MHV in the donor, which forms the main draining vein for S4, is preferred. MHV configuration is crucial for deciding the plane of surgical transection in LDLT and various hepatectomies [2,17]. Retaining MHV within the donor based on S4 venous anatomy often increases donor safety and reduces morbidity in LDLTs [2,17].

The biliary drainage of the left lobe remnant needs to be preserved in LDLT. There is a higher incidence of bile leak in split LDLT than in deceased donor liver transplantation (DDLT) due to resection planes involving S4 and its variant anatomic vascular/biliary configurations [16,18]. Bile leaks can happen from small bile ducts along the hepatic cut surface in S4 that may not be apparent during surgery. Anomalous drainage pathways of the S4 bile duct into the right hepatic or segment 3 ducts could result in significant bile leaks, depending on the resection plane [18]. A new fluid collection in the living donor along the S4 abutting the cut surface of the liver should raise the suspicion of bile leak, and contrast-enhanced MRI with MRCP, especially with the use of Eovist contrast and endoscopic retrograde cholangiopancreatography (ERCP), helps to diagnose bile leaks (Figs. 10 and 11) [16,18].

UNIQUE PATHOLOGIES INVOLVING SEGMENT 4

Pathologies unique to S4 include pseudotumors (focal fat sparing, focal fat infiltration, and abnormal vascular enhancement mimicking neoplasms), developmental conditions (ciliated hepatic foregut cyst [CHFC]), neoplasms (mucinous cystic neoplasm [MCN]), ingested gastric foreign bodies perforating S4, and pathologies directly extending from adjacent organs.

Pseudotumors of Segment 4

Pseudotumors involving S4 could be secondary to vascular etiologies, focal fat deposition, or focal fatty sparing (FFS). Liver parenchyma is typically perfused by a dual blood supply from the portal venous and hepatic arterial systems; however, third-inflow sources resulting in aberrant hepatopetal flow from gastric, cholecystic, paraumbilical, or pancreatic veins may be present. [19,20]. Given its unique vascular supply and location, these pseudolesions are common in segment 4.

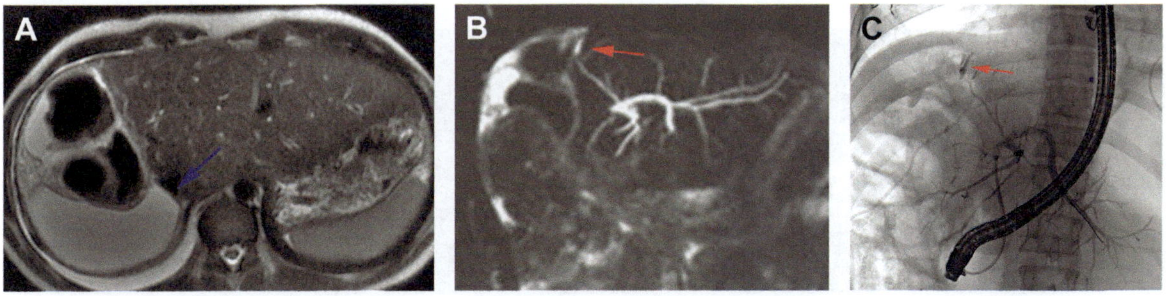

FIG. 10 Images of a patient who underwent donor right hepatectomy 2 weeks prior. Axial T2-weighted MR image (**A**) demonstrates a fluid collection in the right hepatectomy surgical bed (*blue arrow*). 2D MRCP image (**B**) shows the surgical bed collection and a branch of the segment 4 bile duct (*red arrow*) extending to the resection margin. ERCP image (**C**) demonstrates bile leak from the segment 4 bile duct (*red arrow*).

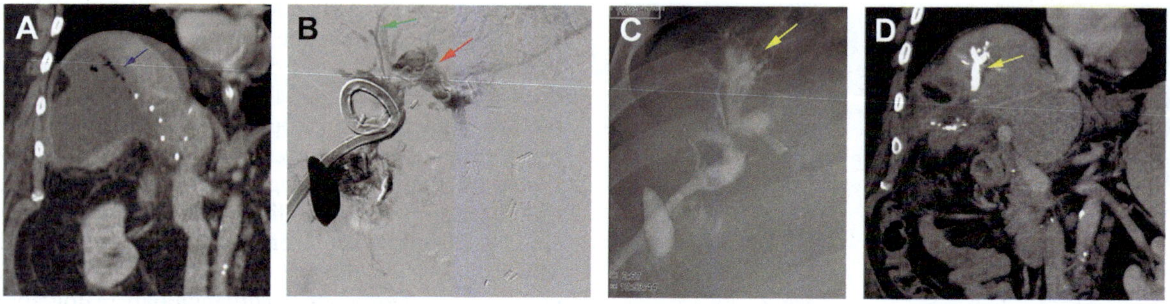

FIG. 11 Status post right hepatectomy for cholangiocarcinoma, the patient developed recurrent surgical bed collections. Coronal post contrast venous phase image (**A**) demonstrates surgical bed collection (*blue arrow*). Digital subtraction image (**B**) post contrast injection through the drainage catheter demonstrates the collection with a tract (*red arrow*) and faint opacification of the segment 4 bile duct (*green arrow*) in the resection margin. Percutaneous approach embolization (**C**) of the tract communicating with the segment 4 duct at the resection margin with the liquid embolic material (N- Butyl Cyanoacrylate liquid agent mixed with ethiodol (*yellow arrow*). Hyperdense embolic agent seen on follow up coronal CT image (**D**) with resolution of the collection. Note that embolic agent is noted in the segmental bile ducts near the resection margin on follow up CT (*yellow arrow*).

ABNORMAL VASCULAR ENHANCEMENT MIMICKING NEOPLASMS

Transient hepatic enhancement differences (THEDs) are perfusion differences evident on arterial/portal venous phase images as an area of hyperenhancement. They are due to potential venous collaterals from the third inflow source [19,20]. THEDs are generally wedge-shaped, subcapsular, and subsegmental but can have variable appearances, including rounded or diffuse geographic areas or seen as areas of peritumoral hyperenhancement (Fig. 12) [19]. THEDs can mimic pathologic lesions when seen on a single phase of contrast-enhanced imaging. Imaging features that help differentiate THED from the hepatic mass are the distribution pattern, lack of mass effect, and presence of normal vessels coursing through the abnormal enhancement area. Additionally, the lack of signal change on other magnetic resonance (MR) sequences supports the diagnosis of THED [19,20].

Although THEDs are not specific for S4, one of the variant abnormal enhancements specific for S4 occurs in the superior vena cava (SVC) obstruction. A focal geographic or wedge-shaped area of S4 arterial and venous hyperenhancement is seen in SVC obstruction. This abnormal enhancement is secondary to abdominal wall collaterals, resulting in portosystemic venous shunting between the SVC and the LPV secondary to SVC obstruction with associated increased third hepatopetal inflow. This phenomenon was initially observed as a hotspot on the Tc99 sulfur colloid nuclear scan and described as a "quadrate lobe hot spot sign" on CT images [21,22]. The characteristic location in the

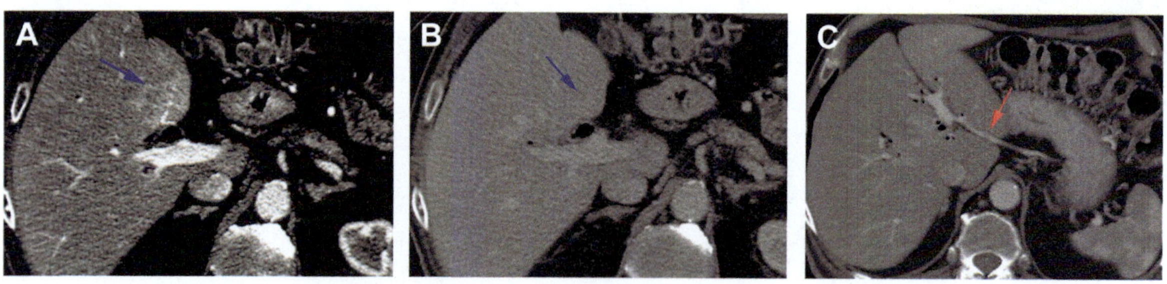

FIG. 12 Axial CT images (**A, B**) demonstrate geographic hyper-enhancing area in segment 4B on late arterial phase (*blue arrow*) that becomes iso-dense to the surrounding liver parenchyma on the venous phase image (*blue arrow*), representing a perfusion anomaly. Axial venous phase CT image (**C**) demonstrates the aberrant left gastric vein draining into distal left portal vein (*red arrow*), likely causing the perfusion anomaly.

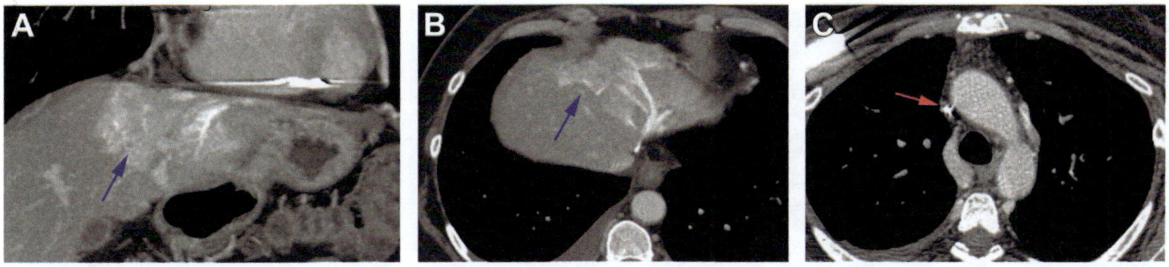

FIG. 13 Coronal and axial contrast enhanced CT images (**A, B**) of the liver and chest (**C**) demonstrate hyper enhancement in segment 4A (*blue arrows*) related to porto-systemic shunt secondary to severe stenosis/ occlusion of the superior vena cava (*red arrow*). This is known as 'hot quadrate lobe sign'.

quadrate lobe of the liver and enhancement in both arterial and venous phase images help differentiate this pseudolesion from other hepatic vascular tumors (Fig. 13) [21,22].

FOCAL FAT DEPOSITION

Focal fatty deposition (FFD) or infiltration is one of the common entities encountered in cross-sectional imaging. It occurs in 30% to 40% of the general population and can be multifocal in up to 20% [23]. The typical locations of FFD include the porta hepatis/posterior aspect of S4, gallbladder fossa, and adjacent to the falciform ligament. The pathophysiology of FFD is related to decreased-focal portal venous flow, which results in nutritional ischemia. The aberrant pancreatoduodenal vein supplies the posterior aspect of S4 instead of the portal vein. It may expose this area of parenchyma to insulin-rich blood from the pancreas, leading to FFD [23].

FFDs are hyperechoic on the US, hypoattenuating on non-contrast CT, and demonstrate hypoenhancement on post-contrast images (Fig. 14). Chemical shift MRI helps demonstrate the areas of FFD as the signal drop on out-of-phase images [20,23]. Areas of FFD are wedge-shaped or geographic, lack mass effect, do not demonstrate restricted diffusion, and have undistorted vessels within [23,24]. An MRI is necessary to diagnose when FFDs are round or nodular in appearance due to concerns about neoplasia (Fig. 15). Fat-containing tumors, including hepatocellular carcinoma, should be differentiated from nodular steatosis. Imaging features that favor the neoplastic process include T2 hyperintensity, heterogenous enhancement pattern, diffusion restriction, pseudocapsule, intratumoral necrosis, or hemorrhage [23,24].

FOCAL FAT SPARING

FFS typically involves the posterior aspect of S4 in an otherwise diffusely steatotic liver and may mimic a liver mass. Anomalous third inflow with the aberrant right gastric vein draining into S4 is thought to cause relative ischemia from the portal venous system and reduced insulin and triglyceride delivery compared to the rest of the liver, resulting in FFS [23,25]. Other

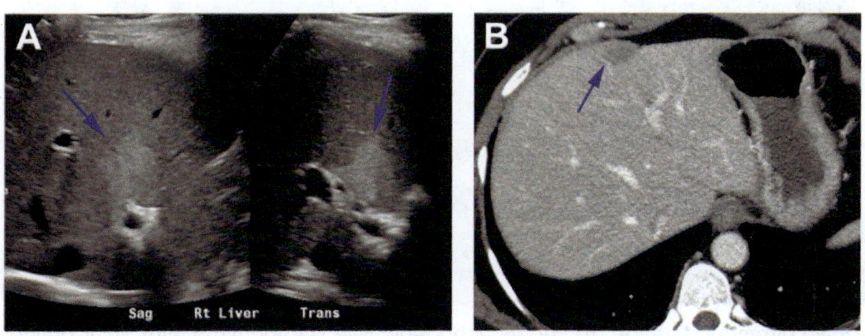

FIG. 14 Grayscale ultrasound image (**A**) shows geographic hyperechoic area in the periportal region, a characteristic site and appearance for focal fatty deposition (FFD) (*blue arrows*). Axial CT image (**B**) of a different patient demonstrating hypodensity near the falciform ligament consistent with FFD (*blue arrow*).

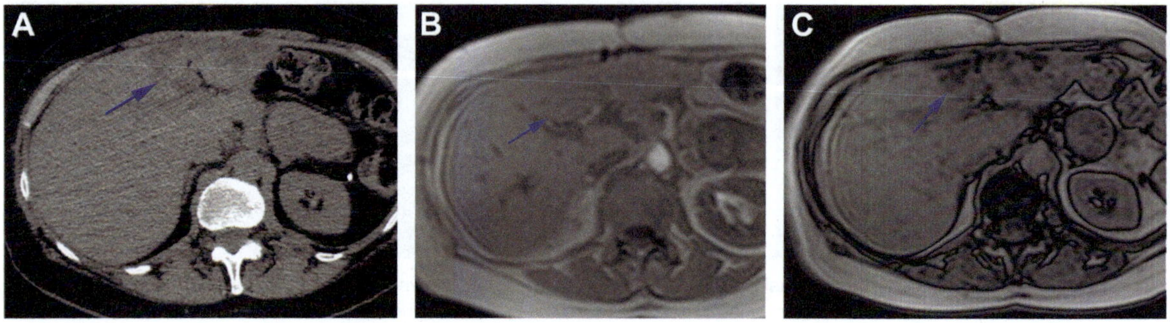

FIG. 15 Axial non contrast CT image (**A**) of a patient with known colorectal malignancy demonstrates ill-defined hypodense lesions (*blue arrows*) in segment 4B and 3 concerning for metastatic disease. Axial T1 in phase (**B**) and out of phase MR images (**C**) clearly depict the signal drop on the out of phase image in this suspicious area consistent with focal fat deposition (*blue arrows*).

areas typical for FFS include the gallbladder fossa, falciform ligament, porta hepatis, and subcapsular regions [23,25].

FFS can mimic a focal intrahepatic hypoechoic mass on the US relative to the hyperechoic steatotic liver. Similarly, the areas of FFS appear relatively hyperdense compared to the surrounding hypoattenuating liver on non-contrast CT. Post-contrast images demonstrate relative heterogeneity in parenchymal enhancement because of FFS [19,23]. MRI, including opposed phase and fat saturation imaging, should be sufficient to establish the diagnosis without needing a biopsy. FFS appears as a T1 isointense area on in-phase images and T1 hyperintense on opposed-phase images relative to the hypointense steatotic background liver (Figs. 16 and 17). Like FFD, features, such as lack of mass effect, undistorted vessel coursing through the area, and no diffusion restriction, favor FFS [19,23].

CILIATED HEPATIC FOREGUT CYST

A ciliated hepatic foregut cyst (CHFC) is a rare cystic lesion of embryologic origin and most commonly occurs in S4. CFHC is a detached hepatic diverticulum or abnormal tracheobronchial bud that may have migrated caudally to be included with the liver. The cyst has 4 layers histologically, including inner ciliated pseudostratified columnar epithelium, lamina propria, smooth muscle, and outer fibrous capsule. The histologic appearance is similar to bronchial and esophageal cysts because of the common embryonic foregut origin of the liver, esophagus, and bronchus [26].

CHFC typically presents as a small subcapsular lesion located in S4. It measures around a mean size of 3 cm, varying between 1 and 12 cm [27,28]. CHFCs are usually incidental findings on imaging or during surgery. On the US, CHFCs are typically seen as a unilocular, hypoechoic lesion. However, they may present

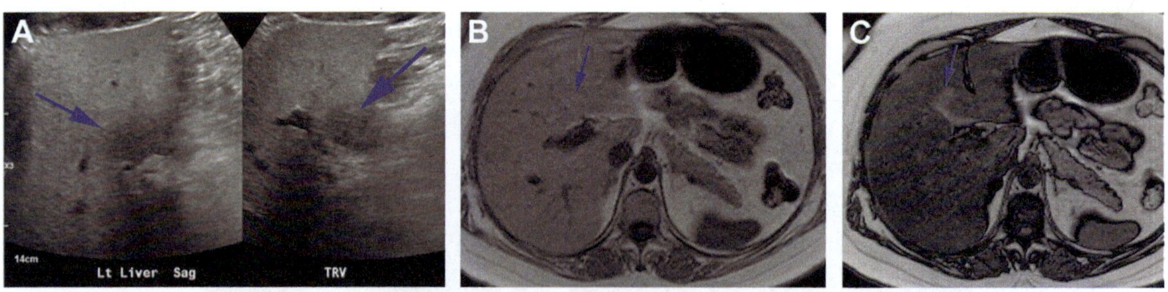

FIG. 16 Grayscale ultrasound image (**A**) shows echogenic liver parenchyma with an ill-defined hypoechoic area in the left hepatic lobe (*blue arrows*). MRI was performed for further evaluation. Axial T1 in phase image (**B**) and T1 out of phase image (**C**) demonstrate the parenchymal signal drop on out of phase image in the rest of the liver parenchyma consistent with focal fat sparing in segment 4B (*blue arrows*).

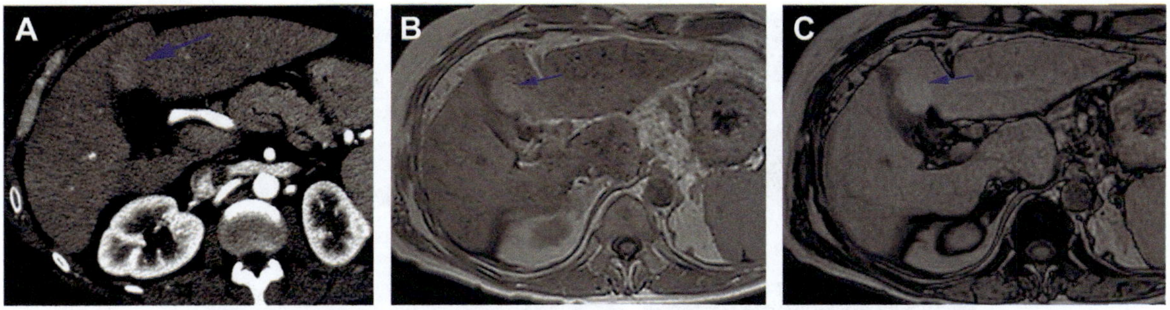

FIG. 17 Axial arterial phase CT image (**A**) demonstrates a hyperdense lesion in segment 4B (*blue arrow*) concerning for a hepatic mass. Axial T1 in phase image (**B**) and T1 out of phase image (**C**) demonstrate subtle signal drop in the surrounding liver parenchyma with relative sparing of the lesion consistent with focal nodular fat sparing (*blue arrows*).

as a solid lesion. On CT, they are hypodense or variable attenuating lesions that do not enhance with contrast (Fig. 18). On MRI, they are T2 hyperintense and variable intensity on T1, depending on the presence of serous material, protein, lipid, or a varying combination of any of these contents [26–28]. There may be fat-fluid levels depending on the amount of lipid content. CHFCs do not demonstrate restricted diffusion or contrast enhancement (see Fig. 18) [27].

CHFCs are clinically and radiologically similar to hepatic cystic neoplasms. The common differentials of the unilocular cyst include simple hepatic cyst, echinococcal cyst, and MCN [27]. While most CHFCs are asymptomatic and incidentally discovered, surgical removal may be necessary due to rare reports of malignant transformation [26–28]. CHFCs should be surgically removed if the cysts exceed 4 to 5 cm in size, present with symptoms, exhibit growth over time, or cysts that display concerning imaging features, like thick septations or focal wall irregularities [27].

MUCINOUS CYSTIC NEOPLASM

MCN of the liver is a rare cystic tumor that accounts for 5% of cystic hepatic neoplasms, predominantly occurring in middle-aged women [29–31]. The World Health Organization's tumor classification system describes MCN as a cyst-forming epithelial tumor, typically lacking communication with the bile ducts. MCN comprises mucin-producing cuboidal to columnar epithelium and is characterized by ovarian-type subepithelial stroma [31,32]. They usually present with non-specific symptoms like abdominal pain, fullness, early satiety, and mass effect. The most common location is the left hepatic lobe, with approximately 54% of the tumors occurring in the S4 [32]. Different hypotheses for the

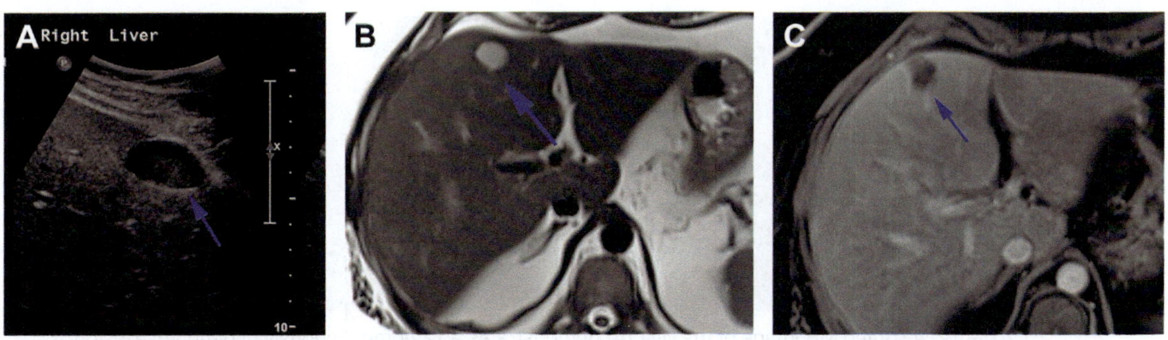

FIG. 18 Grayscale ultrasound image (**A**) shows an echogenic lesion with internal echogenic debris in the left hepatic lobe (*blue arrow*). Axial T2-weighted MR image (**B**) and post contrast T1-weighted axial venous phase MR image (**C**) shows a cystic non-enhancing lesion in segment 4 consistent with ciliated hepatic foregut cyst (*blue arrows*).

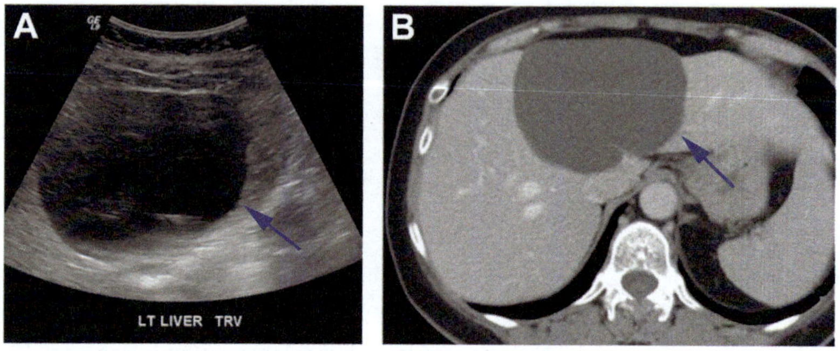

FIG. 19 Grayscale ultrasound image (**A**) and axial post-contrast CT image (**B**) of the liver shows a cystic lesion in the left hepatic lobe (*blue arrows*). There are no septations or solid enhancing components. This lesion was proven to be a mucinous cystic neoplasm on pathology.

histogenesis of MCNs exist, including aberrant descent of primordial germ cells during development or transdifferentiation of the hepatic periductal fetal mesenchyme cells into ovarian stromal cells. The strong predilection of MCN for the S4 supports a developmental origin [31,33].

On imaging, MCNs are often large solitary, multiloculated cystic masses, though sometimes unilocular. The majority of the MCNs are benign (>90%), with malignant change occurring in 3% to 6% [31]. US demonstrates anechoic or hypoechoic lesion depending on the cyst contents associated with internal septations and occasional nodularity. CT shows a low attenuation non-enhancing mass with or without septations and calcifications. The presence of enhancing mural nodules raises the concern for malignancy (Fig. 19) [31]. The cyst demonstrates variable signal intensities on T1 depending on the contents and is hyperintense on T2; septations appear as T2 hypointense linear bands within the cyst. MRI with post-contrast subtraction images depicts the septal, capsular, or nodular enhancement better than CT [29,31]. MRCP demonstrates the presence or absence of biliary communication and upstream biliary dilatation (Fig. 20).

The imaging differentials for MCN would include intraductal papillary neoplasm of the bile duct (IPNB), solitary hepatic/bile duct cyst, cystic metastases, cystic or necrotic hepato cellular carcinoma (HCC), hydatid cyst, and abscesses. The absence of restricted diffusion within the cystic component supports the diagnosis of a cystic or necrotic neoplasm rather than an abscess [29]. The lack of biliary communication or, downstream biliary dilatation, or intraductal mass helps differentiate MCN from IPNB [31]. The treatment for MCN, a premalignant condition, is complete surgical excision. Minimally invasive procedures, such as percutaneous aspiration, sclerotherapy, and surgical fenestration, have a higher recurrence rate than complete resection [29,31].

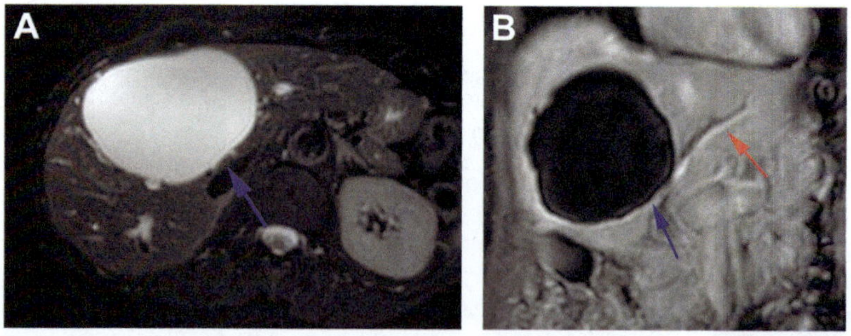

FIG. 20 Axial T2-weighted MR image of the liver (**A**) demonstrates a T2 homogeneously hyperintense lesion in segment 4 (*blue arrow*). Coronal delayed phase post contrast T1-weighted MR image (**B**) demonstrates a non-enhancing cystic lesion in segment 4 (*blue arrow*) causing mass effect and upstream mild intrahepatic biliary dilatation (*red arrow*). There were no septations or solid enhancing components. This cyst was operated due to mass effect and histopathology showed it as mucinous cystic neoplasm

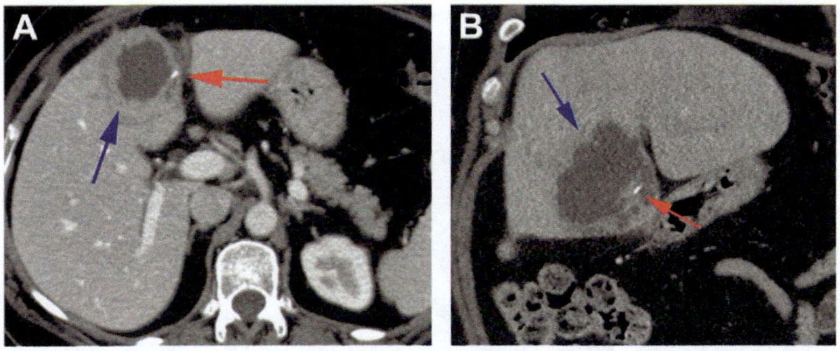

FIG. 21 Axial, and coronal CT venous phase images (**A, B**) demonstrate a peripherally enhancing irregular thick-walled lesion in segment 4B (*blue arrows*) with a linear hyperdense material (*red arrows*) within, consistent with a foreign body related abscess. The patient was operated and found to have a bristle from barbecue grill cleaner brush metal scraper cleaning tool perforating in segment 4 causing abscess

INGESTED FOREIGN BODIES PERFORATING SEGMENT 4

Most ingested foreign bodies in the gastrointestinal (GI) tract pass through uneventfully. However, sharp objects, such as toothpicks, fishbones, shells, chicken bone, grill cleaning brush bristles, and needles, can uncommonly perforate and cause complications like intraperitoneal abscesses. The common perforation sites in the GI tract are the ileocecal junction and rectosigmoid junction [34,35]. Gastric perforation is rare, and further penetration into the liver is even rarer. This leads to a liver abscess formation, commonly in the left hepatic lobe, involving S4B and segment 3 [34,35].

The migrated foreign body may remain silent until an abscess develops. Patients present with nonspecific symptoms, such as abdominal pain, vomiting, fever, anorexia, and uncommon jaundice. Microorganisms isolated from the hepatic abscesses due to foreign body ingestion are usually part of the normal flora of the human GI tract [36]. US may be the initial imaging modality demonstrating a hypoechoic liver lesion with irregular thick walls and septations. CT plays a pivotal role in the diagnosis and helps plan further treatment. CT demonstrates heterogeneously hypodense left hepatic lobe lesion with irregular thick walls with or without enhancing septa. Additionally, CT is sensitive in detecting gastric wall thickening, perigastric/peritoneal inflammation, and specifically linear hyperdense foreign body [35–37]. Coronal and sagittal reformations increase the sensitivity of identifying a thin, sharp foreign body in suspicious cases (Fig. 21). Surgery may be preferable to percutaneous drainage for managing foreign body-related abscesses. The main aim of surgery is to remove the foreign body along with abscess drainage [37]. If not promptly handled, this can result in septic shock, which may be life-threatening.

DIRECT EXTENSION OF PATHOLOGIES FROM ADJACENT ORGANS TO SEGMENT 4

Given the close proximity, gastric, gallbladder, and peritoneal pathologies may spread directly to S4. The gastrohepatic ligament suspends the stomach from the left hepatic lobe. Gastric malignancies from the cardia and lesser curvature or antrum can spread from the stomach to the left hepatic lobe, especially to S4, through the gastrohepatic ligament [38,39]. Gallbladder malignancy can spread directly to S4 because of the proximity (Fig. 22). Rarely, other peritoneal pathologies, such as

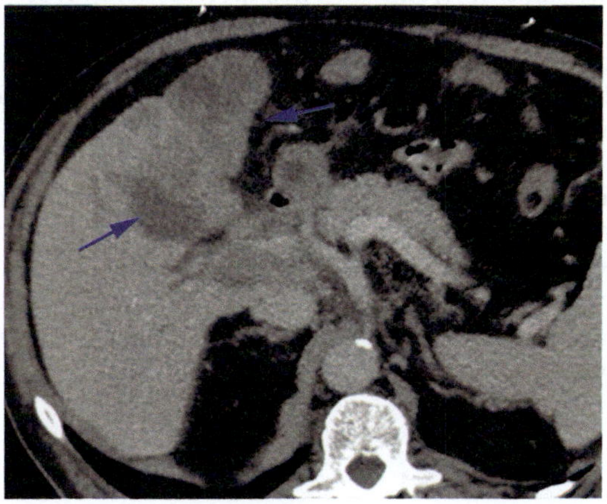

FIG. 22 Axial contrast-enhanced CT image demonstrating gall bladder carcinoma extending into segment 4 (*blue arrows*).

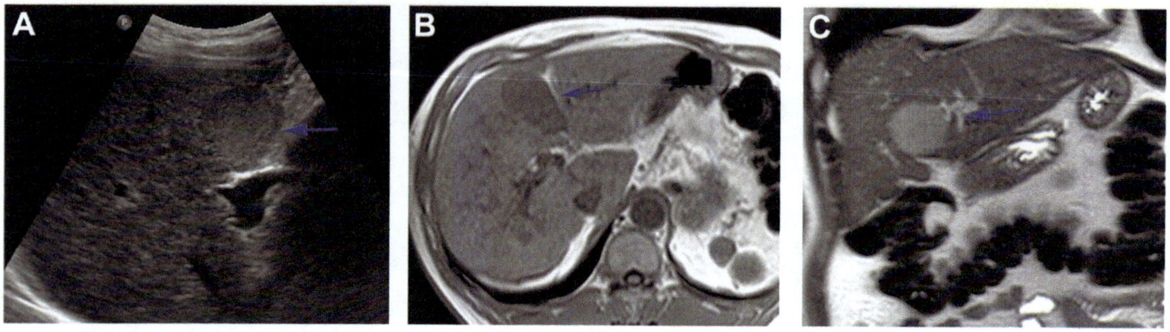

FIG. 23 Grayscale ultrasound image (**A**) shows an echogenic lesion in left hepatic lobe (*blue arrow*). Axial T1-weighted MR image (**B**) shows a T1 hypointense lesion in segment 4B that is hyperintense on coronal T2-weighted image (**C**) (*blue arrows*). This lesion was indeterminate on MRI and hence a biopsy was performed for further evaluation. Histopathology showed this to be splenic tissue consistent with the diagnosis of intrahepatic splenosis.

splenosis, may also involve S4. Rupture or capsular compromise of the spleen results in seeding the splenic pulp on the liver surface, possibly resulting in hepatic splenosis [40]. The diagnosis of hepatic splenosis should be included in the differentials in enhancing lesions on the liver surface or in the subcapsular parenchyma in a patient with prior splenic trauma/rupture (Fig. 23) [40].

SUMMARY

S4, being located centrally in the liver, can have numerous vascular and biliary anatomic variants. Understanding the vascular/biliary anatomy and their variations is crucial in successful liver donor liver transplants, SLTs, and other hepatic resections involving S4. The unique third inflow of S4 makes it a common location for various pseudotumors like FFS, FFD, and THEDs. Pathologic conditions unique to S4 due to its embryologic development include MCN and CHFCs. Additionally, because of the proximity of S4, pathologies may spread from adjacent organs, like penetrating foreign bodies from the stomach and gastric/gall bladder malignancies. Radiologists must understand the imaging characteristics of pathologies frequently affecting S4, as this knowledge plays a pivotal role in patient management.

CLINICS CARE POINTS

- Pre-operative identification of variant arterial/portal venous/hepatic venous anatomy of S4 is very important before living donor liver transplant and other hepatic resections involving S4 and has significant clinical implications.
- Bile leak and S4 infarction are the common complications after hepatic resections involving S4; MRI with eovist contrast is the imaging modality of choice for detecting bile leaks.
- Areas of focal fat infiltration and focal fat sparing are usually wedge-shaped or geographic, lack mass effect, do not demonstrate restricted diffusion, and have undistorted vessels within. Chemical shift MRI, along with other MRI sequences, helps differentiate FFD/FFS from a neoplasm.
- CHFC and hepatic MCNs commonly develop in S4. Contrast-enhanced MRI helps in identification and diagnosis.
- Proximity of S4 makes it prone to involvement from pathologies from adjacent organs, like penetrating foreign bodies from the stomach and gastric/gall bladder malignancies.

DISCLOSURE

The authors have nothing to disclose.

REFERENCES

[1] Soyer P, Bluemke DA, Bliss DF, et al. Surgical segmental anatomy of the liver: demonstration with spiral CT during arterial portography and multiplanar reconstruction. AJR Am J Roentgenol 1994;163(1):99–103.
[2] Shankar SRA, Rela M, Srinivasan P, et al. Surgical anatomy of segment four of liver and its implications in

hepato-biliary surgery and liver transplantation. J Liver Transpl 2022;6:100076:101016/jliver2022100076.
[3] Strasberg SM, Clavien PA, Gadzijev E, et al. The Brisbane 2000 terminology of liver anatomy and resections. HPBVolume 2000;2(3):333–9.
[4] Nagino M, DeMatteo R, Lang H, et al. Proposal of a new comprehensive notation for hepatectomy: the "new World" terminology. Ann Surg 2021;274(1):1–3.
[5] Abdel-Misih SR, Bloomston M. Liver anatomy. Surg Clin North Am 2010;90(4):643–53.
[6] van Gulik TM, van den Esschert JW. James Cantlie's early messages for hepatic surgeons: how the concept of preoperative portal vein occlusion was defined. HPB (Oxford) 2010;12(2):81–3.
[7] Jin GY, Yu HC, Lim HS, et al. Anatomical variations of the origin of the segment 4 hepatic artery and their clinical implications. Liver Transpl 2008;14(8):1180–4.
[8] Deshpande RR, Heaton ND, Rela M. Surgical anatomy of segmental liver transplantation. Br J Surg 2002;89(9):1078–88.
[9] Putta T, John RA, Eapen A, et al. Computed tomography evaluation of the arterial supply to segment 4 of the liver. J Clin Imaging Sci 2018;8:31.
[10] Kamel IR, Kruskal JB, Pomfret EA, et al. Impact of multidetector CT on donor selection and surgical planning before living adult right lobe liver transplantation. AJR Am J Roentgenol 2001;176(1):193–200.
[11] Erbay N, Raptopoulos V, Pomfret EA, et al. Living donor liver transplantation in adults: vascular variants important in surgical planning for donors and recipients. AJR Am J Roentgenol 2003;181(1):109–14.
[12] Borhani AA, Elsayes KM, Catania R, et al. Imaging evaluation of living liver donor candidates: techniques, protocols, and anatomy. Radiographics 2021;41(6):1572–91.
[13] Alghamdi T, Viebahn C, Justinger C, et al. Arterial blood supply of liver segment IV and its possible surgical consequences. Am J Transplant 2017;17(4):1064–70.
[14] Reichert PR, Renz JF, D'Albuquerque LA, et al. Surgical anatomy of the left lateral segment as applied to living-donor and split-liver transplantation: a clinicopathologic study. Ann Surg 2000;232(5):658–64.
[15] Cho A, Okazumi S, Yoshinaga Y, et al. Relationship between left biliary duct system and left portal vein: evaluation with three-dimensional portocholangiography. Radiology 2003;228(1):246–50.
[16] Sarawagi R, Sundar S, Raghuvanshi S, et al. Common and uncommon anatomical variants of intrahepatic bile ducts in magnetic resonance cholangiopancreatography and its clinical implication. Pol J Radiol 2016;81:250–5.
[17] Faitot F, Vibert E, Salloum C, et al. Importance of conserving middle hepatic vein distal branches for homogeneous regeneration of the left liver after right hepatectomy. HPB (Oxford) 2012;14(11):746–53.
[18] Li Z, Rammohan A, Gunasekaran V, et al. Biliary complications after adult-to-adult living-donor liver transplantation: an international multicenter study of 3633 cases. Am J Transplant 2024;24(7):1233–46.
[19] Costa AF, Clarke SE, Stueck AE, et al. Benign neoplasms, mass-like infections, and pseudotumors that mimic hepatic malignancy at MRI. J Magn Reson Imaging 2021;53(4):979–94.
[20] Elsayes KM, Menias CO, Morshid AI, et al. Spectrum of pitfalls, pseudolesions, and misdiagnoses in noncirrhotic liver. AJR Am J Roentgenol 2018;211(1):97–108.
[21] Dickson AM. The focal hepatic hot spot sign. Radiology 2005;237(2):647–8.
[22] Sureka B, Sullere A, Singh Khera P. CT quadrate lobe hot spot sign. Middle East J Dig Dis 2018;10(3):192–3.
[23] Ramanathan S, Raghu V, Virmani V, et al. Unveiling the unreal: comprehensive imaging review of hepatic pseudolesions. Clin Imaging 2021;80:439–53.
[24] Decarie PO, Lepanto L, Billiard JS, et al. Fatty liver deposition and sparing: a pictorial review. Insights Imaging 2011;2(5):533–8.
[25] Kobayashi S. Hepatic pseudolesions caused by alterations in intrahepatic hemodynamics. World J Gastroenterol 2021;27(46):7894–908.
[26] Bishop KC, Perrino CM, Ruzinova MB, et al. Ciliated hepatic foregut cyst: a report of 6 cases and a review of the English literature. Diagn Pathol 2015;10:81.
[27] Ansari-Gilani K, Modaresi Esfeh J. Ciliated hepatic foregut cyst: report of three cases and review of imaging features. Gastroenterol Rep (Oxf) 2017;5(1):75–8.
[28] Fang SH, Dong DJ, Zhang SZ. Imaging features of ciliated hepatic foregut cyst. World J Gastroenterol 2005;11(27):4287–9.
[29] Soni S, Pareek P, Narayan S, et al. Mucinous cystic neoplasm of the liver (MCN-L): a rare presentation and review of the literature. Med Pharm Rep 2021;94(3):366–71.
[30] Fragulidis GP, Pantiora EV, Kontis EA, et al. Biliary mucinous cystic neoplasm of the liver with ovarian stroma and elevated serum and cystic fluid cancer antigen 19-9 levels. Cureus 2017;9(11):e1863.
[31] Lee MH, Katabathina VS, Lubner MG, et al. Mucin-producing cystic hepatobiliary neoplasms: updated nomenclature and clinical, pathologic, and imaging features. Radiographics 2021;41(6):1592–610.
[32] Zen Y, Pedica F, Patcha VR, et al. Mucinous cystic neoplasms of the liver: a clinicopathological study and comparison with intraductal papillary neoplasms of the bile duct. Mod Pathol 2011;24(8):1079–89.
[33] Van Treeck BJ, Lotfalla M, Czeczok TW, et al. Molecular and immunohistochemical analysis of mucinous cystic neoplasm of the liver. Am J Clin Pathol 2020;154(6):837–47.
[34] Panebianco A, Lozito RC, Prestera A, et al. Unusual liver abscess secondary to ingested foreign body: laparoscopic management. G Chir 2015;36(2):74–5.
[35] Santos SA, Alberto SC, Cruz E, et al. Hepatic abscess induced by foreign body: case report and literature review. World J Gastroenterol 2007;13(9):1466–70.
[36] Sim GG, Sheth SK. Retained foreign body causing a liver abscess. Case Rep Emerg Med 2019;2019:4259646.

[37] Minh LHN, Han LTK, Hau NV, et al. Liver abscess caused by the ingested foreign body without sign of gastrointestinal perforation: a case report. Radiol Case Rep 2023;18(12):4404–8.

[38] Gore RM, Newmark GM, Thakrar KH, et al. Pathways of abdominal tumour spread: the role of the subperitoneal space. Cancer Imaging 2009;9(1):112–20.

[39] Young JJ, Pahwa A, Patel M, et al. Ligaments and lymphatic pathways in gastric adenocarcinoma. Radiographics 2019;39(3):668–89.

[40] Vergara D, Ginolfi F, Moscati S, et al. Multiple intrahepatic and abdominal splenosis: an easy call if you know about it. Acta Radiol Open 2018;7(5):2058460118772324.

Advances in Clinical Radiology 7 (2025) 31–43
ADVANCES IN CLINICAL RADIOLOGY

Radiotherapy of Primary Renal Cell Carcinoma

Imaging Considerations Before and After Therapy

Christopher S. Lim, MD, FRCPC[a,*], Patrick Cheung, MD, FRCPC[b], John Hudson, MD, PhD, FRCPC[b], Rachel Glicksman, MD, MSc, FRCPC[c], Satheesh Krishna, MD[d], Nicola Schieda, MD, FRCPC[e]

[a]Department of Medical Imaging, Sunnybrook Health Sciences Centre, University of Toronto, 2075 Bayview Avenue, Toronto, Ontario M4N 3M5, Canada; [b]Department of Radiation Oncology, Sunnybrook Odette Cancer Centre, University of Toronto, 2075 Bayview Avenue, Toronto, ON M4N 3M5, Canada; [c]Radiation Medicine Program, Department of Radiation Oncology, Princess Margaret Cancer Centre, University Health Network, 610 University Avenue, Toronto, ON M5G 2C4, Canada; [d]Department of Medical Imaging, University of Toronto, University Medical Imaging Toronto, University Health Network, Sinai Health System, Women's College Hospital, 610 University Avenue, Toronto, ON M5G 2C4, Canada; [e]Radiation Oncology and Medical Physics, Department of Medical Imaging, The Ottawa Hospital, University of Ottawa, 501 Smyth Road, Ottawa, ON K1H 8L6, Canada

KEYWORDS

• Stereotactic body radiotherapy • Radiation therapy • Renal cell carcinoma • Kidney cancer • Ablation • Computed tomography • MRI

KEY POINTS

- Stereotactic body radiotherapy (SBRT) has emerged as a treatment option for localized renal cell carcinoma in patients that are poor surgical or thermal ablation candidates.
- Pretreatment imaging is crucial for identifying patients who may benefit from treatment of primary RCC with SBRT.
- Imaging appearance of local control and recurrence of primary RCC after SBRT differs considerably compared with the appearance after surgery and TA techniques.

INTRODUCTION

The incidence of renal masses is increasing, related in part to the increased use of cross-sectional imaging [1,2]. The increased detection of renal masses with imaging has led to increasing number of surgical nephrectomies being performed [3]; however, there has not been a substantial decrease in kidney cancer-specific mortality over the same time period, suggesting that RCCs are being overdiagnosed and overtreated [3,4]. Surgical resection, including partial or radical nephrectomy, is the standard of care in management for primary RCC [5]; however, increase the risk of renal insufficiency [6] and include a small but increased risk of mortality [7].

Nonsurgical management for renal masses includes active surveillance (AS), percutaneous thermal ablation (TA) and radiotherapy (RT). AS is an attractive initial management option for small renal masses and should be considered when the risk of intervention (or competing risk of death) outweighs potential benefit of treatment [8]. However, AS may not be desirable in older patients, which have lower cancer-specific survival rate, and with larger tumors, which are typically more aggressive with higher rates of metastasis [8]. Percutaneous TA (microwave, cryoablation, and radiofrequency) has been shown to be useful with similar rates of local recurrence and lower complications compared with partial nephrectomy for small tumors

*Corresponding author. *E-mail address:* cs.lim@utoronto.ca

https://doi.org/10.1016/j.yacr.2025.05.003
www.advancesinclinicalradiology.com
2589-8701/25/

ABBREVIATIONS

AS	active surveillance
CT	computed tomography
OAR	organs at risk
RCC	renal cell carcinoma
RT	radiotherapy
SBRT	stereotactic body radiotherapy
TA	thermal ablation

[9]. However, it may be less effective and have higher complications in larger tumors, central/endophytic masses, and there remains issues of nephron loss related to ablation of the adjacent normal kidney parenchyma [10]. There are also associated risks with anesthesia, which can be more substantial in older, medically frail patients.

In this context, stereotactic body radiotherapy (SBRT), also known as stereotactic ablative body RT, has emerged as another noninvasive curative treatment option for primary RCC. Historically, RCC has been considered a "radioresistant" tumor; however, with technical advancement using SBRT, higher radiobiological effective doses are able to be administered, killing tumor cells while minimizing the damage to surrounding structures and organs at risk (OAR) [11,12]. Recently, SBRT was incorporated into National Comprehensive Cancer Network (NCCN) guidelines for management of localized tumors in patients that are medical inoperable [5]. SBRT has been shown to be effective with high rates of local control and low rates of developing distant metastases in medically inoperable patients [13]. SBRT has been shown to be safe with low rates of serious complication [13,14]. One concern regarding SBRT is damage to the adjacent normal kidney parenchyma, which has been shown to be present but minimal [15]. The concept of limiting renal damage is of importance because there is broad acceptance that any nephron loss, even from conventional management with partial nephrectomy or TA, is associated with risks of renal insufficiency and decreased survival [7].

Imaging plays a crucial role in selecting patients who may be optimally treated with SBRT as well as immediate-term and longer-term postprocedural surveillance after SBRT for primary RCC. Imaging of treatment response and local failure after SBRT differs considerably compared with surgery and TA. The purpose of this article is to provide a rationale and evidence for SBRT in the management of primary RCC and to provide a comprehensive review of the imaging for primary RCC treated with SBRT.

RADIATION TREATMENT OF PRIMARY RENAL CELL CARCINOMA

Stereotactic Body Radiotherapy Mechanism, Planning, and Delivery

Historically, RCC has been considered a "radioresistant" tumor, because RCC tumor cells are able to survive conventional RT treatment [11]. Through technical advancements, SBRT allows the precise delivery of very high radiobiological doses of radiation in a single or few fractions to tumors [11,12]. This highly concentrated ablative radiation treatment has overcome the perceived "radioresistant" of RCC while minimizing the inadvertent damage to surrounding organs [12]. The radiobiologic mechanism of conventional RT, which relies on oxygen-dependent DNA damage, leading to double-strand breaks or mis-repaired breaks, is distinct from effects from SBRT [16]. High doses by SBRT cause endothelial apoptosis, which efficiently destroy tumor vessels/microvasculature and can have improved results particularly in hypervascular tumors, which are dependent on angiogenesis [16]. Furthermore, SBRT can cause immune system activation by inducing the release of tumor-associated antigens and tumor-infiltrating T-lymphocytes causing tumor cell death [12,17]. Another promising but not well understood effect is that administration of high doses of radiation has shown promise in activating immune response against malignant cells, with possible synergistic effect when combined with immunotherapy [18]. Exploring the combination of SBRT with immunotherapy holds potential for improved treatment outcomes using a multimodal therapeutic strategy for primary and metastatic RCC [18].

With conventional RT, which delivers small amounts of radiation usually daily (eg, 2 Gy/fraction for 5–7 week period), SBRT permits higher dose ($\geq$7 Gy) in a few fractions ($\leq$5 fractions) [12]. The basic requirements for delivery of SBRT includes modern treatment machines capable of delivering conformal RT (often with intensity modulation) and having on-board image-guidance capability (cone beam computed tomography [CT] as a minimum), along with appropriate radiation planning software [12]. Delivery methods should be able to compensate for breathing-induced tumor motion which can include the use of breath holding or abdominal compression, respiratory gating and/or tumor tracking using implanted fiducial markers [12]. Using CT, 4-dimensional scanning is routinely utilized to account for breathing-induced motion. In the future, use of MRI for RT will increase, especially with the increasing availability of RT machines with on-board MR imaging.

Several RT techniques exist and the goals of planning regardless of RT technique are similar: to create a conformal high dose region around the target, with rapid dose fall-off beyond the target. Target volumes and OAR are contoured on appropriate image datasets used for RT dose calculations (Fig. 1). Once the gross tumor volume is contoured, often accounting for a volume that encompasses the breathing-induced tumor motion, a small additional margin is typically added ($\leq$5 mm) to account for potential intrafraction motion and residual set-up errors. OAR including ipsilateral and contralateral renal cortex ($\pm$hilum), intestine, stomach, and liver are often contoured, especially if within 5 cm of the target volume (Fig. 1). Typical SBRT doses range from 25 to 48 Gy in 1 to 5 fractions [14].

Evidence of Stereotactic Body Radiotherapy in Primary Renal Cell Carcinoma

The evidence for treating primary RCC with SBRT is evolving. Most studies are comprised of single center trials, which found excellent local control rates ranging from 93% to 100% with generally low rates (0%–9.1%) of moderate or severe treatment-related complications [19–22]. The multicenter individual patient data meta-analysis of 190 patients with median 5-year outcomes found the incidence of local failure at 3, 5, and 7 years of 5.5% (95% CI: 2.8–9.5), 5.5% (2.8–9.5), and 8.4% (4.2–14.3) despite a large pretreatment tumor size of 4.0 cm. Importantly, the 7-year distant failure was only 15.0% (9.1–22.4), and 7-year cancer-specific survival was 92.0% (85.2–95.8) [23]. There were zero grade 3% and 1% grade 4 events. Most patients had baseline kidney dysfunction (median estimated glomerular filtration rate [eGFR] of 60.0 mL/min). There was a median decline in eGFR of 14.2 mL/min at 5 years post-SBRT with only 7 patients (4%) requiring dialysis. More recently, an international multicenter prospective trial involving 70 patients with primary RCC (median tumor size 4.6 cm) treated with SBRT found excellent local control of 100% with a median follow-up time of 43.3 months [13]. Local control was defined as per RECIST version 1.1. There was acceptable toxicity with only 10% grade 3 with no grade 4 reactions. Included patients had pre-existing Chronic Kidney Diseaes (CKD) with mean baseline eGFR of 61.1 mL/min. The average reduction of eGFR at 24 months was 14.6 mL/min after SBRT with only one patient requiring dialysis. This study provides additional prospective evidence that SBRT is an effective therapeutic option for inoperable localized kidney cancer.

The available data make comparison of the oncologic outcomes and treatment-related adverse events between SBRT, surgical resection, and TA difficult. Surgery is the standard of care in the management of localized RCC [5]; however, no randomized studies exist comparing SBRT to surgery. Although there are no head-to-head studies, results of SBRT are similar to TA and partial nephrectomy for small renal masses [24] in oncological outcomes with local recurrence-free survivals with partial nephrectomy, Radiofrequency Ablation (RFA), and cryoablation of 97.7% (96.7–98.6), 95.9% (92.3–99.6), and 95.9% (92.3–99.6), respectively [24]. In comparison, small less than 4 cm renal masses treated with SBRT had similar local failure rate of 95.4% [23]. For larger tumors, SBRT has also shown to be effective with similar rates of local control compared with treatment of small tumors [13,25].

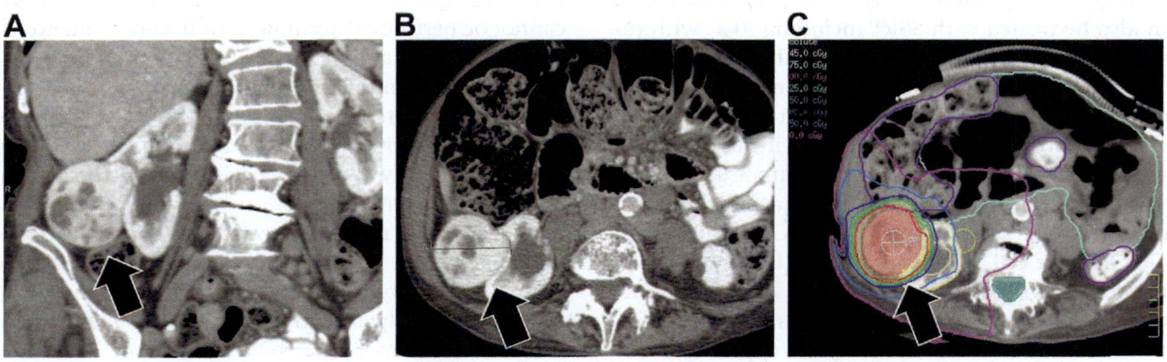

FIG. 1 A 80-year-old male with a right RCC who underwent SBRT with radiation treatment plan. (**A, B**) Coronal (**A**) and axial (**B**) contrast-enhanced CT demonstrates a right renal mass (*black arrow*), biopsy confirmed clear cell RCC. (**C**) Pre-SBRT treatment plan with outlines including gross tumor volume surrounding the tumor as well as the OAR including bowel and kidney.

Conversely, management of larger tumors with TA is limited with higher rates of residual/recurrent tumor [26]. Patients treated with SBRT often have preexisting chronic diseases, such as CKD, which may be a contributing factor as to why patients may not be surgical candidates. CKD is known independent risk factor for poor outcomes and renal disfunction following surgery [7,27]. Therefore, it is difficult to compare changes in eGFR after surgery, TA and SBRT given the distinctly different treated patient populations. Further prospective randomized trials are needed to compare the efficacy and toxicities of SBRT to surgery and TA for local control, complications, and renal function preservation.

Current Indications for Stereotactic Body Radiotherapy in Primary Renal Cell Carcinoma

Currently, SBRT may be indicated in medically inoperable patients with stage 1 (category 2b) or with stage II/III kidney cancer (both category 3) according to 2024 NCCN guidelines [5]. In our own institutions, SBRT for localized RCC is primarily considered in poor surgical candidates and when TA may not provide adequate control, such as in larger masses (>3–3.5 cm) or centrally located tumors. SBRT can also be considered as a form of delayed intervention after an initial management of AS [28]. To our knowledge, there are no precise criteria of medical inoperability and are usually determined in conjunction with urologists considering medical comorbidities, performance status, and suitability for general anesthetic [14]. Individual patient treatment decisions requiring SBRT are often discussed at multidisciplinary rounds [14]. SBRT for primary RCC can also be effective in patients with a solitary kidney with acceptable kidney function loss (Fig. 2) [14]. Additionally, locally advanced RCC can also be treated with SBRT including RCC with tumor thrombus (Fig. 3) [29] and in the neoadjuvant setting prior to surgery [30]. To our knowledge, there are no studies with adequate patient population to describe outcomes of using SBRT specifically for multiple tumors in a single kidney or bilateral kidney tumors. However, it can be inferred that local control rates would be similar to a single RCC treated with SBRT, and the eGFR loss would likely be higher based in part to larger targeted tumor and kidney volume. Previous RT to the retroperitoneum may be a contraindication for renal SBRT; however, this depends on the previous dose delivered to the area in regard to the kidney and OAR's, and the prior radiation treatment plans must be reviewed.

PREABLATION IMAGING AND MANAGEMENT

Pretreatment imaging is essential prior to consideration of radiation therapy to help in the evaluation of tumor characteristics including: differentiation of benign from malignant renal masses, size, location and local extent of tumor, and presence or absence of distant metastases as well as determine optimal treatment modality [31–33].

When identifying a renal mass, assessment of enhancement is essential with renal CT, MRI, or contrast-enhanced ultrasound. If the mass is characterized as cystic with less than 25% enhancing soft tissue, the tumor can be classified according to the Bosniak Classification [34,35]. If the mass is solid (≥25% enhancing soft tissue), identification of macroscopic fat is essential as any noncalcified fat containing solid mass is diagnostic for a benign angiomyolipoma [36]. Advances in imaging have improved our ability to differentiate benign and malignant renal masses, to differentiate the subtypes of RCC and to determinate the grade of RCC and its aggressiveness. Despite these imaging advanced, renal mass biopsy (RMB) is still often required to confirm the diagnosis of cancer [37]. RMB is safe and can impact management decisions in patients found to have a renal mass [37]. The biopsy results may obviate the need for treatment if a benign diagnosis is found [2]. In patients undergoing nonsurgical treatment, RMB provides the only opportunity to make a histologic diagnosis prior to treatment and is recommended [2,14]. If pre-SBRT tissues diagnosis is not obtained, there could be unnecessary treatment of a benign mass and its associated risk of complications and costs stemming from the downstream testing necessitate by the presumptive diagnosis of cancer [2]. There is limited data in scenarios when percutaneous biopsy cannot be performed accurately, or if RMB is attempted but the results are inconclusive. When RMB is not feasible or after initial inconclusive biopsy result, a decision to observe, repeat the biopsy, or initiate presumptive treatment must be decided and the optimal option is usually a shared decision with the patient and medical team [38].

Once a renal mass is detected and confirmed to be malignant, size, location, local, and distant disease extent is necessary to inform treatment decisions. Imaging can also help identify patients who may benefit from treatment by SBRT.

SBRT has been shown to be effective at treatment of larger greater than 4 cm T1b masses (Fig. 4) [25]. In contrast, TA is technically challenging in larger masses

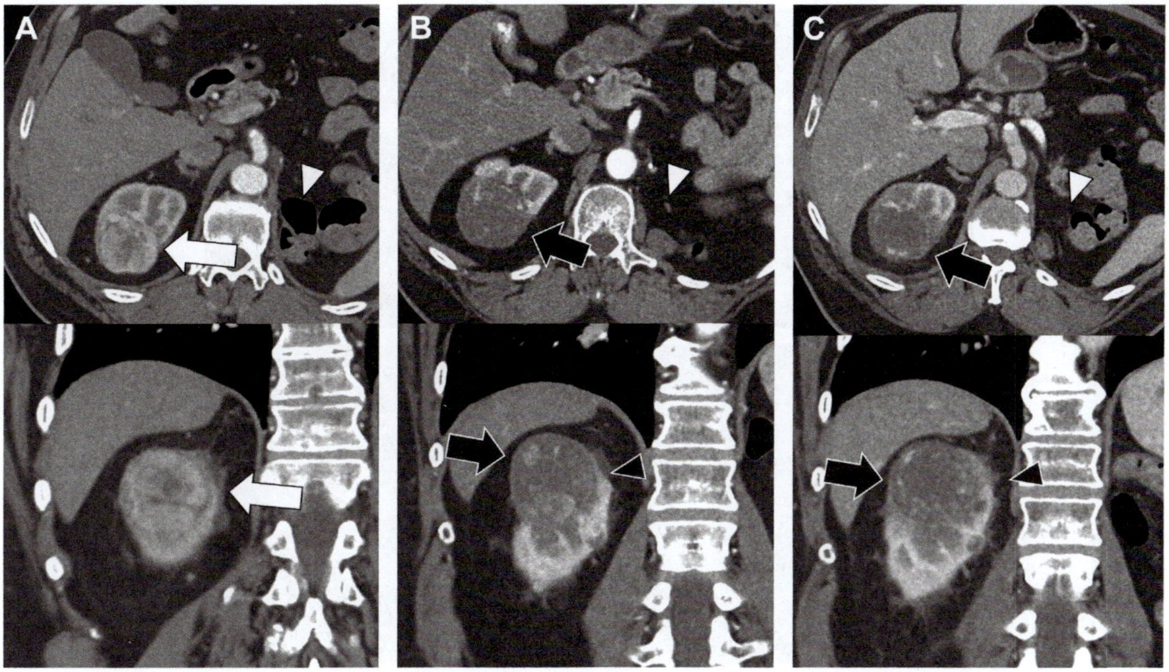

FIG. 2 A 78-year-old male with a solitary right kidney undergoing SBRT for 5 cm clear cell RCC with expected post-SBRT imaging appearance. (**A**) Axial and coronal (top and bottom) contrast-enhanced CT demonstrates a hypervascular biopsy confirmed clear cell RCC (*white arrow*) and left nephrectomy surgical bed from prior xanthogranulomatous pyelonephritis (*white arrowhead*). (**B**) 6-month and (**C**) 12-month post-SBRT axial and coronal CT images demonstrate continued size decrease and decrease in the heterogeneous enhancement (*black arrows*). There is mild adjacent cortical atrophy (*black arrowhead*). Patient's renal function decreased by 10 mL/min and remained stable. Patient remains on routine surveillance at 2 years without local failure or distant metastasis.

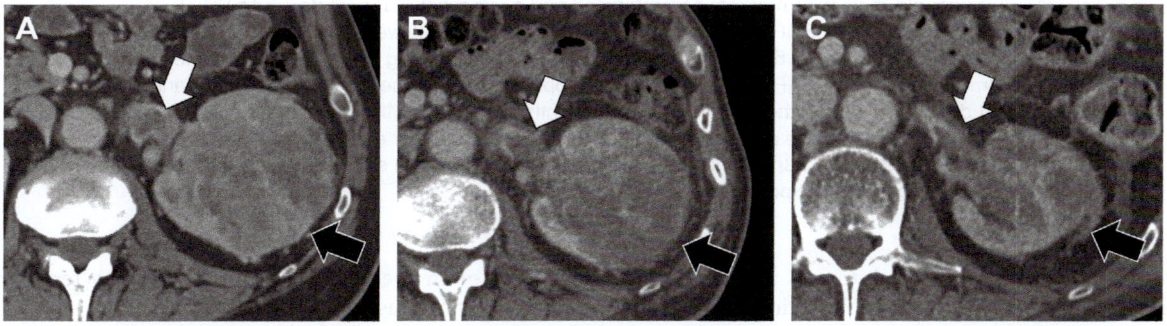

FIG. 3 A 66-year-old male with infiltrating left RCC and tumor thrombus in the main renal vein and inferior vena cava (IVC) (not shown). (**A**) Axial contrast-enhanced CT image demonstrates the left renal mass with left renal vein tumor thrombus (*white arrow*). The patient was treated with SBRT targeting the renal mass and tumor thrombus with post-SBRT imaging demonstrating expected post-SBRT changes at (**B**) 6 months and (**C**) 12 months. The renal mass (*black arrow*) and tumor thrombus (*white arrow*) demonstrated continued decrease in size and enhancement.

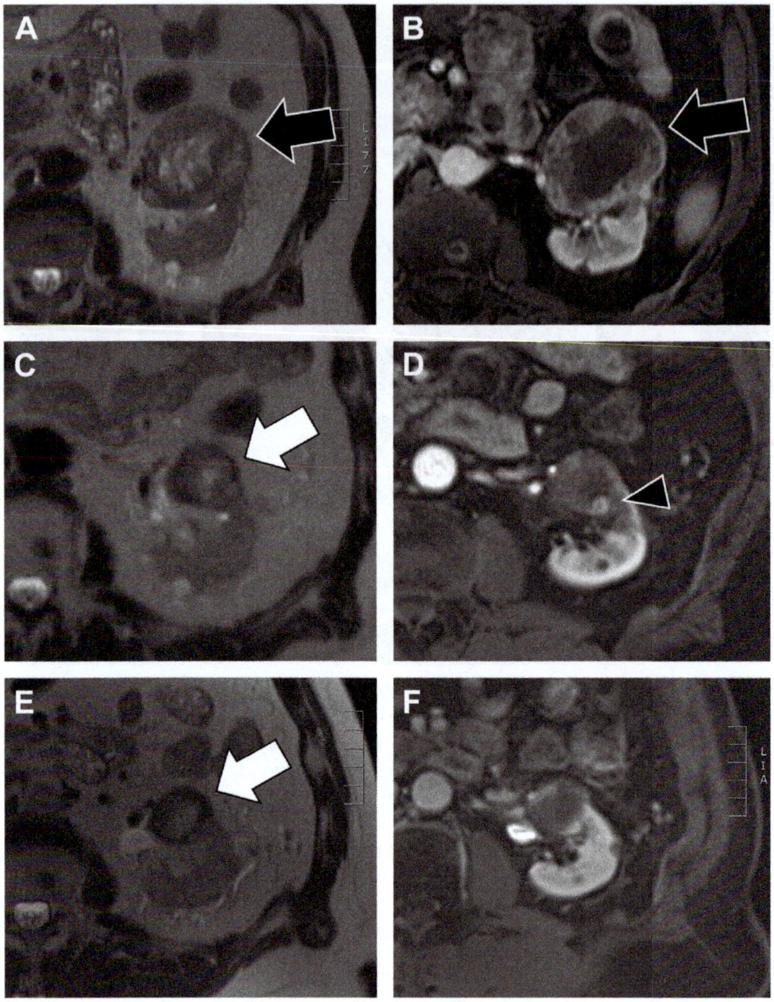

FIG. 4 A 80-year-old male with medical comorbidities and a left renal mass treated with SBRT demonstrating expected post-SBRT appearance on MRI. (**A, B**) Axial T2-weighted (**A**) and corticomedullary phase (**B**) MRI demonstrates a 5.5 cm left renal mass (*black arrow*) arising from the interpolar left kidney, biopsy confirmed clear cell RCC. Patient was deemed inoperable due to medical comorbidities, and TA was not preferred due to the size of the mass. (**C, D**) A 6-month post-SBRT MRI having expected post-SBRT appearance with decrease in size and enhancement, with residual nodular enhancement (*black arrowhead*). (**E, F**) At 12-month post-SBRT surveillance, there was further decrease in size (*white arrow*) and enhancement in keeping with expected post-SBRT changes.

with increased risk of local tumor recurrence and higher rates of postablation complications [10]. Therefore, in a nonoperative patient with a larger tumor, management with SBRT may be preferred; however, this is subject to local institutional experience and preferences. There is no strict renal tumor size cut-off with regards to suitability for treatment with SBRT. Rather than the primary tumor size, the volume of adjacent OAR is often the limiting factor which may result in the decision to use lower SBRT doses.

Tumor location can impact treatment decisions. For example, SBRT may be preferred over TA in endophytic and centrally located tumors. These locations are associated with higher rates of local recurrence and postablation complications with TA (Fig. 5) [39]. Moreover, hilar tumors are less ideal for TA, in part

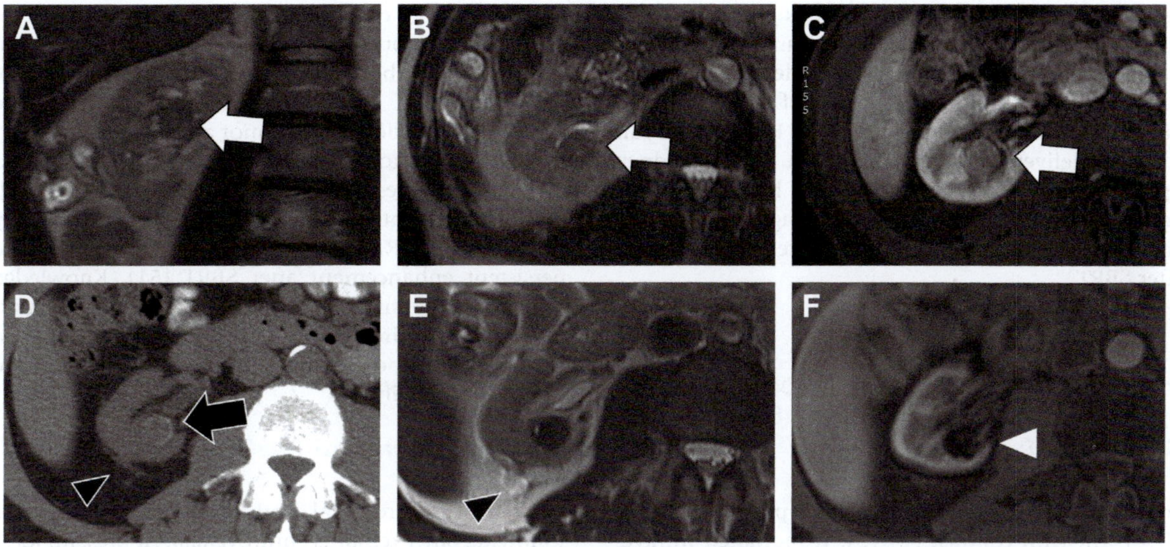

FIG. 5 A 68-year-old male with comorbidities, with a central right renal tumor treated with SBRT. (**A–C**) Coronal (**A**) and axial (**B**) T2-weighted and (**C**) axial corticomedullary phase contrast-enhanced MRI demonstrates a central right renal mass (*black arrow*), located close to the renal pelvis and hilar vessels. RCC was suspected and renal mass biopsy was attempted but was nondiagnostic. Patient was deemed inoperable and referred for SBRT due to the central location, which was preferred over management with TA. Patient could not receive intravenous iodinated contrast due to renal function impairment. (**D**) Unenhanced CT of the kidneys as part of routine chest CT surveillance demonstrated expected post-SBRT appearance with size decrease, areas of calcification within the mass (*black arrow*) and surrounding perinephric stranding (*black arrowhead*). Surveillance MRI performed at 12 months after SBRT with axial T2-weighted (**E**) and corticomedullary phase (**F**) contrast-enhanced images demonstrate continued size decrease from baseline and no significant residual enhancement (*white arrowhead*). Post-SBRT perinephric stranding is also seen (*black arrow*).

due to the heat-sink phenomenon from adjacent large hilar vessels and from concerns relating to damaging the collecting system [40]. Unlike partial nephrectomy and TA, location of tumor is usually not a limiting factor with SBRT. SBRT of centrally located tumors does not result in clinically detectable toxicity to the collecting system based on the anecdotal experience and published literature [23]. Scoring systems have also been developed to characterize the technical challenges and anticipated success of TA [41], which comprises scoring that includes size and location (endo-phytic and closeness to the renal sinus/collecting systems), and has been shown to predict recurrence and complications after TA [41]. Siva and colleagues demonstrated that more complex tumors as graded by these scoring systems could be successfully treated with SBRT, which may not be effectively treated with TA [13].

There are factors that impact SBRT planning, mainly adjacent OAR of radiation-induced injury including: small and large intestines, stomach, and normal renal parenchyma (Fig. 1). For tumors that are immediately adjacent to bowel, efforts are made to limit radiation dose which may result in a slightly lower dose to a portion of the renal mass. It is unclear whether local tumor control is impacted when there is a lower dose provided to a small part of the tumor in efforts to spare adjacent bowel. The published literature for primary renal SBRT includes various dose-fractionation schemes and despite a range of biological effective doses being used, no clear SBRT dose response relationship exists. This suggests that lower SBRT doses may be as effective as higher doses [42]. Overall, the risk of adjacent organ radiation-induced toxicity after SBRT is low but has been observed [15].

Patients should undergo scintigraphy split function to assess the relative function of the kidneys [14]. eGFR declines after SBRT varies but ranges from 5 to 15 mL/min and typically plateaus at 2 years [15] and patients with lower eGFR (<30 mL/min) could be at higher risks of requiring subsequent dialysis after treatment [15]. Furthermore, renal function can also decrease from underlying comorbidities, independent renal damage from SBRT. The overall risk of needing subsequent dialysis is very low after SBRT. Renal SBRT can still be delivered to patients with severe kidney dysfunction, but they should ideally be followed by nephrology for optimal medical management of CKD and counseled about the potential of requiring dialysis after SBRT.

POST-STEREOTACTIC BODY RADIOTHERAPY IMAGING AND MANAGEMENT OF PRIMARY RENAL CELL CARCINOMA

Expected Imaging Findings

Local treatment response after SBRT is performed using CT or MR with contrast [14,15]. If iodinated intravenous (IV) contrast cannot be administered due to allergy or concern of contrast-associated acute kidney injury, MR with gadolinium can be performed safely as risks of nephrogenic systemic fibrosis with group 1 gadolinium-based contrast agents are ~0% even in at risk patients [43]. Noncontrast enhanced CT can also be utilized to evaluate the renal mass size and can be performed with concurrent chest CT.

Expected post-SBRT imaging findings include progressive tumor shrinkage and atrophy of the adjacent kidney parenchyma (Figs. 2-5) [44,45]. Central necrosis or nonenhancing areas are common, and areas of calcification have been observed (Fig. 5) [14,19]. Surrounding perinephric stranding is also seen (Fig. 5). Continued size decrease over serial examinations has been consistently observed following treatment with SBRT [44]. For example, Hannan and colleagues found mean change in tumor growth rate 1 year after treatment of −1.3 cm/year [19] and size is known to slowly decrease in size over many years [14,46,47]. A pitfall in imaging assessment of size in the early post-treatment interval is "pseudoprogression." "Pseudoprogression" after SBRT occurs when there is a paradoxic initial increase in tumor size, typically around 1 to 5 months, which subsequently resolves and is related to treatment-related inflammation (Fig. 6) [22,48,49].

Unlike with TA, persistent tumor enhancement is an expected finding post-SBRT [50] and cannot be used solely in the assessment of residual tumor (Figs. 2, 3, and 6). This is a major difference in post-treatment imaging comparing SBRT to TA where the presences of enhancement indicates residual untreated tumor [50]. Enhancement after SBRT is expected to slowly evolve over time and often decreases; however, persistent enhancement, or even, initial increase, can be seen and is not a reliable indicator of treatment failure alone [14,46]. For TA, cell death occurs due to immediate physical destruction of the tumor and vascular architecture as oppose to the mechanism of SBRT, described earlier, which results in progressive cell death [44]. This is consistent with other tumors within the body treated with SBRT, which are known to demonstrate persistent enhancement after SBRT [51]. Knowledge that persistent enhancement is an expected finding after SBRT is required by interpreting radiologists to not incorrectly diagnosis residual tumor when size is the same or improving.

Imaging Findings of Residual and Local Failure

Assessment of residual and local failure/recurrence following SBRT remains controversial. At present, local tumor control is determined using RECIST 1.1 size criteria [14]. Local failure can be diagnosed when there is progressive size increase over serial scans (Fig. 7). At our institutions, local failure is also raised when there is new or larger area of enhancement, which was previously not enhancing, when it is progresses over serial examinations. Pseudoprogression, described earlier, is a pitfall in the early post-SBRT period (Fig. 6). When interpreting post-SBRT imaging, knowledge of when SBRT treatment was completed is required. Post-SBRT primary RCC imaging assessment must be interpreted with caution understanding the possibility of "pseudoprogression" and routine immediate (<6 month) imaging is not typically performed to avoid this pitfall [14]. There are limitations to RECIST 1.1, which does not incorporate enhancement of tumors treated with SBRT and other therapies. Attempts to overcome these limitations have led to the development of other reporting system such as mRECIST and CHOI criteria; however, none have been primary developed or validated for RCC after SBRT. There is ongoing need for image standardization and refinement of radiographic response after SBRT [15]. Given the limitations of RECIST 1.1 size assessment, imaging biomarkers with MRI and novel PET techniques have shown promise [46,52,53]; however, require further multicenter and prospective validation.

Assessment of residual disease with imaging is further complicated as the reference standard (histopathology) is limited at correctly identifying residual viable aggressive tumors post-SBRT. Residual tumor cells are commonly identified on biopsy 6 to 12 months following SBRT; however, these positive biopsies do not appear to be associated with subsequent radiographic

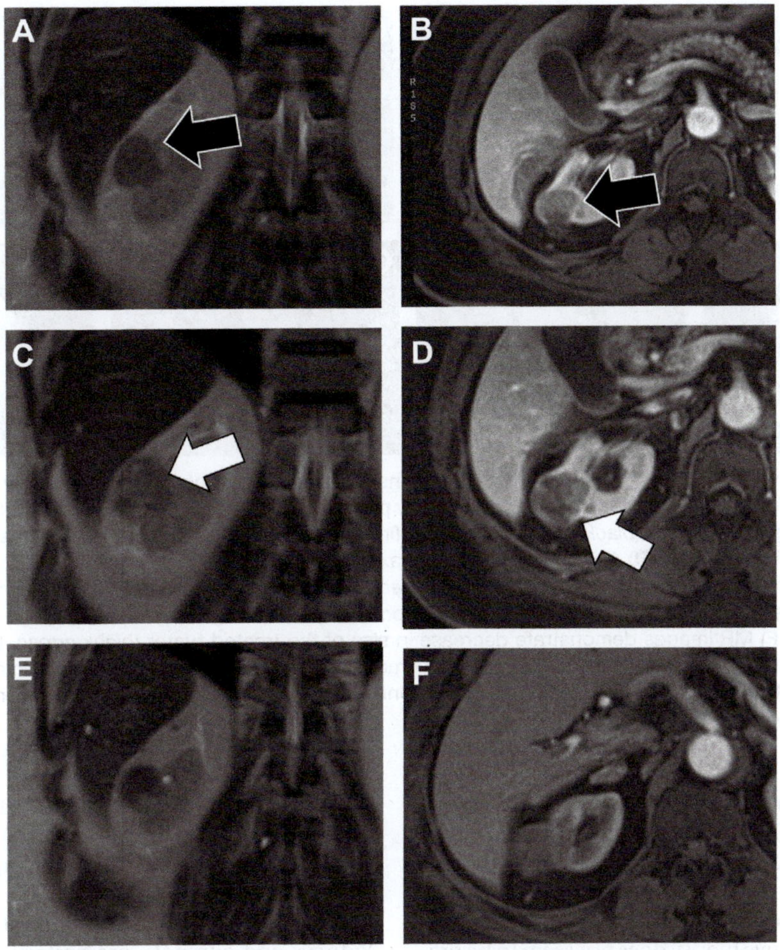

FIG. 6 A 77-year-old female with medical comorbidities treated with SBRT demonstrating pseudoprogression on short-term follow-up MRI after SBRT. (**A, B**) Coronal T2-weighted (**A**) and axial corticomedullary phase (**B**) contrast-enhanced MR images demonstrate right upper pole renal mass (*black arrow*), biopsy confirmed papillary RCC. Patient was deemed inoperable and treated with SBRT. (**C, D**) A 1-month post-SBRT MRI, performed for surveillance of a 1-cm pancreatic neuroendocrine tumor (not shown), coronal T2-weighted (**C**) and axial corticomedullary phase (**D**) contrast-enhanced MR images demonstrate paradoxic enlargement of the renal mass with new heterogeneous signal intensity on T2-weighted images and enhancement (*white arrow*). (**E, F**) A 6-month post-SBRT coronal T2-weighted (**E**) and axial corticomedullary phase (**F**) contrast-enhanced MR images show the renal mass has decreased in size and enhancement. Although the mass shows persistent enhancement, this can be expected after SBRT and continued follow-up was performed. The patient remains on surveillance after 5 years without local failure or distant metastasis.

progression or treatment failure [14]. Hannan and colleagues performed histologic and molecular analysis on post-treatment biopsies 1 year after SBRT, and most tumors showed expected findings of decreased cellularity, increased hyalinization, increased fibrosis, which is consistent with expected post-SBRT imaging appearance [19]. When positive tumor cells were identified, the cells were scarce and expressed p16, a marker of cellular senescence, and a marker of terminal (permanent nonreplicative) differentiated state. Furthermore, in a study by Ponsky and colleagues, 64% (7/11) of patients with post-SBRT biopsies identified positive tumor cells. In one of these patients, a subsequent biopsy identified no tumor cells without interim treatment. Five other patients

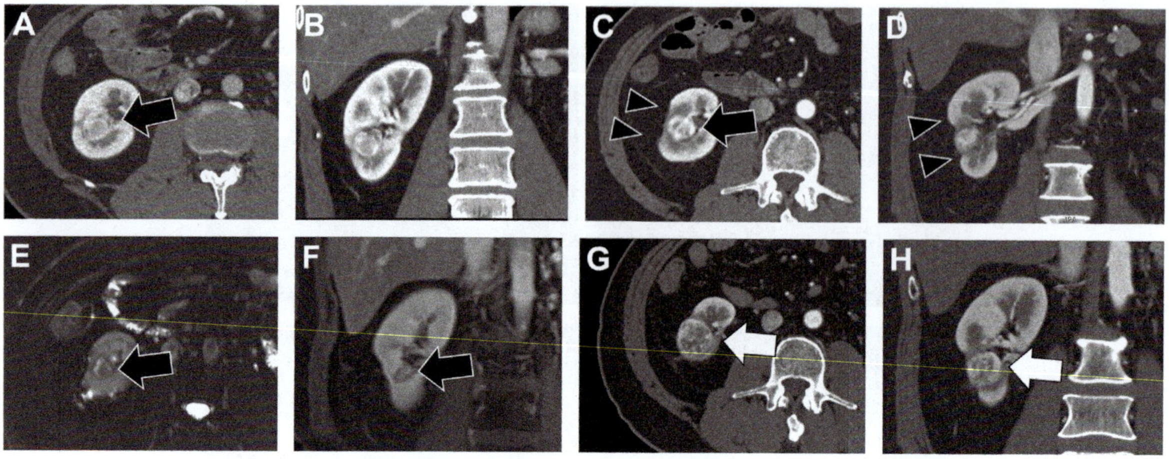

FIG. 7 A 70-year-old male treated with SBRT demonstrating post-treatment local failure 15 months after SBRT. (**A, B**) Axial (**A**) and coronal (**B**) corticomedullary phase contrast-enhanced CT images demonstrate an endophytic right renal mass (*black arrow*), biopsy confirmed clear cell RCC. Patient was deemed inoperable and treated with SBRT. (**C, D**) A 6-month post-SBRT axial (**C**) and coronal (**D**) demonstrates slight decrease in size with similar enhancement of the renal mass (*black arrow*). There is post-SBRT cortical thinning of the adjacent cortex (*black arrowhead*). (**E, F**) A 9-month post-SBRT T2-weighted fat-saturated (**E**) and coronal postcontrast (**F**) MR images demonstrate decrease in size of the treated tumor (*black arrow*). (**G, H**) A 15-month post-SBRT contrast-enhanced CT images demonstrate interval growth and enhancement (*white arrow*). Given the time period (15 months after treatment), increased tumor growth and enhancement, patient was diagnosed with post-treatment local recurrence.

underwent salvage procedures with no evidence of progression/failure [22]. These findings suggest that SBRT induces cell death in most cells; however, a minority of cells enters senescence, a state of irreversible cell arrest, which are thought to be "nonviable" tumor cells [19]. To this end, given that a positive biopsy does not seem to be predictive of subsequent local tumor and progression, routine post-SBRT biopsy does not seem to contribute to local response evaluation and is not recommended unless there are imaging findings concerning for local recurrence [14]. The limitations of post-SBRT biopsy further emphasize the importance of imaging assessment of recurrence and the need for identification of improved imaging biomarkers.

The rates of moderate and severe treatment-related toxicity after SBRT are low; however, when present, can be identified on imaging. The adjacent stomach, small and large bowel can be close to the primary tumor and are at risk of radiation-induced injury. Features of bowel injury include thickening, adjacent inflammatory changes and free air. The collecting system and ureters are also at theoretic risk of radiation toxicity; however, no reports of SBRT-related collecting system injuries exist to date [23]. Adjacent renal damage is expected post-SBRT, and a lower volume of renal cortex spared from exposure to RT doses may be associated with decreased renal function loss [28].

After SBRT treatment, follow-up imaging is often performed approximately every 6 months [14]. Cross-sectional imaging of the abdomen, including kidneys and adrenals, are performed and chest imaging (CT or radiograph) should also be performed to assess for distant metastasis. Based on a consensus statement from high volume centers, all institutions used CT to assess response with some also using MRI [54]. CT has the advantage of being more accessible and has decreased cost compared with MRI. Another advantage is that chest CT imaging can be performed at the same time as the CT of the abdomen and may be more convenient for the patient. MRI has improved contrast resolution and may be more beneficial, particularly if MR imaging biomarkers are validated in clinical practice. Early follow-up cross-sectional imaging is limited and is confounded by the possibility of "pseudoprogression" and, therefore, may not be clinically beneficial [14]. Duration of follow-up is not specified; however, surgical guidelines recommend follow-up for at least 5 years. There is paucity of data to direct frequency of follow-up after 5 years; however, imaging beyond 5 years can be performed at the discretion of the clinician and shared decision making with the patients.

SUMMARY

RT for primary RCC is increasingly utilized in clinical practice and SBRT has overcome the perception that RCC is "radioresistant." SBRT has shown to be effective in medically inoperable patients with low rates of toxicity. Pretreatment imaging is crucial in identifying RCC, determine the extent and presence of metastasis and determine the optimal treatment modality. Knowledge that the expected post-SBRT imaging findings differ from TA is essential. Typical post-SBRT appearances include continued size decrease. Unlike with TA, persistent tumor enhancement is an expected finding post-SBRT. Knowledge that the imaging pitfall of "pseudoprogression" immediately after SBRT is crucial. This article provides a comprehensive overview of SBRT mechanism, evidence and current indication of SBRT in primary RCC, the pre-SBRT imaging and management as well as the expected post-SBRT appearances, and findings of residual and local failure.

CLINICS CARE POINTS

- Stereotactic body radiotherapy (SBRT) has emerged as a treatment option for localized renal cell carcinoma (RCC) in patients that are considered poor surgical or thermal ablation (TA) candidates.
- Pretreatment imaging is crucial for identifying patients who may benefit from treatment of primary RCC with SBRT.
- Imaging appearance of local control and recurrence of primary RCC after SBRT differs considerably compared with the appearance after surgery and TA techniques.

DISCLOSURE

C.S. Lim: Collaborative Research Agreement with IBM Watson Health Imaging, Honorarium from AstraZeneca. R.M. Glicksman: honoraria from Bayer, TerSera, Tolmar, and Knight Therapeutics, and research funding from Astellas and TerSera. All other authors have no relevant disclosures.

REFERENCES

[1] Capitanio U, Bensalah K, Bex A, et al. Epidemiology of renal cell carcinoma. Eur Urol 2019;75:74.

[2] Lim CS, Schieda N, Silverman SG. Update on indications for percutaneous renal mass biopsy in the era of advanced CT and MRI. AJR Am J Roentgenol 2019; 1–10. https://doi.org/10.2214/ajr.19.21093.

[3] Johnson DC, Vukina J, Smith AB, et al. Preoperatively misclassified, surgically removed benign renal masses: a systematic review of surgical series and United States population level burden estimate. J Urol 2015;193(1): 30–5.

[4] Wong MCS, Goggins WB, Yip BHK, et al. Incidence and mortality of kidney cancer: temporal patterns and global trends in 39 countries. Sci Rep 2017;7(1):15698. https://doi.org/10.1038/s41598-017-15922-4.

[5] Motzer RJ, Jonasch E, Agarwal N, et al. NCCN Guidelines® insights: kidney cancer, version 2.2024. J Natl Compr Canc Netw 2024;22(1):4–16.

[6] Patel HD, Pierorazio PM, Johnson MH, et al. Renal functional outcomes after surgery, ablation, and active surveillance of localized renal tumors: a systematic review and meta-analysis. Clin J Am Soc Nephrol 2017;12:1057.

[7] Go AS, Chertow GM, Fan D, et al. Chronic kidney disease and the risks of death, cardiovascular events, and hospitalization. N Engl J Med 2004;351(13):1296–305.

[8] Schieda N, Krishna S, Pedrosa I, et al. Active surveillance of renal masses: the role of radiology. Radiology 2022; 302(1):11–24.

[9] Rivero JR, De La Cerda J 3rd, Wang H, et al. Partial nephrectomy versus thermal ablation for clinical stage T1 renal masses: systematic review and meta-analysis of more than 3,900 patients. J Vasc Interv Radiol 2018; 29(1):18–29.

[10] Ljungberg B, Albiges L, Abu-Ghanem Y, et al. European association of urology guidelines on renal cell carcinoma: the 2022 update. Eur Urol 2022;82(4):399–410.

[11] Zaorsky NG, Louie AV, Siva S. Radiation therapy options in kidney cancer. Curr Opin Support Palliat Care 2023; 17(4):308–14.

[12] Swaminath A, Chu W. Stereotactic body radiotherapy for the treatment of medically inoperable primary renal cell carcinoma: current evidence and future directions. Can Urol Assoc J 2015;9(7–8):275–80.

[13] Siva S, Bressel M, Sidhom M, et al. Stereotactic ablative body radiotherapy for primary kidney cancer (TROG 15.03 FASTRACK II): a non-randomised phase 2 trial. Lancet Oncol 2024;25(3):308–16.

[14] Siva S, Louie AV, Kotecha R, et al. Stereotactic body radiotherapy for primary renal cell carcinoma: a systematic review and practice guideline from the International Society of Stereotactic Radiosurgery (ISRS). Lancet Oncol 2024;25(1):e18–28.

[15] Barbour AB, Upadhyay R, Anderson AC, et al. Stereotactic body radiation therapy for primary renal cell carcinoma: a case-based radiosurgery society practice guide. Pract Radiat Oncol 2024. https://doi.org/10.1016/j.prro.2024.06.012.

[16] De Meerleer G, Khoo V, Escudier B, et al. Radiotherapy for renal-cell carcinoma. Lancet Oncol 2014;15(4):e170–7.

[17] Singh AK, Winslow TB, Kermany MH, et al. A pilot study of stereotactic body radiation therapy combined with cytoreductive nephrectomy for metastatic renal cell carcinoma. Clin Cancer Res 2017;23(17):5055–65.

[18] Jiang A, Liu Y, Cai C, et al. Re: stereotactic ablative body radiotherapy for primary kidney cancer (TROG 15.03 FASTRACK II): a non-randomised phase 2 trial. Eur Urol 2024;86(2):188–9.

[19] Hannan R, McLaughlin MF, Pop LM, et al. Phase 2 trial of stereotactic ablative radiotherapy for patients with primary renal cancer. Eur Urol 2023;84(3):275–86.

[20] Grubb WR, Ponsky L, Lo SS, et al. Final results of a dose escalation protocol of stereotactic body radiotherapy for poor surgical candidates with localized renal cell carcinoma. Radiother Oncol 2021;155:138–43.

[21] Siva S, Pham D, Kron T, et al. Stereotactic ablative body radiotherapy for inoperable primary kidney cancer: a prospective clinical trial. BJU Int 2017;120(5):623–30.

[22] Ponsky L, Lo SS, Zhang Y, et al. Phase I dose-escalation study of stereotactic body radiotherapy (SBRT) for poor surgical candidates with localized renal cell carcinoma. Radiother Oncol 2015;117(1):183–7.

[23] Siva S, Ali M, Correa RJM, et al. 5-year outcomes after stereotactic ablative body radiotherapy for primary renal cell carcinoma: an individual patient data meta-analysis from IROCK (the International Radiosurgery Consortium of the Kidney). Lancet Oncol 2022;23(12):1508–16.

[24] Andrews JR, Atwell T, Schmit G, et al. Oncologic outcomes following partial nephrectomy and percutaneous ablation for cT1 renal masses. Eur Urol 2019;76(2): 244–51.

[25] Correa RJM, Louie AV, Zaorsky NG, et al. The emerging role of stereotactic ablative radiotherapy for primary renal cell carcinoma: a systematic review and meta-analysis. Eur Urol Focus 2019;5(6):958–69.

[26] Ali M, Acosta Ruiz V, Psutka SP, et al. Ablative therapies for localized primary renal cell carcinoma. Société Internationale d'Urologie Journal 2022;3(6):437–49.

[27] Patel HD, Pierorazio PM, Johnson MH, et al. Renal functional outcomes after surgery, ablation, and active surveillance of localized renal tumors: a systematic review and meta-analysis. Clin J Am Soc Nephrol 2017;12(7): 1057–69.

[28] Glicksman RM, Cheung P, Korol R, et al. Stereotactic body radiotherapy for renal cell carcinoma: oncological and renal function outcomes. Clin Oncol (R Coll Radiol) 2023;35(1):20–8.

[29] Freifeld Y, Pedrosa I, McLaughlin M, et al. Stereotactic ablative radiation therapy for renal cell carcinoma with inferior vena cava tumor thrombus. Urol Oncol 2022;40(4):166.e9–13.

[30] Raj RK, Upadhyay R, Wang SJ, et al. Incorporating stereotactic ablative radiotherapy into the multidisciplinary management of renal cell carcinoma. Curr Oncol 2023;30(12):10283–98.

[31] Krishna S, Leckie A, Kielar A, et al. Imaging of renal cancer. Semin Ultrasound CT MR 2020;41(2):152–69.

[32] Siddaiah M, Krishna S, McInnes MDF, et al. Is ultrasound useful for further evaluation of homogeneously hyperattenuating renal lesions detected on CT? AJR Am J Roentgenol 2017;209(3):604–10.

[33] Sadoughi N, Krishna S, Macdonald DB, et al. Diagnostic accuracy of attenuation difference and iodine concentration thresholds at rapid-kilovoltage-switching dual-energy CT for detection of enhancement in renal masses. AJR Am J Roentgenol 2019;213(3):619–25.

[34] Silverman SG, Pedrosa I, Ellis JH, et al. Bosniak classification of cystic renal masses, version 2019: an update proposal and needs assessment. Radiology 2019;292(2): 475–88.

[35] Narayanasamy S, Krishna S, Prasad Shanbhogue AK, et al. Contemporary update on imaging of cystic renal masses with histopathological correlation and emphasis on patient management. Clin Radiol 2019;74:83.

[36] Silverman SG, Israel GM, Trinh QD. Incompletely characterized incidental renal masses: emerging data support conservative management. Radiology 2015;275(1):28–42.

[37] Marconi L, Dabestani S, Lam TB, et al. Systematic review and meta-analysis of diagnostic accuracy of percutaneous renal tumour biopsy. Eur Urol 2016;69:660.

[38] Silverman SG, Israel GM, Herts BR, et al. Management of the incidental renal mass. Radiology 2008;249(1): 16–31.

[39] McClure TD, Chow DS, Tan N, et al. Intermediate outcomes and predictors of efficacy in the radiofrequency ablation of 100 pathologically proven renal cell carcinomas. J Vasc Interv Radiol 2014;25(11):1682–8, quiz 1689.

[40] Gervais DA, McGovern FJ, Arellano RS, et al. Radiofrequency ablation of renal cell carcinoma: part 1, Indications, results, and role in patient management over a 6-year period and ablation of 100 tumors. AJR Am J Roentgenol 2005;185(1):64–71.

[41] Camacho JC, Kokabi N, Xing M, et al. R.E.N.A.L. (Radius, exophytic/endophytic, nearness to collecting system or sinus, anterior/posterior, and location relative to polar lines) nephrometry score predicts early tumor recurrence and complications after percutaneous ablative therapies for renal cell carcinoma: a 5-year experience. J Vasc Interv Radiol 2015;26(5):686–93.

[42] Huang RS, Chow R, Chopade P, et al. Dose-response of localized renal cell carcinoma after stereotactic body radiation therapy: a meta-analysis. Radiother Oncol 2024; 194:110216.

[43] Schieda N, van der Pol CB, Walker D, et al. Adverse events to the gadolinium-based contrast agent gadoxetic acid: systematic review and meta-analysis. Radiology 2020;200073.

[44] Abou Elkassem AM, Lo SS, Gunn AJ, et al. Role of imaging in renal cell carcinoma: a multidisciplinary perspective. Radiographics 2021;41(5):1387–407.

[45] Yamamoto T, Kadoya N, Takeda K, et al. Renal atrophy after stereotactic body radiotherapy for renal cell carcinoma. Radiat Oncol 2016/05/26 2016;11(1):72.

[46] Sun MR, Brook A, Powell MF, et al. Effect of stereotactic body radiotherapy on the growth kinetics and enhancement pattern of primary renal tumors. AJR Am J Roentgenol 2016;206(3):544–53.

[47] Nomiya T, Tsuji H, Hirasawa N, et al. Carbon ion radiation therapy for primary renal cell carcinoma: initial clinical experience. Int J Radiat Oncol Biol Phys 2008;72(3):828–33.

[48] Aghdam N, Hall E, Bennett L, et al. Transient radiographic pseudoprogression following fractionated SBRT for primary renal cell carcinoma. Int J Radiat Oncol Biol Phys 2023;117(2):e362–3.

[49] Chang JH, Cheung P, Erler D, et al. Stereotactic ablative body radiotherapy for primary renal cell carcinoma in non-surgical candidates: initial clinical experience. Clin Oncol (R Coll Radiol) 2016;28(9):e109–14.

[50] Haroon M, Sathiadoss P, Hibbert RM, et al. Imaging considerations for thermal and radiotherapy ablation of primary and metastatic renal cell carcinoma. Abdom Radiol (NY) 2021/07/10 2021. https://doi.org/10.1007/s00261-021-03178-6.

[51] Low RN, Fuller DB, Muradyan N. Dynamic gadolinium-enhanced perfusion MRI of prostate cancer: assessment of response to hypofractionated robotic stereotactic body radiation therapy. AJR Am J Roentgenol 2011;197(4):907–15.

[52] Muselaers S, Erdem S, Bertolo R, et al. PSMA PET/CT in renal cell carcinoma: an overview of current literature. J Clin Med 2022;11(7). https://doi.org/10.3390/jcm11071829.

[53] Reynolds HM, Parameswaran BK, Finnegan ME, et al. Diffusion weighted and dynamic contrast enhanced MRI as an imaging biomarker for stereotactic ablative body radiotherapy (SABR) of primary renal cell carcinoma. PLoS One 2018;13(8):e0202387.

[54] Siva S, Ellis RJ, Ponsky L, et al. Consensus statement from the international radiosurgery oncology consortium for kidney for primary renal cell carcinoma. Future Oncol 2016;12(5):637–45.

Advances in Clinical Radiology 7 (2025) 45–56
ADVANCES IN CLINICAL RADIOLOGY

Curative Intent Percutaneous Thermal Ablation for Colorectal Liver Metastases

State of the Art 2025 Update

Dimitrios Xenos, MD, Vlasios S. Sotirchos, MD, Constantinos T. Sofocleous, MD, PhD*
Department of Radiology, Interventional Radiology Service, Memorial Sloan Kettering Cancer Center, New York, NY, USA

KEYWORDS
• Curative intent • Percutaneous thermal ablation • Colorectal liver metastases

KEY POINTS
- Thermal ablation is recommended as a standalone therapy for potentially resectable small colorectal liver metastases as long as all visible tumors can be eradicated with adequate margins.
- Split-dose PET/ computed tomography (CT) and CT hepatic arteriography can optimize tumor localization and targeting and significantly improve intraprocedural ablation monitoring.
- Three-dimensional (3D) software-based assessment of the ablation zone is superior to the two-dimensional side-by-side assessment and helps detect areas of insufficient coverage by the ablation zone.
- Reliable real-time 3D evaluation of the ablation zone on cross-sectional and metabolic imaging as well as through tissue assessments allows reablation when insufficient minimal ablation margins (<5 mm) or detection of residual viable tissue is detected, improving local tumor control.

INTRODUCTION

Colorectal cancer (CRC) constitutes the fourth most commonly diagnosed malignancy worldwide and the leading cause of cancer-related death in the United States for men, and the second etiologic factor for women under the age of 50 years [1]. Patients with colorectal liver metastases (CLM) have worse prognosis.

Current international guidelines recommend thermal ablation (TA) as a standalone therapy or in conjunction with surgery and/or chemotherapy for potentially resectable CLM for select patients with small-volume disease, as long as all visible tumors can be eradicated [2]. The recent COLLISION randomized controlled trial (NCT03088150) further supports TA instead of resection for small CLM (≤3 cm) that can be ablated with minimal ablation margins (MM) ≥5 mm, as it is associated with fewer complications, shorter hospital stay, no compromise in disease control and overall survival, and better per treated tumor control [3]. Eradication of CLM is achieved through the application of lethal temperatures in the form of heat using radiofrequency (RFA) or microwave ablation (MWA), or in the form of freezing using cryoablation. Several publications have indicated that the MM is the most important predictive factor of local tumor progression (LTP) -free survival. MM of at least 5 mm has been suggested by many studies and proposed by the National Comprehensive Cancer Network (NCCN) as a critical ablation

*Corresponding author. Interventional Oncology/ Radiology Service, Memorial Sloan Kettering Cancer Center, New York, NY. *E-mail address:* sofoclec@mskcc.org

https://doi.org/10.1016/j.yacr.2025.05.004 www.advancesinclinicalradiology.com
2589-8701/25/

ABBREVIATIONS

2D	two-dimensional
3D	three-dimensional
ceCT	contrast-enhanced computed tomography
ceMRI	contrast-enhanced MRI
ceUS	contrast-enhanced ultrasound
CLM	colorectal liver metastases
CRC	colorectal cancer
CT	computed tomography
CTHA	computed tomography hepatic arteriography
DIR	deformable image registration
FDG	fluorodeoxyglucose
LTP	local tumor progression
MM	minimal ablation margin
MWA	microwave ablation
NCCN	National Comprehensive Cancer Network
RFA	radiofrequency ablation
RIR	rigid image registration
SUV	standardized uptake value
TA	thermal ablation
US	ultrasound

technical endpoint to achieve satisfactory local tumor control rates when considering curative intent ablation for CLM [2,4–20]. It is important to note that in *KRAS* mutant CLM the prognosis is worse, with higher LTP rates, consequently requiring an MM greater than 10 mm in order to achieve acceptable local tumor control [21,22].

PREABLATION IMAGING

Contrast-enhanced computed tomography (ceCT) is widely available and the most commonly used imaging modality offering high-quality information about tumor location and anatomy, necessary for ablation planning [23]. The method is associated with per tumor detection sensitivity of 84% but is significantly decreased to 35% for smaller CLM with a diameter less than 1 cm [24]. MRI with hepatobiliary contrast agent is recommended for the detection of smaller tumors, especially those less than 1 cm in largest diameter [25]. Fluorodeoxyglucose (FDG)- PET/computed tomography (CT) is also recommended for restaging before ablation, not only to confirm the presence of hypermetabolic activity of known tumors but also more importantly to rule out occult extrahepatic metastases.

MRI constitutes the imaging modality of choice for accurate diagnosis of CLM with high per tumor specificity ranging from 86.9% to 100% [26]. A recent international trial evaluating the added value of contrast-enhanced MRI (ceMRI) to ceCT, in patients with CLM scheduled for local treatment, demonstrated that ceMRI changed the treatment plan in 31% of patients (CAMINO: NL8039) [25]. Because of the superiority of ceMRI over ceCT, the current NCCN guidelines recommend liver ceMRI for exact evaluation of the number and distribution of CLMs for treatment planning [2]. For CLM undergoing curative intent ablation, ceCT and ceMRI within 30 days of the procedure are required [2].

Although PET/CT is not recommended at the initial routine patient evaluation, in patients considered for locoregional image-guided interventions or surgery, baseline PET/CT evaluation can be considered according to the latest NCCN guidelines, as it demonstrates high sensitivity in the detection of extrahepatic disease and can alter patient management [2]. Maffione and colleagues [27] reported a change in the management of a mean of 24% of the patients and a mean incidence of extrahepatic disease detection in 32%. PET/CT is also recommended in the presence of contraindications to intravenous contrast administration and in cases of ambiguous ceCT or ceMRI results [2]. Main limitations of this approach include decreased sensitivity for patients concurrently receiving chemotherapy or for target tumors smaller than 1 cm [28]. PET/CT is recommended with anatomic imaging ceCT and/or ceMRI. The authors advocate all 3 imaging modalities when assessing the eligibility of patients with CLM, for curative intent TA, as supported by the NCCN guidelines [2].

The time interval between the ablation and image acquisition is critical for proper ablation evaluation. CLM can demonstrate rapid growth within short time periods; therefore, current guidelines suggest updated anatomic and metabolic imaging within the preceding month before any locoregional treatment with curative intent as an absolute requirement for accurate disease restaging [2].

DAY OF ABLATION

Immediate preablation imaging

A preprocedural multiphase ceCT is the minimum requirement for tumor delineation, segmentation, and confirmation of the ablation plan. The authors recommend triphasic liver CT examination with thin cuts and reconstructions before and immediately after TA. In cases where the scan cannot provide a satisfactory resolution of the target tumor, tumor border editing can be applied at the most recent contrast-enhanced scan (CT or MRI) available within 30 days from ablation. Real-time ultrasound (US) guidance for ablation electrode placement and real-time ablation zone monitoring are recommended for tumors visible with this modality. Real-time FDG-PET is also highly recommended for tumor detection and segmentation, as previously described [28]. The authors strongly recommend the use of the split-dose PET/CT technique for ablation guidance, monitoring, and confirmation for FDG-avid tumors, as detailed in later discussion.

Split-dose PET/computed tomography–guided ablation

In short, with this technique, the first FDG dose equal to -third (4 mCi) of the diagnostic dose (4 mCi) is administered within 30 to 60 minutes before ablation. This allows tumor localization for targeting, typically for the subsequent 60 to 120 minutes. Once the ablation is considered complete, the second FDG injection, equal to the two-thirds of the diagnostic dose (8 mCi), is administered, followed by repeat PET/CT acquisition 30 minutes later. During the time, between the second FDG injection and the image acquisition, a postablation ceCT is repeated and used for ablation zone (AZ)/MM assessments. Additional confirmatory biopsies of the AZ can be performed at this time point [28].

Computed tomographic hepatic arteriography

CT hepatic arteriography (CTHA) includes selective catheter placement in common or proper hepatic artery, enabling repeated administration of small amounts of contrast [29]. The method allows clear depiction of intrahepatic arterial constructure and has demonstrated statistically significant improvement in the accuracy of CLMs [30]. The tumors appear as either a contrast-enhancing ring with hypoattenuating core or, in cases of LTP (after local treatment), as an incomplete hyperattenuating ring [29,30]. At the end of each ablation cycle, repeated contrast injection demonstrates enhancement of the ablation zone and potential residual tumor. The clear depiction of preprocedural tumor contours and postprocedural AZ allows for image registration and MM assessment. Disadvantages of this method include the increased radiation exposure and iodine contrast use [29,30].

Ablation monitoring

The position of the ablation electrode before applying lethal heat energy is confirmed with CT and US imaging. If the tumor is not visible by CT or US, the CT and US can be fused with ceMRI, ceCT, or PET/CT within 30 days of the ablation day. The authors strongly advocate the use of intraprocedural real-time PET/CT for CLM localization using the split-dose technique as described above. This technical capability has the unique advantage of continuous visualization of the PET-avid tumor with repeated short real-time PET/CT breath-hold acquisitions, before and during the ablation procedure. Real-time PET can detect most of the CLMs, even those that are not visible by non-ceCT. In a prior publication, 32.1% of CLM were either poorly conspicuous or undetectable by unenhanced CT alone; however, with the addition of real-time PET/CT, only 2.1% remained undetectable [31]. Moreover, the split-dose PET/CT technique allows intraprocedural accurate localization and target tumor visualization with electrodes in place, even after hydrodissection or target tumor mobilization. The method overcomes limitations of real-time US monitoring of the AZ, where the AZ is often obscured by the air generated during ablation. It also provides continuous visualization of the target tumor, allowing accurate electrode repositioning in order to create an AZ completely encompassing the target tumor with the desired MM. CTHA is an alternative option that provides repeated target tumor depiction before initiation of each ablation cycle [29,30].

Ablation confirmation

Technical success of ablation is assessed at least with triphasic ceCT. The tumor should be completely ablated with the AZ covering the entire tumor and an additional stereotactic rim of at least 5 mm MM around the target CLM [32]. Assessment of ablation completeness can be improved when the split-dose PET technique is used [31]. Detection of residual FDG-avid foci within the ablation zone can be sampled as needed for further confirmation and re-ablated within the same setting (Fig. 1) [23,31,33]. Assessment of technical completeness with PET/CT is accompanied by challenges [33]. Immediate postablation bleeding or tissue inflammation and minimal distortion may decrease the reliability of residual viable tumor detection [34]. Shyn and colleagues [12] evaluated the AZ by combining preprocedural FDG-PET/CT and immediate postablation Nitrogen-13 ammonia perfusion PET. This method was efficient in AZ delineation and confirmation of technically successful ablation but failed to directly assess residual viable tumor metabolic activity. Tumor viability assessment is feasible with

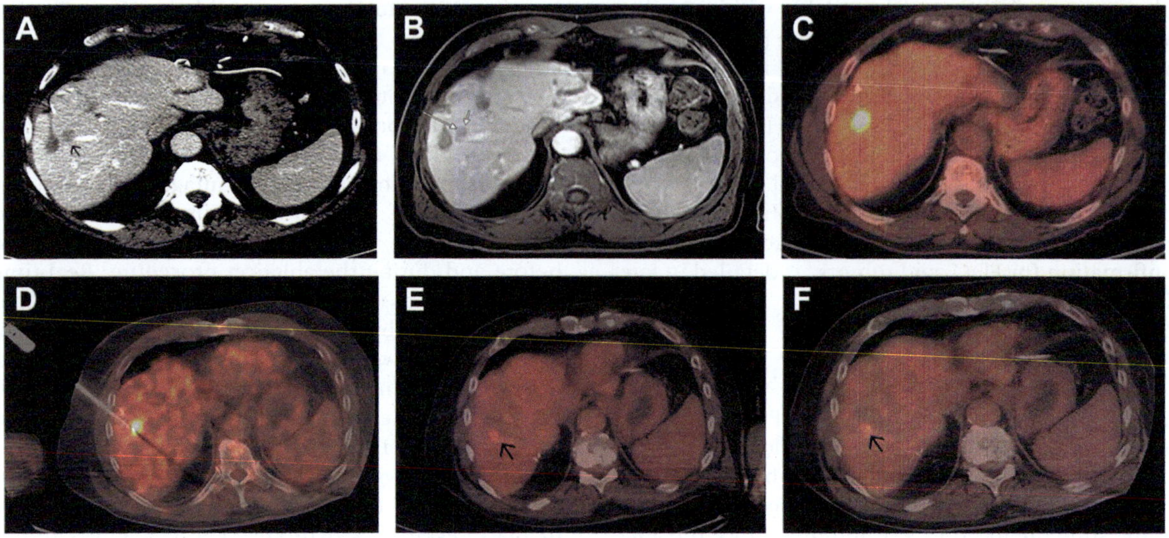

FIG. 1 A 79-year-old man with history of CLMs managed with chemotherapy and liver resections underwent MWA for new metastasis at segment 8 demonstrated on preprocedural anatomic (**A**; *arrowhead*; **B**; *arrowhead*) and metabolic (**C**) imaging. The tumor presented avid FDG uptake on the ablation day and was successfully targeted under PET/CT guidance using the split-dose PET/CT technique (**D**; first dose of 4 mCi). Postablation PET/CT showing FDG uptake along the posterior margin (**E**, **F**; *arrowhead*) after the injection of the second dose (8 mCi), indicating residual viable tumor. This area was subsequently re-treated in the same session with ablation.

real-time split-dose FDG-PET [28]. The partition of the 2 doses takes into account the FDG decay, so that approximately 10% of the initial dose is present at the final postablation scan, hours after the first FDG injection, minimizing background activity from the original injection. The largest second FDG injection allows an accurate depiction of the AZ and increases the sensitivity of detecting hypermetabolic activity originating from residual viable tumor postablation (Fig. 2). An additional advantage associated with PET/CT utilization is the calculation of the standardized uptake value (SUV) ratio. SUV ratio has demonstrated significant predictive value for LTP in patients with MM $\geq$5 mm and negative biopsy specimens from the AZ center and margin [35].

Another imaging modality used for intraprocedural ablation monitoring and immediate confirmation of ablation completeness is contrast-enhanced ultrasound (ceUS). Utilization of ceUS is associated with the inability to provide clear visualization of the electrode and the target tumor because TA generates gas bubbles that obscure the AZ (Fig. 3). According to Dietrich and colleagues [36], for immediate postablation assessment, ceUS should be performed after 5 to 10 minutes, to allow the hyperechoic gas to be diffused into the surrounding tissue. The modality is also suboptimal in the assessment of patients with increased body habitus or with hepatic steatosis.

Ablation zone and minimal ablation margin assessment

Historically, assessment of the ablation technique efficacy and AZ margins was performed on the first follow-up cross-sectional imaging scan, typically after 4 to 8 weeks [32]. The MM calculated on the first follow-up ceCT imaging (4–8 weeks after ablation) was found to be a strong independent predictor of LTP [4,14]. The methodology of MM measurement proposed by Wang and colleagues [14] relied on the use of hepatic anatomic landmarks on ceCT that were graded for their reliability. The difference between the distance of a specific landmark from the tumor border subtracting the distance of the same landmark from the edge of the AZ was used to estimate the MM and AZ tumor coverage. The results of the study indicated that MM constitutes a predictor of LTP, and postablation MM greater than or equal to 5 mm was associated with a significant decrease (of 46%) in LTP rate [14]. The investigators also pointed out the necessity of development and application of image registration and fusion

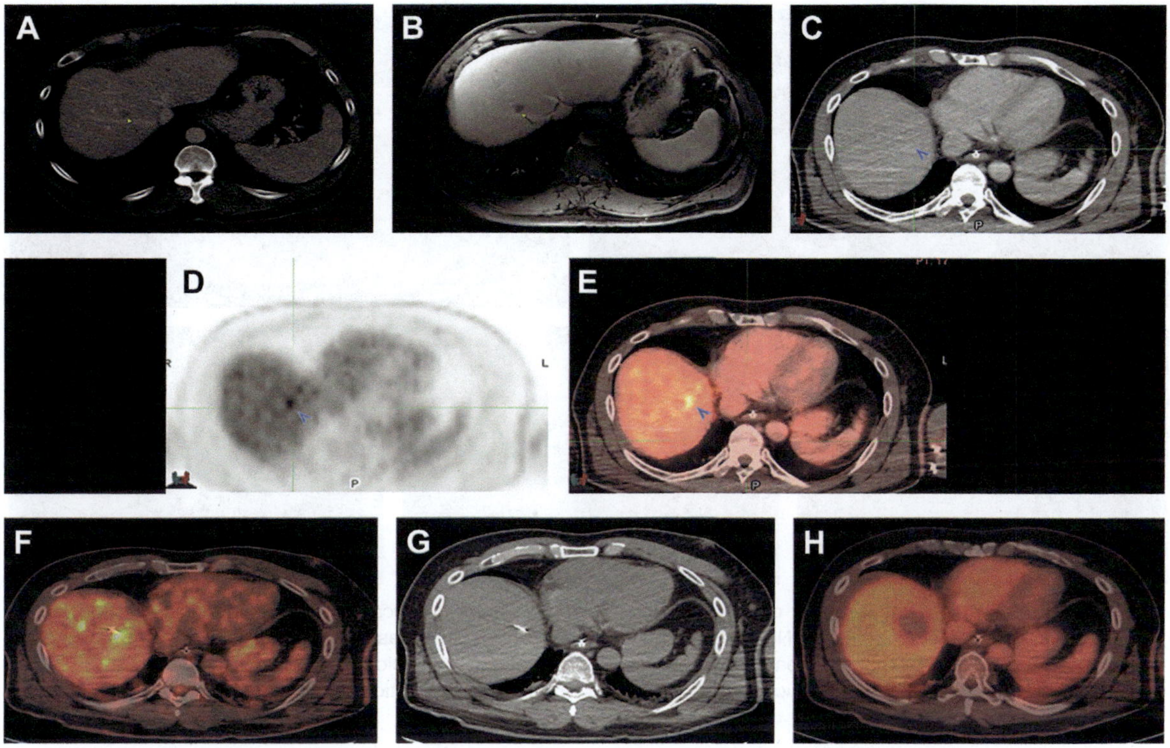

FIG. 2 A 56-year-old man with a history of upper rectal adenocarcinoma after robotic laparoscopic resection and CAPOX chemotherapy. A new segment 8 tumor suspicious for metastasis was detected on preprocedural anatomic imaging (**A, B**; *yellow arrowhead*) in the setting of increasing carcinoembryonic antigen (CEA) (from 4.3 to 7.8) investigation. The target tumor was not visible on the ceCT on ablation day imaging (**C**: *blue arrowhead* indicates the target tumor location). Intraprocedural PET (**D**) and PET/CT (**E**) show the FDG-avid tumor (*blue arrowhead*). Real-time breath-hold PET/CT (**F**) and corresponding CT (**G**) confirm accurate targeting of the tumor for ablation. Repeat PET/CT following administration of the second FDG dose with the split-dose protocol shows the photopenic ablation zone, which covers the target tumor with adequate margins (**H**).

software in order to calculate MM immediately within the procedure room at the time of ablation, as the methods available at that time could not provide the desirable information in a timely manner.

Although this two-dimensional (2D) method can easily be performed without advanced fusion software, it is prone to registration errors and is time-consuming [14]. Postablation liver distortion, tissue dehydration, contraction and subsequent displacement, variations in patient positioning, and respiratory phases make the evaluation of the AZ and MM challenging. Finally, this method presents challenges for assessment of the MM in the coronal and sagittal planes.

The need of reliable MM of 5-mm assessment around the treated tumor that indicates the extent and the exact location of the tissue at risk for LTP has led to the evolution of several platforms providing quantitative three-dimensional (3D) software-based analysis for precise evaluation of the tumor and the AZ and improved discrimination power for the calculation of postablation margin volumes and areas of insufficient coverage and at risk for LTP [5,13,19].

TARGET TUMOR CONTOURING

The current assessment of the AZ and MM is recommended to take place on the immediate postablation ceCT using advanced imaging processing software, reconstructing 3D volumetric margins for technical success confirmation ceCT [5,8,13,19,20]. The same method is recommended at the 4- to 8-week postablation ceCT for technical efficacy evaluation [32].

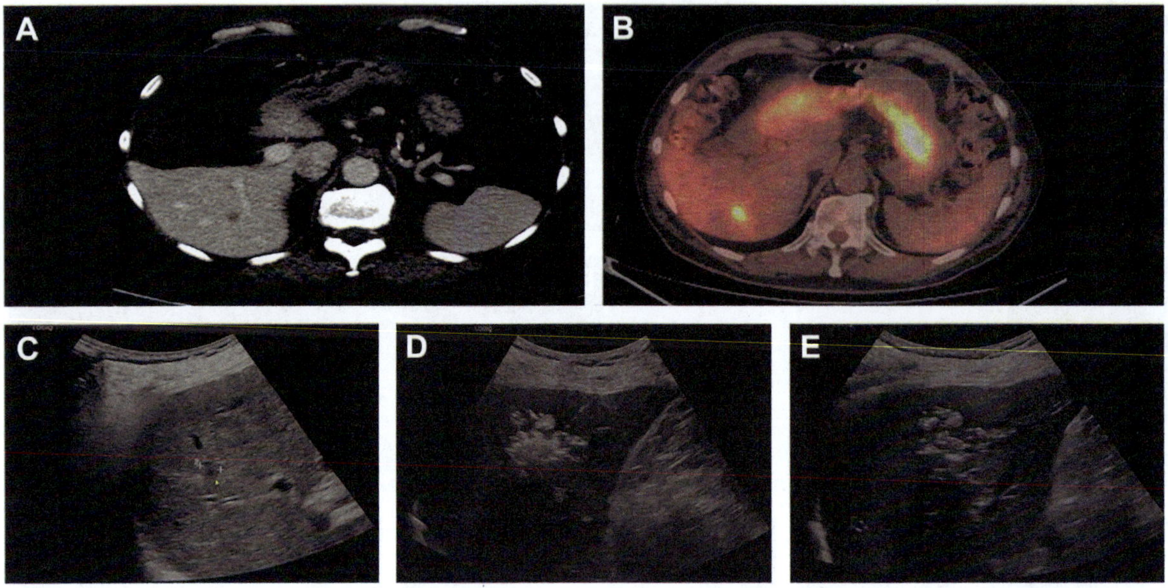

FIG. 3 Ablation day of a 77-year-old woman with a history of rectal adenocarcinoma treated with resection, radiation therapy chemotherapy. New segment 6 tumor suspicious for metastasis on preprocedure anatomic (**A**) and metabolic (**B**) imaging. Real-time US demonstrates solid hypoechoic target tumor (**C**). The electrode is placed, and the artifacts produced secondary to air bubble during ablation obscure real-time monitoring (**D**, **E**).

Three-dimensional software-based assessments

The currently available methods for image registration include rigid image registration (RIR) and nonrigid or intensity-based deformable image registration (DIR) [13,19]. The RIR does not account for tissue deformation or positioning changes and often requires manual manipulation to correct image misregistration [13]. In contrast, DIR algorithms account for these alterations, allowing for tumor-contouring adjustments in the preablation liver imaging along with the corresponding 5-mm and 10-mm theoretic margin contours around the target tumor. The workflows of the software in both categories constitute a stepwise process, including automatic, semiautomatic, and manually adjusted steps. Advanced biomechanical platforms with DIR allow both deformable and rigid registration.

There are 2 options for tumor segmentation: (1) a semiautomatic option that contours the target tumor in all planes based on voxel difference between tumor and normal liver parenchyma, and (2) a manual option where the operator detects and manually contours the target tumor in all planes. Once segmentation on the axial plane is performed, the tumor is reviewed in the coronal and the sagittal planes to complete 3D tumor rendering and to include areas not covered by the axial contours. After the tumor contours are confirmed, reliable liver parenchymal landmarks are used to ensure satisfactory semiautomatic registration and proper alignment of the preablation to the postablation images. The bifurcation of intrahepatic vessels represents the most reliable landmark constituting a fixed 3D point within the liver parenchyma. Smooth vessel segments, surgical clips, and liver capsule or organ ligaments constitute less reliable fixed 2D points that are prone to dislocation secondary to tissue scarring, respiration, and positioning [14]. The preablation ceCT depicting vascular structures and in particular portal venous branching is used for proper tumor and corresponding ablation zone registrations.

The workflow automatically generates 5-mm and 10-mm regions of interest around the tumor boundaries visualized as differently colored concentric curved closed lines, representing the theoretic AZ margins. Once the workflow fuses the theoretic images with the actual AZ, it provides the operator the opportunity to visually evaluate the registration accuracy with pseudo-colored overlay of the preablation and postablation ceCT and allows for minimal adjustments based on the liver contour and anatomic landmarks whenever

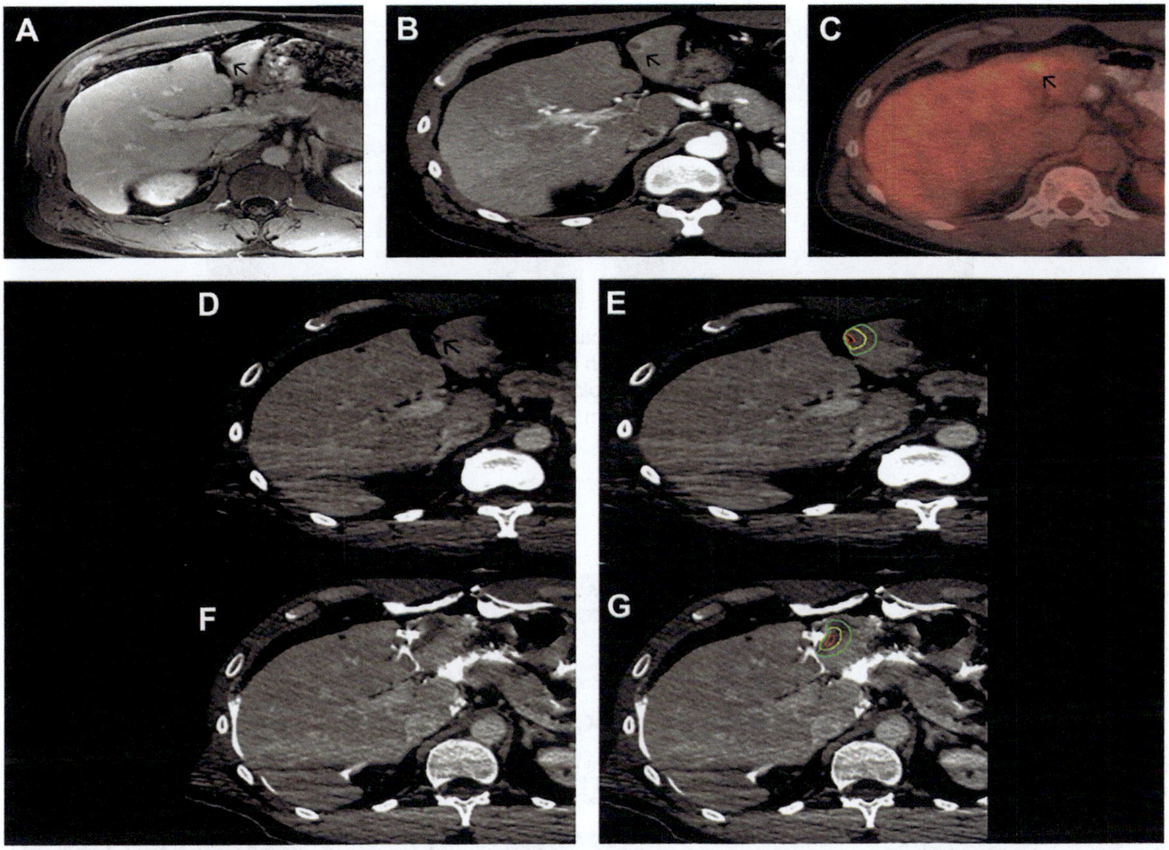

FIG. 4 A 52-year-old male patient with a history of CRC under chemotherapy treatment presented with new synchronous segment 3 liver metastasis on anatomic (**A, B**) and metabolic (**C**). Target tumor at segment 3 was visible at the ceCT on the ablation day (**D**), and the imaging modality was used for lesion contouring (**E**). *Red circle* represents the tumor contours, *yellow circle* and *green circle* represent the 5 and10 millimeters (mm) margins around the target tumor, respectively. Real-time hydrodissection with water-soluble contrast was conducted to buffer the nearby stomach diaphragm and colon (**F, G**). Hydrodissection causes deformation of the edge of the organ requiring manual adjustments to ensure proper preablation and postablation image registration for MM evaluation (**G**).

necessary. This is an extremely important step in the process, as alignment and registration can be very challenging, especially in cases of hydrodissection, subcapsular or perihepatic hematoma as well as tumor mobilization secondary to organ contraction and deformation as a result of the thermal injury (Fig. 4). Once the registration is satisfactory, the margins are visually assessed. Volumetric 3D assessment and the volume of the insufficient coverage, wherever the desirable MM is not achieved, are also automatically estimated (Fig. 5). In cases of incomplete coverage of the critical 5 mm, the interventional oncologist/radiologist evaluates the images, and if feasible and safe, offers additional ablation to achieve technically successful ablation (Fig. 6) [4,5,9,13,17,20,28,32,37,38].

Laimer and colleagues [15] and Sibinga Mulder and colleagues [6] assessed intraprocedural 3D volumetric MM using semiautomatic nonrigid registration with utilization of preablation and postablation ceCT. Vasiniotis Kamarinos and colleagues [13] similarly assessed the MM and compared intraprocedural 3D assessments with the 4- to 8-week postablation 2D assessment, establishing the superiority of the stereotactic approach. Anderson and colleagues [37] evaluated the implementation of biomechanical model-based DIR registration and compared it with RIR. Using the same principle,

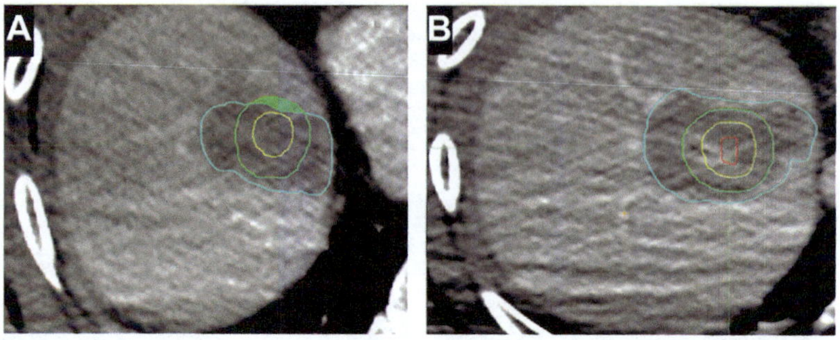

FIG. 5 The same patient as in Fig. 1. Ablation technical success confirmation on postablation ceCT. (**B**) (*red circular line*) The tumor contours; (*yellow*) 5-mm region of interest (minimal margin); (*green*) 10-mm region of interest (minimal margin); (*blue*) the margins of the ablation zone. Green-colored parenchyma represents volume of insufficiant coverage (VIC) for MM ≥10 mm (**A**).

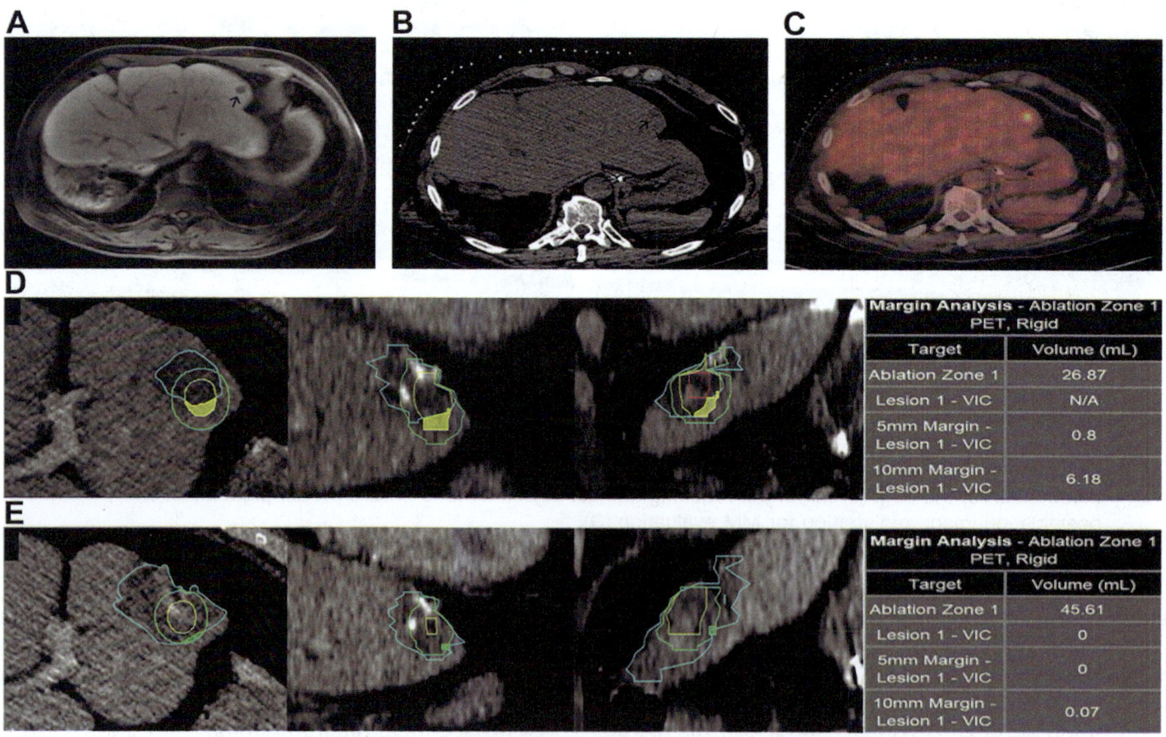

FIG. 6 A 70-year-old woman with metastatic colon cancer, history of left hemicolectomy, hepatic resections, and prior chemotherapy underwent liver ablation (MWA) for recurrent tumor in segment 2 demonstrated at preprocedural anatomic imaging (**A**; *arrowhead*) and on anatomic (**B**; *arrowhead*) and metabolic (**C**) imaging at the procedure day. Intraprocedural margin assessment demonstrating MM ≤5 mm (**D**; yellow-colored parenchyma), indicating the need for supplementary ablation. Technical success after additional ablation uniformly reaching MM ≥5 mm around the target tumor (**E**; green-colored parenchyma corresponds to MM ≤10 mm). The tables at the end of each image demonstrate the automatically calculated VIC. N/A, not applicable. *Yellow colored* areas indicate areas of insufficiant coverage of the ablation zone with required minimal margins of 5 mm

Lin and colleagues [5,7] reproduced the same comparison using the same software with the addition of artificial intelligence–based tumor and AZ contouring. All the investigators reported manual contour correction for preablation and postablation image registration whenever appropriate. Despite minimal technical differences between investigators with regards to target tumor contouring, all indicated superiority of DIR versus RIR for the detection of areas with insufficient coverage being at risk for LTP. All studies highlighted the importance of immediate intraprocedural assessment as an objective and standardized evaluation of tumor coverage and ablation success, in addition to the 4- to 8-week postablation efficacy evaluation. As a matter of fact, Zirakchian and colleagues [19] demonstrated higher sensitivity of the intraprocedural 3D margin assessment in terms of predictive value for LTP compared with the 4- to 8-week postablation assessment. Methodologies proposing utilization of ceMRI in preprocedural and 72-hours postablation settings are not currently recommended, as they do not offer immediate ablation completeness assessment [10]. Recently, Paolucci and colleagues [20] proposed biomechanical model-based DIR software using artificial intelligence–based autosegmentation as a reliable and obligatory ablation completeness validation method after associating intraprocedural MM of 5-mm confirmation with less than 1% LTP risk. Implementation of this method is further supported by the recently published results of a randomized phase II trial (COVER-ALL; NCT04083378) demonstrating statistically significant superiority in achieving MM $\geq$5 mm with software utilization in comparison to visual assessment for primary and secondary hepatic tumors [39].

In this context, the ongoing international multicenter single-arm phase II/III clinical trial ACCLAIM (Ablation with Confirmation of Colorectal Liver Metastasis; NTC05265169) aims to prove that more than 90% local tumor control rates can be achieved with intraprocedural 3D minimal margin confirmation of at least 5 mm, or immediate re-ablation to achieve MM $\geq$5 mm.

ABLATION COMPLETENESS CONFIRMATION WITH INTRAPROCEDURAL TISSUE SAMPLING

One important limitation of image-guided tumor ablation in comparison to surgery is the lack of pathologic evidence of complete tumor eradication. Imaging evaluation of the AZ and margins presumes that the entire hypoattenuating area covered by the AZ represents coagulative necrosis. Micrometastases undetectable by current imaging methods adjacent to the target CLM as well as residual microscopic viable tumor, within or adjacent to the AZ, can lead to recurrent tumor. Earlier work by Sofocleous and colleagues [40] assessed tissue on RFA electrodes with morphologic stains and Ki67 immunohistochemistry showing a strong association between postablation-detected Ki67-positive tumor cells and an increased risk of LTP and shorter overall survival. Snoeren and colleagues [41] similarly analyzed the viability of tissue adherent to the electrode by autofluorescence method using glucose-6-phosphate diaphorase staining. The investigators concluded that the presence of viable tumor cells adherent to the needle electrode represents an independent risk factor for LTP [40,41].

Subsequent prospective work by Sotirchos and colleagues [38] showed that biopsy confirmation of complete necrosis at the center and suspected minimal margin of the AZ was an independent predictor of LTP. Vasiniotis and colleagues [4] more recently reported results of a prospective, single-group, phase II clinical trial (NCT01494324) that combined both tissue and imaging tests performed immediately after TA, validating the predictive value of the MM and pathologic confirmation of complete treatment after TA for CLM.

The same group described the use of fluorescent tissue staining for the immediate intraprocedural assessment of ablation zone biopsy specimens. Tissue samples were evaluated with mitochondrial viability (MitoTracker Red) and nuclear (Hoechst) stains, and composite images with confocal microscopy within 30 minutes were obtained. Tissue assessment using this method demonstrated high concordance with standard morphologic and immunohistochemical assessment of tumor viability, allowing their application as a real-time biomarker of residual tumor viability and detection of tumors at risk for LTP [42,43]. This approach allows intraprocedural identification of patients at high risk for LTP and permits re-ablation in the same setting. The AZ biopsy targets are ideally planned using 3D software. Whenever feasible, at least one biopsy sample is obtained from the AZ center (where the tumor used to be) and one from the suspected MM. In cases of either incomplete coverage of the CLM with a 5-mm MM, detection of residual FDG-avid tumor and/or presence of viable tumor cells on AZ biopsies, the procedure is considered incomplete and repeat ablation is offered in the same setting, sparing the patient future additional procedures.

Follow-up imaging for local tumor control surveillance

After establishment of ablation efficacy with the first postablation imaging at 4 to 8 weeks from the procedure, continued imaging surveillance to detect subsequent LTP is mandatory. The current guidelines for disease surveillance include anatomic cross-sectional imaging with ceCT and/or ceMRI with the addition of FDG-PET/CT every 2 to 4 months for the first year, and every 3 to 6 months thereafter [2]. The first postablation imaging serves as the new baseline for further assessment of the ablation zone and prompt detection of LTP in subsequent imaging.

SUMMARY

Current medical imaging and equipment, software, and tissue examinations are available on site in the image registration suite, enabling the immediate confirmation of complete ablation and optimization of ablation outcomes. There is still, however, a lack of universal consensus on the application of all available confirmatory methods as part of the standard ablation practice.

Standardization of preablation and postablation imaging for AZ evaluation and MM calculation and localization with 3D software-based validation is underway through ongoing trials. Additional AZ histopathologic confirmation of ablation completeness is feasible and can help improve oncologic outcomes after ablation, especially when ablation is offered instead of resection as a local cure for CLM.

DISCLOSURE

There is no conflict of interest during the conduction of this review article.

REFERENCES

[1] Siegel RL, Giaquinto AN, Jemal A. Cancer statistics, 2024. CA Cancer J Clin 2024;74(1):12–49.
[2] Benson AB, Venook AP, Adam M, et al. Colon cancer, version 3.2024, NCCN clinical practice guidelines in oncology. J Natl Compr Canc Netw 2024;22(2 D). https://doi.org/10.6004/jnccn.2024.0029.
[3] van der Lei S, Puijk RS, Dijkstra M, et al. Thermal ablation versus surgical resection of small-size colorectal liver metastases (COLLISION): an international, randomised, controlled, phase 3 non-inferiority trial. Lancet Oncol 2025;26(2):187–99.
[4] Vasiniotis KN, Vakiani E, Gonen M, et al. Biopsy and margins optimize outcomes after thermal ablation of colorectal liver metastases. Cancers (Basel) 2022;14(3). https://doi.org/10.3390/cancers14030693.
[5] Lin Y-M, Paolucci I, Albuquerque MSJ, et al. Ablative margin quantification using deformable versus rigid image registration in colorectal liver metastasis thermal ablation: a retrospective single-center study. Eur Radiol 2024;34(9):5541–50.
[6] Sibinga Mulder BG, Hendriks P, Baetens TR, et al. Quantitative margin assessment of radiofrequency ablation of a solitary colorectal hepatic metastasis using MIRADA RTx on CT scans: a feasibility study. BMC Med Imaging 2019;19(1). https://doi.org/10.1186/s12880-019-0360-2.
[7] Lin Y-M, Paolucci I, O'Connor CS, et al. Ablative margins of colorectal liver metastases using deformable CT image registration and autosegmentation. Radiology 2023;307(2):e221373.
[8] Lin Y-M, Paolucci I, Albuquerque MSJ, et al. Intraprocedural versus initial follow-up minimal ablative margin assessment after colorectal liver metastasis thermal ablation: which one better predicts local outcomes? Investig Radiol 2024;59(4):314–9.
[9] Chlorogiannis D-D, Sotirchos VS, Georgiades C, et al. The importance of optimal thermal ablation margins in colorectal liver metastases: a systematic review and meta-analysis of 21 studies. Cancers (Basel) 2023;15(24). https://doi.org/10.3390/cancers15245806.
[10] Tani S, Tatli S, Hata N, et al. Three-dimensional quantitative assessment of ablation margins based on registration of pre- and post-procedural MRI and distance map. Int J Comput Assist Radiol Surg 2016;11(6):1133–42.
[11] Andreou A, Aloia TA, Brouquet A, et al. Margin status remains an important determinant of survival after surgical resection of colorectal liver metastases in the era of modern chemotherapy. Ann Surg 2013;257(6):1079–88.
[12] Shyn PB, Casadaban LC, Sainani NI, et al. Intraprocedural ablation margin assessment by using ammonia perfusion PET during FDG PET/CT-guided liver tumor ablation: a pilot study. Radiology 2018;288(1):138–45.
[13] Vasiniotis Kamarinos N, Gonen M, Sotirchos V, et al. 3D margin assessment predicts local tumor progression after ablation of colorectal cancer liver metastases. Int J Hyperth 2022;39(1):880–7.
[14] Wang X, Sofocleous CT, Erinjeri JP, et al. Margin size is an independent predictor of local tumor progression after ablation of colon cancer liver metastases. Cardiovasc Interv Radiol 2013;36(1):166–75.
[15] Laimer G, Jaschke N, Schullian P, et al. Volumetric assessment of the periablational safety margin after thermal ablation of colorectal liver metastases. Eur Radiol 2021;31(9):6489–99.
[16] Kurilova I, Bendet A, Petre EN, et al. Factors associated with local tumor control and complications after thermal ablation of colorectal cancer liver metastases: a 15-year retrospective cohort study. Clin Colorectal Cancer 2021;20(2):e82–95.

[17] Puijk RS, Ruarus AH, Vroomen LGPH, et al. Colorectal liver metastases: surgery versus thermal ablation (COLLISION) - a phase III single-blind prospective randomized controlled trial. BMC Cancer 2018;18(1):821.
[18] Shady W, Petre EN, Gonen M, et al. Percutaneous radiofrequency ablation of colorectal cancer liver metastases: factors affecting outcomes–A 10-year experience at a single center. Radiology 2016;278(2):601–11.
[19] Zirakchian ZM, Sotirchos VS, Kirov A, et al. Three-Dimensional margin as a predictor of local tumor progression after microwave ablation: intraprocedural versus 4-8-week postablation assessment. J Vasc Interv Radiol 2024;35(4):523–32.e1.
[20] Paolucci I, Albuquerque Marques Silva J, Lin Y-M, et al. Identification of A0 minimum ablative margins for colorectal liver metastases: multicentre, retrospective study using deformable CT registration and artificial intelligence-based autosegmentation. Br J Surg 2024; 111(9). https://doi.org/10.1093/bjs/znae165.
[21] Kitsel Y, Cooke T, Sotirchos V, et al. Colorectal cancer liver metastases: genomics and biomarkers with focus on local therapies. Cancers (Basel) 2023;15(6). https://doi.org/10.3390/cancers15061679.
[22] Shady W, Petre EN, Vakiani E, et al. Kras mutation is a marker of worse oncologic outcomes after percutaneous radiofrequency ablation of colorectal liver metastases. Oncotarget 2017;8(39):66117–27.
[23] Chlorogiannis D-D, Moussa AM, Zhao K, et al. Imaging considerations before and after liver-directed locoregional treatments for metastatic colorectal cancer. Diagnostics (Basel, Switzerland) 2024;14(7). https://doi.org/10.3390/diagnostics14070772.
[24] Tsili AC, Alexiou G, Naka C, et al. Imaging of colorectal cancer liver metastases using contrast-enhanced US, multidetector CT, MRI, and FDG PET/CT: a meta-analysis. Acta Radiol 2021;62(3):302–12.
[25] Gїgec B, Hansen IS, Kemmerich G, et al. MRI in addition to CT in patients scheduled for local therapy of colorectal liver metastases (CAMINO): an international, multicentre, prospective, diagnostic accuracy trial. Lancet Oncol 2024;25(1):137–46.
[26] Qiu Q-S, Zhu K, Wang J-H, et al. Diagnostic performance of contrast enhanced CT alone or in combination with (Non-)Enhanced MRI for colorectal liver metastasis. Acad Radiol 2023;30(9):1856–65.
[27] Maffione AM, Lopci E, Bluemel C, et al. Diagnostic accuracy and impact on management of (18)F-FDG PET and PET/CT in colorectal liver metastasis: a meta-analysis and systematic review. Eur J Nucl Med Mol Imaging 2015;42(1):152–63.
[28] Ryan ER, Sofocleous CT, Schїder H, et al. Split-dose technique for FDG PET/CT-guided percutaneous ablation: a method to facilitate lesion targeting and to provide immediate assessment of treatment effectiveness. Radiology 2013;268(1):288–95.
[29] Puijk RS, Nieuwenhuizen S, van den Bemd BAT, et al. Transcatheter CT hepatic arteriography compared with conventional CT fluoroscopy guidance in percutaneous thermal ablation to treat colorectal liver metastases: a single-center comparative analysis of 2 historical cohorts. J Vasc Interv Radiol 2020;31(11):1772–83.
[30] van der Lei S, Opperman J, Dijkstra M, et al. The added diagnostic value of transcatheter CT hepatic arteriography for intraprocedural detection of previously unknown colorectal liver metastases during percutaneous ablation and impact on the definitive treatment plan. Cardiovasc Interv Radiol 2023;46(9):1257–66.
[31] Zirakchian ZM, Yeh R, Kunin HS, et al. Real-time split-dose PET/CT-Guided ablation improves colorectal liver metastasis detection and ablation zone margin assessments without the need for repeated contrast injection. Cancers (Basel) 2022;14(24). https://doi.org/10.3390/cancers14246253.
[32] Ahmed M, Solbiati L, Brace CL, et al. Image-guided tumor ablation: standardization of terminology and reporting criteria–a 10-year update. Radiology 2014; 273(1):241–60.
[33] Dzaye O, Cornelis FH, Kunin HS, et al. Advancements and future outlook of PET/CT-Guided interventions. Tech Vasc Interv Radiol 2023;26(3):100916.
[34] Vandenbroucke F, Vandemeulebroucke J, Ilsen B, et al. Predictive value of pattern classification 24 hours after radiofrequency ablation of liver metastases on CT and positron emission tomography/CT. J Vasc Interv Radiol 2014;25(8):1240–9.
[35] Cornelis FH, Petre EN, Vakiani E, et al. Immediate post-ablation (18)F-FDG injection and corresponding SUV are surrogate biomarkers of local tumor progression after thermal ablation of colorectal carcinoma liver metastases. J Nucl Med 2018;59(9):1360–5.
[36] Dietrich CF, Nolsøe CP, Barr RG, et al. Guidelines and good clinical practice recommendations for contrast-enhanced ultrasound (CEUS) in the liver-update 2020 WFUMB in cooperation with EFSUMB, AFSUMB, AIUM, and FLAUS. Ultrasound Med Biol 2020;46(10): 2579–604.
[37] Anderson BM, Lin Y-M, Lin EY, et al. A novel use of biomechanical model-based deformable image registration (DIR) for assessing colorectal liver metastases ablation outcomes. Med Phys 2021;48(10):6226–36.
[38] Sotirchos VS, Petrovic LM, Gїnen M, et al. Colorectal cancer liver metastases: biopsy of the ablation zone and margins can Be used to predict oncologic outcome. Radiology 2016;280(3):949–59.
[39] Odisio BC, Albuquerque J, Lin Y-M, et al. Software-based versus visual assessment of the minimal ablative margin in patients with liver tumours undergoing percutaneous thermal ablation (COVER-ALL): a randomised phase 2 trial. Lancet Gastroenterol Hepatol 2025. https://doi.org/10.1016/S2468-1253(25)00024-X.
[40] Sofocleous CT, Garg S, Petrovic LM, et al. Ki-67 is a prognostic biomarker of survival after radiofrequency ablation of liver malignancies. Ann Surg Oncol 2012;19-(13):4262–9.

[41] Snoeren N, Huiskens J, Rijken AM, et al. Viable tumor tissue adherent to needle applicators after local ablation: a risk factor for local tumor progression. Ann Surg Oncol 2011;18(13):3702–10.
[42] Vasiniotis Kamarinos N, Vakiani E, Fujisawa S, et al. Immunofluorescence assay of ablated colorectal liver metastases: the frozen section of image-guided tumor ablation? J Vasc Interv Radiol 2022;33(3):308–15.e1.
[43] Sotirchos VS, Fujisawa S, Vakiani E, et al. Fluorescent tissue assessment of colorectal cancer liver metastases ablation zone: a potential real-time biomarker of complete tumor ablation. Ann Surg Oncol 2019;26(6):1833–40.

Advances in Clinical Radiology 7 (2025) 57–69
ADVANCES IN CLINICAL RADIOLOGY

Current Status of Pulmonary Embolism Intervention

Joshua Tublin, MD, Oussama Metrouh, MD, Julie C. Bulman, MD, RPVI, Jeffrey L. Weinstein, MD, FSIR*
Section of Interventional Radiology, Department of Radiology, Beth Israel Deaconess Medical Center-Harvard Medical School, One Deaconess Road, Rosenburg 3, Boston, MA 02215, USA

KEYWORDS
• Pulmonary embolism • PE • Thrombectomy • Thrombolysis • Catheter-directed thrombectomy
• Catheter-directed thrombolysis

KEY POINTS

- The classification systems and available treatments for pulmonary embolism are evolving.
- Determining which patients would benefit from intervention is unclear, but scoring systems are being investigated to help determine which patients may benefit based on their presentation.
- The utilization of pulmonary embolism response teams (PERT) can help make clinical decisions for individual patients through consensus because guidelines lag in this rapidly evolving space.

INTRODUCTION

Epidemiology

Pulmonary embolism (PE) is a major cause of morbidity and mortality in the United States and worldwide. In the US alone, it is estimated that around 100,000 deaths per year are due to PE, and between 5% to 10% of all inpatient deaths result from PE [1]. It is the third most common cause of cardiovascular death [2]. The overall severity, presentation, and morbidity of each patient with a PE vary. The majority of cases resolve and are uncomplicated after treatment with anticoagulation (AC), often in the outpatient setting [3,4]. Typical presenting symptoms are chest pain, cough, hemoptysis, dyspnea, and often in retrospect, up to 95% of cases are due to venous thromboembolism of the lower extremity or pelvic veins [5].

Complications and Public Health Burden

Large acute PE can lead to right ventricular (RV) dysfunction, arrhythmia and ultimately hemodynamic instability and shock. In addition to the immediate complications, "Postpulmonary embolism syndrome" is a broad-encompassing term used to describe multiple long-term complications of PE, which include chronic thromboembolic pulmonary hypertension, chronic thromboembolic disease, or PE-related dyspnea (functional limitations due to dyspnea without an identifiable vascular cause). Approximately one-third of the patients with a PE diagnosis report persistent symptoms of exercise intolerance and dyspnea [6]. Treating patients with PE is also a significant cost burden, with the average cost of treating a single impatient reported to be approximately $8763 [7].

RISK STRATIFICATIONS

Two main systems are used to stratify PE severity.

1. The American Heart Association: massive, submassive, and low-risk.
2. The European Society of Cardiology: high, intermediate–high, intermediate–low, and low–risk.

*Corresponding author. *E-mail address:* jlweinst@bidmc.harvard.edu

https://doi.org/10.1016/j.yacr.2025.05.005 www.advancesinclinicalradiology.com
2589-8701/25/

ABBREVIATIONS

AC	anticoagulation
BNP	brain natriuretic peptide
CDT	catheter-directed thrombolysis
DOACs	direct oral anticoagulants
EKOS	EkoSonic Endovascular System
FDA	Food and Drug Administration
FLARE trial	FlowTriever Pulmonary Embolectomy Clinical Study
HI-PEITHO	Higher Risk Pulmonary Embolism Thrombolysis
ICH	intracranial hemorrhage
ICU	intensive care unit
LBMT	large-bore mechanical thrombectomy
MT	mechanical thrombectomy
PE	pulmonary embolism
PERT	pulmonary embolism response team
PESI	pulmonary embolism severity index
RV	right ventricule
RV/LV	right ventricle to left ventricle
sPESI	simplified PESI
ULTIMA trial	Ultrasound-Assisted Catheter-Directed Thrombolysis for Acute Intermediate-Risk PE
USCDT	ultrasound-assisted CDT

Risk stratification for PE involves evaluating the severity of the condition and identifying patients at high-risk of mortality or complications to guide clinical management. This process includes evaluating clinical presentations, hemodynamic stability, imaging findings, and biomarkers, specifically troponin and other markers such as brain natriuretic peptide (BNP). Patients with massive PE, characterized by sustained hypotension or shock, are classified as high-risk and often require immediate treatment, either with systemic thrombolysis, catheter-directed thrombolysis (CDT), catheter-directed thrombectomy, or surgical intervention [8]. Submassive PE, associated with right ventricular dysfunction or elevated cardiac biomarkers without hypotension, represents an intermediate-risk category and may necessitate closer monitoring or catheter-directed therapies (Fig. 1) [9]. Low risk-PE patients are hemodynamically stable without evidence of right heart strain or elevated biomarkers, and can often be managed with anticoagulation alone, sometimes in an outpatient setting [10]. Tools such as the pulmonary embolism severity index (PESI) or simplified PESI (sPESI) aid in risk stratification by incorporating clinical parameters to predict mortality and adverse outcomes [11]. PESI is a scoring system based on 11 clinical variables, including demographic factors, comorbidities, and clinical signs. These variables include age, sex, comorbidities, vital signs, and clinical signs to determine where a patient falls into 5 risk categories. The sPESI was developed to simplify risk assessment and improve practicality in clinical settings [12]. It includes 6 binary variables including age, history of cancer, history of chronic cardiopulmonary disease, systolic blood pressure under 100 mm Hg, tachycardia over 110 bpm, and oxygen saturation under 90% to determine if a patient is high-risk or low-risk.

Additional stratification scoring systems have been applied in deciding when advanced therapies are indicated such as the Bova score, which uses 4 variables including heart rate greater than or equal to 110 bpm, systolic blood pressure 90 to 100 mm Hg, elevated cardiac troponin and right ventricle dysfunction on echocardiography. This scoring system stratifies patients into stages 1 through 3, with stage 3 being the highest risk [13,14]. A stage 3 Bova score has been correlated with a 42% PE-related complication rate and can be used to justify additional monitoring and interventions. Despite being normotensive, stage 3 patients have been shown to have a 6.5-fold increased risk of an adverse outcome, supporting the concept of *normotensive shock* [15].

Normotensive shock is an emerging area of investigation. While a patient with acute PE can be normotensive, they can be in a more precarious state than those with similar biomarkers that are not in normotensive shock. In the FLASH registry, normotensive shock was defined as a cardiac index less thanor equal to 2.2 L/min/m^2. In these patients with a systolic blood pressure greater than or equal to 90 mm Hg, there was a significant improvement in cardiac output after mechanical thrombectomy (MT) as opposed to those patients with similar biometric parameters but with a cardiac index over 2.2 L/min/m^2. This suggests that some patients with intermediate-risk PE features may benefit more than others from intervention [16]. Identifying PE patients in normotensive shock can guide providers in determining those that need interventions beyond systemic anticoagulation. While measuring cardiac index is an invasive means of measuring cardiac function, researchers have used this data to create a composite shock score that uses elevated troponin, elevated BNP, reduced RV function, saddle PE, concomitant deep venous thrombosis, and tachycardia

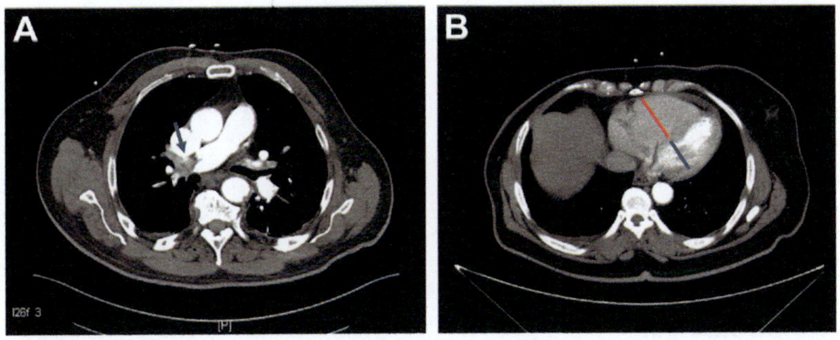

FIG. 1 CTA of the Chest with Acute PE and evidence of right heart strain. (**A**) Intravenous contrast enhanced axial CT image demonstrating thrombus in the distal right main pulmonary artery (blue arrow). (**B**) Axial CT image from a different patient showing the right ventricle (red bar) being larger than the left ventricle (blue bar), indicating elevated right heart pressure.

to determine those who are in normotensive shock [17]. The role of intervention in patients with normotensive shock will continue to evolve and is an area of ongoing investigation.

STANDARD THERAPY AND ITS LIMITATIONS

Anticoagulation, the Mainstay of Treatment

Anticoagulation is the gold standard treatment for PE, aimed at preventing clot growth and propagation, recurrence, and associated mortality. The benefits of anticoagulation include reducing the risk of recurrent venous thromboembolism by up to 90% when initiated promptly and often for an extended period of time [18]. Limitations include contraindications to anticoagulation, such as active bleeding or severe thrombocytopenia, and challenges in monitoring/dose adjustments [19,20]. Direct oral anticoagulants (DOACs) offer significant advantages, including fixed dosing and fewer monitoring requirements, but their cost and dependence on renal clearance may limit use in patients with altered kidney function without dose adjustment. While anticoagulation is highly effective for most patients with low-risk and some intermediate-risk PE, an individualized risk-benefit assessment, often performed by a multispecialty team, is critical to optimize outcomes [21].

Systemic Thrombolysis

Systemic thrombolysis has been used since the 1960s as a treatment for acute PE, particularly in high-risk cases involving hemodynamic instability. However, systemic thrombolysis carries significant risks, with major bleeding rates of 10% to 20% and intracranial hemorrhage (ICH) occurring in approximately 2% to 5% of patients [22]. These risks often outweigh benefits in intermediate-risk PE without hemodynamic compromise, limiting its routine use in such cases. Despite these risks, systemic thrombolysis has demonstrated efficacy in reducing mortality in high-risk PE, although it is less effective at preventing recurrence compared to anticoagulation alone [8]. Current guidelines advocate a tailored approach, reserving systemic thrombolysis for patients with high-risk PE or although rare, selected cases of intermediate-risk PE where a patient's clinical and hemodynamic status may decompensate imminently [10,23]. For these reasons, systemic thrombolysis is rarely used in the high-risk population, reported in only 16.1% of eligible unstable patients [24].

CATHETER-BASED THERAPIES

Catheter-based thrombolysis and thrombectomy have emerged as alternative treatments for PE, offering targeted approaches to manage high-risk and selected intermediate-risk cases [25]. Introduced in the 1990s, these techniques were developed to address the limitations of systemic thrombolysis, particularly the high-risk of major bleeding. CDT involves delivering a thrombolytic agent (e.g., alteplase) directly into the thrombus, allowing for lower drug doses and reduced systemic exposure [26]. MT, performed with devices like aspiration catheters or rotational systems, removes thrombi without relying on thrombolytics, which is advantageous in patients with contraindications to systemic anticoagulation or thrombolysis [27]. Suction-based aspiration systems provide direct emboli removal, while rotational thrombectomy devices combine clot fragmentation and extraction.

The earliest Interventional Radiology techniques for aspirating pulmonary embolism emerged in the 1970s, using rigid catheter-based systems to physically extract clots. Initial methods, such as aspiration embolectomy using rigid catheters, were often limited by incomplete clot removal, technical complexity, and significant risks [21,22].Despite these challenges, these early interventions laid the groundwork for modern catheter-based approaches.

Catheter-Directed Thrombolysis

Standard catheter-directed thrombolysis techniques

Two commonly used CDT systems are the Uni-Fuse (Angiodynamics) and Cragg-McNamara catheter (Medtronic); however, only the Uni-Fuse has Food and Drug Administration (FDA) approval for the treatment of PE. Both catheters are 4 to 5 Fr with multiple distal side holes to allow for even delivery of a thrombolytic agent to a region of thrombus. The Cragg-McNamara infusion catheter specifically allows for infusion without a guidewire in place [28]. CDT allows for a significant reduction (often >50%) in the typical bolus dose of tPA given during systemic thrombolysis, thus reducing the risk for bleeding and ICH. This decreased dose is administered slowly over several hours, and prolonged infusion times often require continuous intensive care unit (ICU) monitoring [29].

Ultrasound facilitated catheter-directed thrombolysis

In ultrasound-assisted CDT (USCDT), the device consists of an infusion catheter capable of emitting ultrasound waves. These ultrasound waves help disrupt the clot, enhancing the diffusion of the thrombolytic drug [30]. This combination of mechanical and pharmacological effects accelerates the process of clot lysis, leading to faster restoration of pulmonary perfusion. Most prospective studies on CDT have been conducted using USCDT, which has built an evidence base among interventional therapies for acute PE [31–33]. EkoSonic Endovascular System (EKOS) was the first FDA approved lysis catheter specifically for PE.

As with standard CDT, the USCDT catheter can be placed in one or both pulmonary arteries depending on the extent of the thrombus on CT angiography and real-time fluoroscopy (Fig. 2). The optimal thrombolytic dose, ultrasound delivery adjustments and treatment duration remains uncertain and may vary depending on institutional protocols and patient factors, with data from the OPTALYSE trial suggesting equivalence between regimens from 4 mg to 12 mg of tPA for RV functional improvement but a dose-dependent response in PAP and clot burden [32]. Results from the recently published prospective KNOCOUT PE registry (489 patients from 64 sites with acute intermediate–high or high-risk PE treated with USCDT) showed lower major bleeding events rates (1.6%) than previously reported [34].

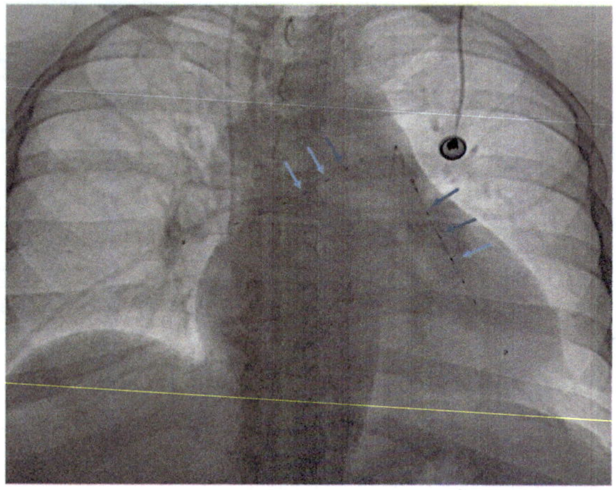

FIG. 2 Fluoroscopic image of EKOS catheters within bilateral pulmonary arteries. AP fluoroscopic image of the chest depicting bilateral EKOS lysis catheters in the right and left pulmonary arteries. Note the beaded appearance related to the ultrasound component (*arrows*).

Mechanical fragmentation with thrombolysis

The Bashir Endovascular Catheter is a device used in the treatment of intermediate–high-risk PE, designed to improve clot dissolution by combining MT with targeted thrombolysis. The catheter features an expandable, multi-segmented infusion basket that mechanically creates channels within the clot, allowing for better penetration of thrombolytic agents and restoration of blood flow [35]. This design aims to enhance the efficiency of clot breakdown while aiming to reduce the dosage of thrombolytic drugs, presumably lowering the risk of bleeding complications commonly associated with systemic thrombolysis.

Although preliminary studies have reported favorable safety and efficacy outcomes, current evidence is limited to smaller clinical trials and observational studies [36,37]. Large, randomized controlled trials are needed to establish definitive clinical guidelines, determine long-term safety and efficacy, and compare the Bashir catheter to other available catheter-directed therapies. Protocols using short infusion times and even performing the entire lysis while the patient is in the procedure (on the table lysis) is being studied in the RESCUE II study and the presently enrolling RAPID-PE trial.

Aspiration Thrombectomy

Aspiration thrombectomy devices have revolutionized the management of PE by offering rapid clot removal without the need for thrombolytics. The Indigo Aspiration System with Lightning (Penumbra), FlowTriever (Inari), AlphaVac (Angio Dynamics), and AngioVac (Angio Dynamics) are the current FDA approved devices and each have unique characteristics that influence their clinical use. Below is a comparison of these devices based on design, mechanism of action, procedural considerations, and clinical outcomes. Table 1.

The Lightning Indigo Aspiration system is a medium-bore catheter, available in 12Fr or 16Fr and provides a lower-profile venous access than other FDA approved devices. Its mechanism is grounded in computer-assisted vacuum modulation to control aspiration strength to control blood loss when the catheter is not engaged in clot [38,39]. A smaller catheter provides easier maneuverability especially around the heart to gain access into pulmonary arteries and proximal segmental branches (Fig. 3).

The FlowTriever system is a medium to large bore system with catheters ranging in size from 16Fr, 20Fr, and 24Fr. It uses manual aspiration and can be used in conjunction with an optional blood filtration system whereby the clot can be filtered from the aspirated blood and returned to the patient. It is typically used over a wire, allowing access to be maintained in the selected pulmonary vessel. This system is commonly used for large burden proximal thrombi [40,41] (Fig. 4). This device can also be used for clot-in-transit and right atrial thrombus.

AngioVac is an additional aspiration thrombectomy and bypass system used primarily for right atrial clot (Fig. 5), PE clot with associated right atrial clot-in-transit, and central venous clot. The system is composed of a 22 Fr suction catheter, and a 16Fr–20Fr outflow cannula (inserted at the internal jugular or contralateral femoral vein) to limit blood loss [42]. Ultimately, the system is advantageous for large clots, but there are practical considerations including the need for anesthesia, a perfusionist, and possibly additional imaging including trans-esophageal ultrasound [43].

AlphaVac, is another MT device that utilizes manual aspiration. Recently the Alpha Vac F18 (18 Fr Cannula) received FDA clearance for the treatment of acute PE in April of 2024 [42]. Clinical efficacy and safety were demonstrated in the APEX-AV trial for the treatment of intermediate–high-risk PE with significant improvement in RV function as a clinical endpoint [44].The choice of aspiration thrombectomy device for pulmonary embolism should be based on patient-specific factors, operator comfort/experience, clot burden, hemodynamic status, and procedural risk tolerance.

CLINICAL TRIALS SHAPING THE FIELD

ULTIMA trial (Published in 2014)

The ULTIMA trial (Ultrasound-Assisted Catheter-Directed Thrombolysis for Acute Intermediate-Risk PE), published in 2014, represented a pivotal moment in the evolution of PE management. This randomized controlled trial assessed the efficacy of USCDT with low-dose alteplase in comparison to anticoagulation alone in patients with intermediate-risk PE. The trial demonstrated that USCDT significantly reduced the right ventricle to left ventricle (RV/LV) diameter ratio within 24 hours, without increasing the risk of major bleeding [31]. These findings provided evidence supporting the safety and efficacy of targeted thrombolysis, particularly in patients at risk of clinical deterioration but who may not qualify for systemic thrombolysis due to bleeding concerns. The ULTIMA trial catalyzed a shift in PE management by reinforcing the role of catheter-directed therapies in intermediate-risk PE, driving the adoption of minimally invasive interventions tailored to patient-specific risk profiles. It also served as a cornerstone for subsequent trials evaluating catheter-based interventions, contributing to the integration of these techniques into contemporary treatment algorithms for PE [9,10,25].

SEATTLE II Trial (Published in 2015)

Bringing additional evidence after the ULTIMA trial, the SEATTLE II trial was a prospective, single-arm, multicenter study that evaluated the safety and efficacy of USCDT using the EKOS (Bothell, Washington) for patients with acute high and intermediate–high-risk PE. The trial demonstrated significant reductions in the RV/LV ratio on CT, pulmonary artery systolic pressure, and thrombus burden within 48 hours, with no reported cases of ICH. Major bleeding events occurred in 10% of patients, primarily related to vascular access [33]. SEATTLE II was a pivotal study that reinforced USCDT use as a safer alternative to systemic thrombolysis, particularly for patients at risk of bleeding complications. It contributed to the growing body of evidence for catheter-directed therapies in PE management, paving the way for additional trials and the FDA approval of the device for PE treatment.

TABLE 1
List of mechanical aspiration thrombectomy devices and some distingushing features

Device	Mechanism of action	Advantages	Things to consider	Ideal use cases
Indigo Aspiration System with Lightning (Penumbra)	Computer-assisted vacuum aspiration through a flexible catheter.	Medium-bore for a lower profile access (12Fr, 16Fr); different distal catheter shapes.	May require multiple passes; aspirated blood cannot be returned	Fresh, acute clot. Multiple segmental PE, preference for a medium-bore catheter.
FlowTriever System (Inari Medical)	MT using aspiration.	Medium and large bore (16Fr, 20Fr, and 24Fr), curved and straight catheters; blood return system available. Used over a wire.	Larger catheter sizes limit use in smaller vessels.	High central clot burden
AlphaVac System (Angio-Dynamics)	Hybrid mechanical aspiration with an expandable funnel-shaped tip for clot capture.	Large bore (18Fr and 22Fr); different distal angles; controlled volume of aspiration.	Larger catheter size limits use in smaller vessels	High central clot burden
AngioVac System (Angio-Dynamics)	Extracorporeal circulation with continuous filtration of thrombi.	Continuous circulation; large bore without concern for aspiration blood loss.	Requires large bore access; need for perfusionist	Right heart thrombi, large proximal clots.

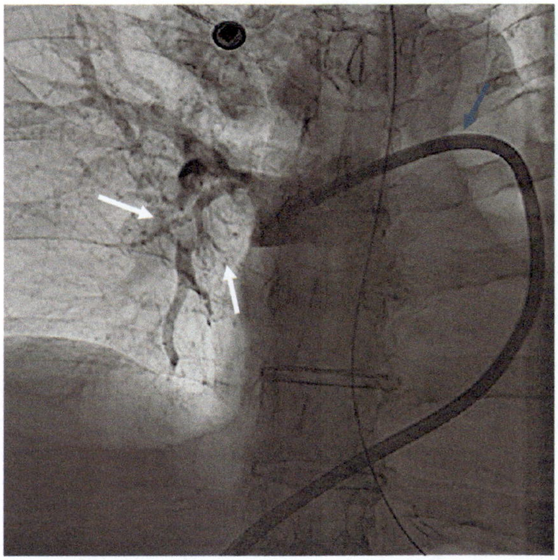

FIG. 3 Right pulmonary angiogram through 16Fr Penumbra Lightning Flash catheter (*blue arrow*) showing filling defect in the distal right main pulmonary artery (*white arrows*) with decreased perfusion to the right lower lobe.

FLARE trial (Published in 2019)

FLARE (FlowTriever Pulmonary Embolectomy Clinical Study) trial evaluated the safety and efficacy of the FlowTriever System for the treatment of acute intermediate-risk and high-risk PE. This prospective, single-arm, multicenter study demonstrated significant improvements in RV/LV diameter ratio, with a mean reduction of 25% at 48 hours compared to baseline [27]. The absence of systemic thrombolytics minimized bleeding risks, with no device-related deaths and a low rate of major complications reported. These findings supported the use of percutaneous MT as a standalone therapy, particularly for patients contraindicated for thrombolysis or at heightened risk of bleeding. The FLARE trial significantly influenced PE management by providing robust evidence for catheter-based MT as a viable and safe alternative to systemic therapies, expanding treatment options for patients with intermediate-risk and high-risk PE [9,10].

EXTRACT PE (Published in 2021)

The EXTRACT-PE study evaluated the Safety and Efficacy of the Indigo CAT8 mechanical aspiration thrombectomy system for the treatment of acute PE. This prospective, single-arm, multicenter trial demonstrated a significant reduction in the RV/LV diameter ratio by an average of 27% at 48 hours. Pulmonary artery pressure reduced by 7.9%, and there was a reduction in the mean CT obstruction index of 11.3% ($P<.0001$ for both). No patients required CDT within 48 hours after the procedure, and the rate of major bleeding events was 1.7%. The study also reported a high procedural success rate with minimal blood loss, no device-related deaths, and a low rate of major adverse events, emphasizing the safety profile of the system [39].

The EXTRACT-PE study reinforced the growing role of MT as a potential frontline treatment for intermediate-risk PE, particularly for patients contraindicated for thrombolysis. It further validated the efficacy of

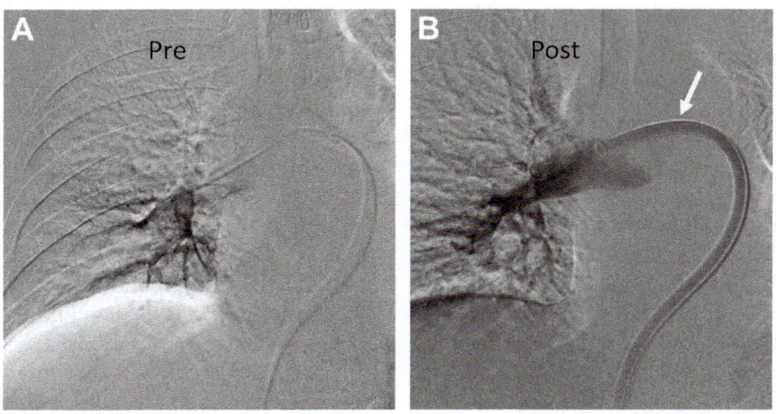

FIG. 4 Images depicting aspiration thrombectomy using the Inari FlowTriever device. (**A**) Preaspiration pulmonary angiogram of right lower lobe pulmonary artery demonstrating filling defect. (**B**) Postaspiration pulmonary angiogram demonstrating significantly increased flow to the lower lobe with 24Fr Inari device in the right pulmonary artery (*white arrow*).

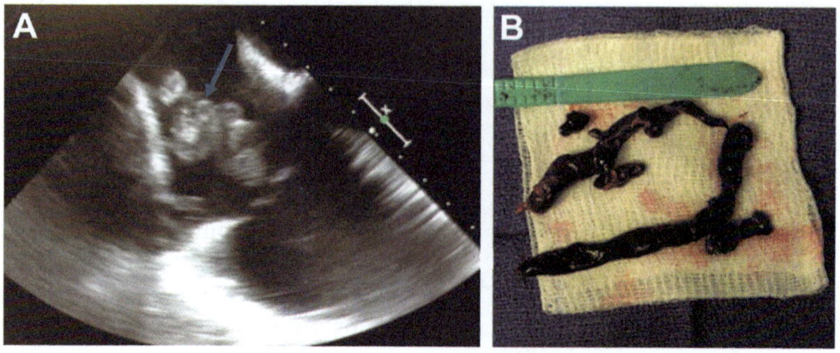

FIG. 5 (**A**) Echocardiography image depicting echogenic thrombus in the right atrium (*arrow*), representing clot in transit. (**B**) Tubular thrombus post aspiration using the AngioVac device.

aspiration thrombectomy in rapidly restoring pulmonary perfusion and paved the way for broader adoption of catheter-based strategies in multidisciplinary approaches to PE management.

RESCUE study (Published in 2022)

It was a multicenter prospective study that assessed the safety and efficacy of pharmaco-mechanical CDT (using the Bashir catheter) in acute intermediate–high-risk PE [36]. Significant RV reduction was seen at 48 hours post procedure. With an average procedure time of 15 minutes and 4 serious adverse events (total of 109 patients), the Bashir catheter was shown to be a quick, effective and safe option for the treatment of intermediate–high-risk PE, providing clinicians with another effective tool for the treatment of acute PE. A subsequent RESCUE II study used the Bashir catheter to administer 4 mg of tPA to each lung during an on-the-table protocol with no infusion afterward. This small sample study demonstrated the feasibility of using the device for intraprocedural-only lysis that is being further evaluated in a new RESCUE-PE trial that aims to enroll 500 patients across 50 centers.

The FLASH registry (Published in 2023)

This multicenter, prospective registry evaluated the safety and efficacy of the FlowTriever system in acute PE treatment and further validated MT as a standalone treatment [45]. The registry included 800 patients and results showed significant reductions in RV strain and pulmonary artery pressure, coupled with a low rate of adverse events, highlighting the system's safety and efficacy without thrombolytic use for the treatment of intermediate and high-risk PE.

STRIKE PE study (Published in 2024)

Similarly, recent interval analysis of the STRIKE PE study; aimed at determining the efficacy and safety using computer-assisted vacuum thrombectomy—Indigo Aspiration system (Penumbra), show significant reduction in PA pressure, RV/LV ratio, and low number of major adverse events (2.7%) of those 109 total patients treated. The majority of PE's within this study fall into the intermediate–high-risk category (~95%). The study also has measured quality of life outcomes, with promising result; significant improvement in Borg dyspnea scale at 90 days [46].

PEERLESS trial (Published in 2024)

This recently published trial evaluated the safety and efficacy of large-bore mechanical thrombectomy (LBMT) compared to CDT for the treatment of acute intermediate-risk PE [47]. The primary endpoint of this prospective, multicenter, randomized controlled trial was a hierarchical win ratio that assessed the following clinical outcomes: (1) all-cause mortality, (2) ICH, (3) major bleeding, (4) clinical deterioration and/or escalation to bailout therapy, and (5) postprocedural ICU admission and length of stay, evaluated at the sooner discharge or 7 days postprocedure. Overall, out of 550 patients, the primary endpoint occurred significantly less frequently with LBMT compared to CDT. LBMT was associated with lower rates of clinical deterioration and/or escalation to bailout therapy (1.8% vs 5.4%; $P = .04$) and significantly less postprocedural ICU utilization (41.6% vs 98.6%; $P < .001$). Importantly, there were no significant differences in mortality or major bleeding between the 2 strategies, supporting LBMT as a safe and effective alternative to CDT, particularly for patients at higher risk of bleeding or contraindicated for thrombolysis.

Importantly, and a major takeaway, PEERLESS trial highlights the potential of LBMT to improve acute outcomes while minimizing resource utilization, specifically ICU length of stay (often required during prolonged catheter thrombolysis infusion). One major limitation is that lysis patients at many centers, by default, are monitored in the ICU, which was a significant factor in the *win* for LBMT. It is also unclear what constituted deterioration and bailout in the lysis cohort and that a given center may have a preference and expertise in one treatment strategy over the other.

REAL-PE Registry (Published in 2024)

The REAL-PE registry was a real-world big data analysis project that compared the safety and efficacy of USCDT and MT for treating acute PE. Using an electronic health record platform, the study analyzed data from over 83 million patients across 16 U.S. health systems, identifying 2259 patients treated with USCDT (EKOS) or MT (FlowTriever). The primary analysis revealed that MT was associated with significantly higher rates of major bleeding, including hemoglobin reduction (>2 g/dL and >5 g/dL) and transfusion requirements, compared to USCDT. Intracranial hemorrhage was also more common in MT-treated patients. However, in-hospital mortality, length of stay, and 30-day readmission rates were similar between the 2 groups [48]. The REAL-PE registry suggests that EKOS may be a safer option than FlowTriever in real-world settings, particularly due to its lower bleeding risk.

However, with the recent publication of the PEERLESS trial results supporting MT over CDT for PE treatment, some ambiguity may arise regarding the optimal treatment strategy. As companies seek to demonstrate the superiority of their devices, and trials vary in design with different inclusion and exclusion criteria, it is crucial for physicians to thoroughly understand all relevant studies and their limitations and potential for bias. For this reason, a popular method for making treatment decisions is utilizing a pulmonary embolism response team (PERT) framework, ensuring individualized patient discussions without bias toward any specific device or treatment strategy.

APEX-AV study (Published in 2024)

The APEX AV study was an additional prospective single arm study that evaluated the outcomes, safety, and efficacy of the AlphaVac aspiration system for treatment of patients with acute intermediate–high-risk PE [44]. With 122 total patients treated across 25 states, there was significant reduction in RV/LV ration and overall clot burden 48 hours post procedure. No deaths were reported with a total of 5 major adverse events (all bleeding related).

As described, numerous preliminary efficacy/safety studies have shown promising data and likely have influenced the widespread use and adoption of aspiration thrombectomy within the space of interventional radiology.

Upcoming trials

PE-TRACT trial (National Institutes of Health funded, enrolling). PE-TRACT [49] is an ongoing trial that is a response, and necessary critical pause, to the fast advancement of catheter-directed treatment with only industry-sponsored single arm studies evaluating primary efficacy and safety. PE-TRACT sets itself apart as an independent, investigator-initiated trial to investigate outcomes of different catheter-therapies. The intervention group will be catheter-directed therapies (eg, CDT and MT) and AC compared to a control group of AC. Primary outcomes will be peak oxygen consumption at 3 months, New York Heart Association (NYHA) classification at 12 months, Major Adverse Event (MAE) at 7 days.

STORM PE trial (industry funded, enrolling). In a similar take, the ongoing STORM PE trial [50] aims to evaluate the safety and efficacy of Computer Assisted Vacuum Thrombectomy (using the Indigo Aspiration System from Penumbra) plus anticoagulation versus anticoagulation alone in patients with acute intermediate–high-risk PE. The primary outcomes will focus on change in the RV/LV ratio assessed by CT at 48 hours, major adverse events within 7 days, and quality of life and functional outcomes at 90 days.

HI-PEITHO study (industry funded, enrolling). The Higher Risk Pulmonary Embolism Thrombolysis (HI-PEITHO) study is an ongoing multinational, multicenter randomized controlled trial to evaluate short and long term clinical outcomes of intermediate–high-risk PE treated with either ultrasound facilitated CDT plus anticoagulation or anticoagulation alone [51]. The HI-PEITHO trial is distinct from previously published USCDT trials in its specific focus on intermediate–high-risk PE patients and its primary clinical composite outcome that includes (1) Pulmonary PE-related mortality, (2) cardiorespiratory decompensation or collapse, or (3) nonfatal symptomatic and objectively confirmed recurrence of PE. The study will contribute further evidence to the existing data on the long term clinical outcomes of acute PE patients in the intermediate–high-risk category.

PEITHO-3 (assistance publique—hôpitaux de Paris funded, enrolling). This randomized, placebo-controlled, double-blind, multicenter, multinational trial aims to evaluate the efficacy and safety of a reduced-dose thrombolytic therapy combined with low-molecular-weight heparin in patients with intermediate–high-risk PE. Patients are randomized to receive alteplase (0.6 mg/kg, max 50 mg) or placebo within the first 6 hours of diagnosis. The primary objective is to assess the efficacy of reduced-dose thrombolysis in preventing adverse outcomes at 30 days, while secondary objectives include evaluation of safety, net clinical benefit, and long-term clinical outcomes at 6 months and 2 years [52]. The study also examines the impact on health care resource utilization at 30 and 180 days. In summary, the PEITHO 3 trial aims to investigate whether a reduced thrombolytic dose therapy can balance efficacy and bleeding risks for intermediate–high-risk PE patients.

Ongoing investigational device approval studies (industry funded, enrolling). New technologies have emerged in the management of PE, and multiple trials are currently underway to validate these devices and seek FDA approval, including Symphony-PE, ENGULF, AVENTUS, QUADRA-PE, TRUST, SPIRARE II, and others. As evidence from these studies continues to evolve, it is essential for clinicians to stay informed and prepared to integrate these emerging therapies into practice. Understanding the strengths and limitations of each device, along with engaging in multispecialty, patient-centered discussions, will be critical in determining the most effective therapeutic approach to achieve the best outcomes.

PULMONARY EMBOLISM RESPONSE TEAM AND ITS IMPORTANCE

PERT is an interdisciplinary team composed of specialists from various clinical fields, dedicated to improving care and outcomes for patients with acute PE, particularly those in the intermediate–high and high-risk categories. Specialties involved include, but are not limited to, pulmonary and critical care medicine, cardiology, vascular medicine, vascular surgery, hematology, diagnostic radiology, interventional radiology, emergency medicine, cardiac surgery, and pharmacy.

The cornerstone of the PERT model is based on team activation via a single contact number (or pager) notification system and, if available, the utilization of a virtual web-based conference program that enables all clinicians to review data, discuss cases and potential treatment options in real time. The primary goal is to reach consensus on the optimal, individualized care plan for each complex PE case.

PERT allows efficient decision-making and facilitates treatment protocol implementation [53]. The exact composition and operating mode of PERT are not fixed and vary between different institutions depending on the available expertise and resources. Multiple studies have shown that the institution of a PERT can reduce adverse events and mortality in PE patients [54,55]. Nevertheless, challenges exist, and despite this complex physician work, there is a gap in coding accurately for these conferences, leading to inadequate or absent reimbursement for multidisciplinary PERT consultations [56]. Additionally, with many different physicians involved in the care team, it is still unclear who will be accountable for any medico-legal responsibility, and multiple physicians can be subject to litigation [57].

Although current guidelines recommend the implementation of a PERT for acute PE management, these recommendations are based on a low level of evidence [10]. More rigorous multi-center and prospective studies are needed to evaluate PERT outcomes on patients and cost-effectiveness within the health care system.

Part of the reliance, implementation, and widespread use of PERTs when evaluating patients presenting with intermediate–high and high-risk PE is in some part due to the *gray* areas. There are many therapy options in the PE population (e.g. anticoagulation, systemic thrombolysis, CDT, MT, surgery), each with their own benefits, risks, efficiency, and practicality, but a clear treatment algorithm with data to support long term benefits has not been implemented.

STATE OF THE EVIDENCE AND FUTURE DIRECTIONS

Significant advancements in catheter-directed therapies have transformed the management of acute PE, with multiple trials demonstrating their safety and efficacy in restoring pulmonary perfusion and improving hemodynamics in intermediate to high-risk PE patients. However, many devices used are cleared through the FDA's 510(k) process, which allows for approval based on their equivalence to existing devices rather than rigorous long-term efficacy studies. This raises questions about their sustained benefits compared to anticoagulation alone, particularly regarding long-term outcomes such as chronic thromboembolic pulmonary hypertension, quality of life, and mortality. Ongoing trials like PE-TRACT aim to address some of the gaps by evaluating medium-term and long-term outcomes of these treatment modalities. Additionally, the lack of standardized endpoints for assessing procedural success complicates efforts to measure the true effectiveness of these therapies.

Another challenge lies in the heterogeneity of patient presentations, imaging findings, and risk stratification systems, coupled with the wide range of treatment modalities and devices. This variability, along with a scarcity of comparative data supporting each therapeutic option, creates a complex decision-making landscape.

Finally, the economic implications of catheter-directed therapies remain underexplored. While these therapies have the potential to reduce hospital stays and lower health care costs by avoiding prolonged hospitalization, their high upfront costs and variability in reimbursement policies pose barriers to widespread adoption. Results from a multicenter cost analysis study that compared the costs associated with CDT over MT did not reveal a clear cost advantage of one treatment over the other for intermediate-risk PE. The observed nonsignificant cost differences were influenced by variations in practice patterns across the study period among the participating institutions [58]. More cost-effectiveness research should be focused on strategies to reduce length of stay, improve efficiency and minimize the overall cost related to acute PE management.

In summary, identifying which patients would benefit from intervention for PE, what tools and clinical parameters that can identify these patients, and what treatment strategy or strategies would be the most efficacious, both immediately and long term, remains elusive. Presently, PERT teams play a vital role in developing individualized and local treatment algorithms as evidence and the number of treatment options continues to evolve.

DISCLOSURE

None of the authors have any relevant financial disclosures.

REFERENCES

[1] Zghouzi M, Mwansa H, Shore S, et al. Sex, racial, and geographic disparities in pulmonary embolism–related mortality nationwide. Annals ATS 2023;20(11):1571–7.

[2] Goldhaber SZ, Bounameaux H. Pulmonary embolism and deep vein thrombosis. Lancet 2012;379(9828):1835–46.

[3] Erkens PMG, Gandara E, Wells P, et al. Safety of outpatient treatment in acute pulmonary embolism. J Thromb Haemostasis 2010;8(11):2412–7.

[4] Rivera-Lebron B, McDaniel M, Ahrar K, et al. Diagnosis, treatment and follow up of acute pulmonary embolism: consensus practice from the PERT consortium. Clin Appl Thromb Hemost 2019;25:1076029619853037. https://doi.org/10.1177/1076029619853037.

[5] Ishaaya E, Tapson VF. Advances in the diagnosis of acute pulmonary embolism. F1000Res 2020;9:44.

[6] Pugliese SC, Kawut SM. The post–pulmonary embolism Syndrome: real or ruse? Annals ATS 2019;16(7):811–4.

[7] Fanikos J, Rao A, Seger AC, et al. Hospital costs of acute pulmonary embolism. Am J Med 2013;126(2):127–32.

[8] Jaff MR, McMurtry MS, Archer SL, et al. Management of massive and submassive pulmonary embolism, iliofemoral deep vein thrombosis, and chronic thromboembolic pulmonary hypertension: a scientific statement from the American heart association. Circulation 2011; 123(16):1788–830.

[9] Giri J, Sista AK, Weinberg I, et al. Interventional therapies for acute pulmonary embolism. Circulation 2019;140(20). https://doi.org/10.1161/CIR.0000000000000707.

[10] Konstantinides SV, Meyer G, Becattini C, et al. 2019 ESC Guidelines for the diagnosis and management of acute pulmonary embolism developed in collaboration with the European Respiratory Society (ERS). Eur Heart J 2020;41(4):543–603.

[11] Leidi A, Bex S, Righini M, et al. Risk stratification in patients with acute pulmonary embolism: current evidence and perspectives. JCM 2022;11(9):2533.

[12] Aujesky D, Obrosky DS, Stone RA, et al. Derivation and validation of a prognostic model for pulmonary embolism. Am J Respir Crit Care Med 2005;172(8):1041–6.

[13] Fernández C, Bova C, Sanchez O, et al. Validation of a model for identification of patients at intermediate to high risk for complications associated with acute symptomatic pulmonary embolism. Chest 2015;148(1):211–8.

[14] Bova C, Vanni S, Prandoni P, et al. A prospective validation of the Bova score in normotensive patients with acute pulmonary embolism. Thromb Res 2018;165:107–11.

[15] Chen X, Shao X, Zhang Y, et al. Assessment of the Bova score for risk stratification of acute normotensive pulmonary embolism: a systematic review and meta-analysis. Thromb Res 2020;193:99–106.

[16] Bangalore S, Horowitz JM, Beam D, et al. Prevalence and predictors of cardiogenic shock in intermediate-risk pulmonary embolism. JACC Cardiovasc Interv 2023;16(8):958–72.

[17] Zhang RS, Yuriditsky E, Zhang P, et al. Impact of time to catheter-based therapy on outcomes in acute pulmonary embolism. Circ: Cardiovascular Interventions 2025; 18(1). https://doi.org/10.1161/CIRCINTERVENTIONS.124.014499.

[18] Chopard R, Albertsen IE, Ecarnot F, et al. Extended anticoagulation after pulmonary embolism: a multicenter observational cohort analysis. JAHA 2022;11(13):e024425.

[19] Stevens SM, Woller SC, Kreuziger LB, et al. Antithrombotic therapy for VTE disease. Chest 2021;160(6):e545–608.

[20] Schulman S, Kearon C, Subcommittee on Control of Anticoagulation of the Scientific and Standardization Committee of the International Society on Thrombosis and Haemostasis. Definition of major bleeding in clinical investigations of antihemostatic medicinal products in non-surgical patients. J Thromb Haemostasis 2005; 3(4):692–4.
[21] Becattini C, Agnelli G. Risk stratification and management of acute pulmonary embolism. Hematology 2016; 2016(1):404–12.
[22] Daley MJ, Murthy MS, Peterson EJ. Bleeding risk with systemic thrombolytic therapy for pulmonary embolism: scope of the problem. Ther Adv Drug Saf 2015; 6(2):57–66.
[23] Marti C, John G, Konstantinides S, et al. Systemic thrombolytic therapy for acute pulmonary embolism: a systematic review and meta-analysis. Eur Heart J 2015;36(10): 605–14.
[24] Stein PD, Matta F, Hughes PG, et al. Nineteen-year trends in mortality of patients hospitalized in the United States with high-risk pulmonary embolism. Am J Med 2021; 134(10):1260–4.
[25] Kuo WT, Sista AK, Faintuch S, et al. Society of interventional radiology position statement on catheter-directed therapy for acute pulmonary embolism. J Vasc Intervent Radiol 2018;29(3):293–7.
[26] Tapson V, Jimenez D. Catheter-based approaches for the treatment of acute pulmonary embolism. Semin Respir Crit Care Med 2017;38(01):073–83.
[27] Tu T, Toma C, Tapson VF, et al. A prospective, single-arm, multicenter trial of catheter-directed mechanical thrombectomy for intermediate-risk acute pulmonary embolism. JACC Cardiovasc Interv 2019;12(9):859–69.
[28] Cragg-McNamara™ valved infusion catheter. Available at: https://www.medtronic.com/en-us/healthcare-professionals/products/cardiovascular/infusion-therapy/cragg-mcnamara-valved-infusion-catheter.html. Accessed January 27, 2025.
[29] Furfaro D, Stephens RS, Streiff MB, et al. Catheter-directed thrombolysis for intermediate-risk pulmonary embolism. Annals ATS 2018;15(2):134–44.
[30] Braaten JV, Goss RA, Francis CW. Ultrasound reversibly disaggregates fibrin fibers. Thromb Haemost 1997; 78(3):1063–8.
[31] Kucher N, Boekstegers P, Müller OJ, et al. Randomized, controlled trial of ultrasound-assisted catheter-directed thrombolysis for acute intermediate-risk pulmonary embolism. Circulation 2014;129(4):479–86.
[32] Tapson VF, Sterling K, Jones N, et al. A randomized trial of the optimum duration of acoustic pulse thrombolysis procedure in acute intermediate-risk pulmonary embolism. JACC Cardiovasc Interv 2018;11(14):1401–10.
[33] Piazza G, Hohlfelder B, Jaff MR, et al. A prospective, single-arm, multicenter trial of ultrasound-facilitated, catheter-directed, low-dose fibrinolysis for acute massive and submassive pulmonary embolism. JACC Cardiovasc Interv 2015;8(10):1382–92.
[34] Sterling KM, Goldhaber SZ, Sharp ASP, et al. Prospective multicenter international registry of ultrasound-facilitated catheter-directed thrombolysis in intermediate-high and high-risk pulmonary embolism (KNOCOUT PE). Circ: Cardiovascular Interventions 2024;17(3). https://doi.org/10.1161/CIRCINTERVENTIONS.123.013448.
[35] BASHIR™ Endovascular Catheter. Thrombolex. Available at: https://thrombolex.com/bashir-endovascular-catheter/. Accessed January 27, 2025.
[36] Bashir R, Foster M, Iskander A, et al. Pharmacomechanical catheter-directed thrombolysis with the Bashir endovascular catheter for acute pulmonary embolism. JACC Cardiovasc Interv 2022;15(23):2427–36.
[37] First-in-Human study to assess the safety and feasibility of the Bashir endovascular catheter for the treatment of acute intermediate-risk pulmonary embolism. Circ Cardiovasc Interv 2021. https://doi.org/10.1161/CIRCINTERVENTIONS.120.009611.
[38] Lightning Indigo system | peripheral thrombectomy | Penumbra. Penumbra, inc. Available at: https://www.penumbrainc.com/products/peripheral-thrombectomy-cavt/. Accessed January 27, 2025.
[39] Sista AK, Horowitz JM, Tapson VF, et al. Indigo aspiration system for treatment of pulmonary embolism. JACC Cardiovasc Interv 2021;14(3):319–29.
[40] FlowTriever® system for the treatment of pulmonary embolism (PE) - Inari medical - patients first. Always. Available at: https://www.inarimedical.com/flowtriever-system. Accessed January 27, 2025.
[41] Mojibian HR, Chow E, Pollak J. FlowTriever system for mechanical thromboembolectomy. Future Cardiol 2021; 17(4):585–92.
[42] The AlphaVac System. Angiodynamics. Available at: https://www.angiodynamics.com/product/alphavac/. Accessed January 27, 2025.
[43] Moriarty JM, Rueda V, Liao M, et al. Endovascular removal of thrombus and right heart masses using the AngioVac system: results of 234 patients from the prospective, multicenter registry of AngioVac procedures in detail (RAPID). J Vasc Intervent Radiol 2021;32(4): 549–57.e3.
[44] Ranade M, Foster MT, Brady PS, et al. Novel mechanical aspiration thrombectomy in patients with acute pulmonary embolism: results from the prospective APEX-AV trial. J Soc Cardiovasc Angiogr Interv 2024;102463. https://doi.org/10.1016/j.jscai.2024.102463.
[45] Toma C, Jaber W, Weinberg M, et al. Acute outcomes for the full US cohort of the FLASH mechanical thrombectomy registry in pulmonary embolism. EuroIntervention 2023. https://doi.org/10.4244/EIJ-D-22-00732.
[46] Moriarty JM, Dohad SY, Schiro BJ, et al. Clinical, functional, and quality-of-life outcomes after computer assisted vacuum thrombectomy for pulmonary embolism: interim analysis of the STRIKE-PE study. J Vasc Intervent Radiol 2024;35(8):1154–65.e6.
[47] Jaber WA, Gonsalves CF, Stortecky S, et al. Large-bore mechanical thrombectomy versus catheter-directed

thrombolysis in the management of intermediate-risk pulmonary embolism: primary results of the PEERLESS randomized controlled trial. Circulation 2025;151(5). https://doi.org/10.1161/CIRCULATIONAHA.124.072364.
[48] Monteleone P, Ahern R, Banerjee S, et al. Modern treatment of pulmonary embolism (USCDT vs MT): results from a real-world, big data analysis (REAL-PE). J Soc Cardiovasc Angiogr Interv 2024;3(1):101192.
[49] RePORT RePORTER. Available at: https://reporter.nih.gov/search/I05Wh0xOe0agNBNSR5guhg/project-details/9748145#description. Accessed January 27, 2025.
[50] STORM-PE TRIAL. Penumbra inc. Penumbra, Inc. 2023. Available at: https://www.penumbrainc.com/storm-pe-trial/. Accessed January 27, 2025.
[51] Klok FA, Piazza G, Sharp ASP, et al. Ultrasound-facilitated, catheter-directed thrombolysis vs anticoagulation alone for acute intermediate-high-risk pulmonary embolism: rationale and design of the HI-PEITHO study. Am Heart J 2022;251:43–53.
[52] Assistance Publique - Hôpitaux de Paris. A reduced dose of thrombolytic treatment for patients with intermediate high-risk acute pulmonary embolism: a randomized controled trial. clinicaltrials.gov. 2024. Available at: https://clinicaltrials.gov/study/NCT04430569. Accessed February 20, 2025.
[53] Dudzinski DM, Piazza G. Multidisciplinary pulmonary embolism response teams. Circulation 2016;133(1):98–103.
[54] Porres–Aguilar M, Anaya-Ayala JE, Heresi GA, et al. Pulmonary embolism response teams: a novel approach for the care of complex patients with pulmonary embolism. Clin Appl Thromb Hemost 2018;24(9_suppl):48S–55S.
[55] Wright C, Goldenberg I, Schleede S, et al. Effect of a multidisciplinary pulmonary embolism response team on patient mortality. Am J Cardiol 2021;161:102–7.
[56] Porres-Aguilar M, Jiménez D, Porres-Muñoz M, et al. Pulmonary embolism response teams: purpose, evidence for efficacy, and future research directions. Res Pract Thromb Haemost 2019;3(4):769.
[57] Monteleone PP, Rosenfield K, Rosovsky RP. Multidisciplinary pulmonary embolism response teams and systems. Cardiovasc Diagn Ther 2016;6(6):662–7.
[58] Tran A, Toma C, Jaber W, et al. Cost-comparison of mechanical thrombectomy and catheter-directed thrombolysis in intermediate-risk pulmonary embolism. J Soc Cardiovasc Angiogr Interv 2024;3(2):101187.

Advances in Clinical Radiology 7 (2025) 71–81
ADVANCES IN CLINICAL RADIOLOGY

Rapid MRI for Acute Pediatric Emergencies

Increasing Efficiency with Noninvasive Imaging

Jillian Krauss, MD, Jonathan D. Samet, MD*
Department of Medical Imaging, Northwestern University Feinberg School of Medicine, Ann and Robert H. Lurie Children's Hospital of Chicago, 225 East Chicago Avenue, Chicago, IL 60611, USA

KEYWORDS
• Fast or rapid or accelerated MRI • Noncontrast • Pediatric MRI • Pediatric emergencies

KEY POINTS
- Advancements in MRI technology have allowed for better accessibility of MRI for pediatric patients secondary to decreased scan times and improvement in motion sensitivity.
- Rapid, noncontrast, nonsedated MRI techniques have been successfully employed to various degrees in pediatric body, brain, and musculoskeletal imaging in the emergency setting.
- Rapid MRI protocols often replace the need for CT, especially for acute brain pathologies, which decreases radiation exposure, particularly in patients who may require frequent imaging.
- Diffusion-weighted sequences can act as a "substitute" for contrast administration and can be incredibly helpful in abscess detection.

INTRODUCTION

Pediatric patients present to the emergency department (ED) for a variety of different reasons, ranging from abdominal pain to headache, and the clinical picture can often be confusing. Overall, there has been a trend toward increased use of imaging by ED physicians and midlevel providers in evaluating and diagnosing these patients [1]. Although traditionally imaging mostly consisted of radiographs, ultrasound (US), and when appropriate, computed tomography (CT) to help determine a patient's diagnosis, over the years, there has been increased utilization of MRI. Increased awareness on the part of health care providers and by patients/families regarding the potential carcinogenic risks of ionizing radiation has largely driven this trend [1,2].

Traditionally the performance of MRI in pediatric patients had been relatively prohibitive in the emergent setting, in part, due to the lengthy scan times often necessitating the use of anesthesia or sedation, and the potential need for intravenous contrast. Over the years, MRI has become more accessible and emerged as an alternative cross-sectional imaging modality to evaluate pediatric patients in the ED attributable to several factors including reduced scan times, decreased motion sensitivity, and improved spatial resolution [1,3,4]. Additionally, the development and optimization of rapid, noncontrast, nonsedated MRI techniques and protocols has been a focus of recent pediatric MRI research, allowing for these examinations to accurately diagnose many commonly encountered emergent pediatric pathologies.

*Corresponding author. *E-mail address:* jsamet@luriechildrens.org

https://doi.org/10.1016/j.yacr.2025.05.006 www.advancesinclinicalradiology.com
2589-8701/25/

ABBREVIATIONS

CT	computed tomography
DWI	diffusion-weighted imaging
ED	emergency department
FOV	field of view
MRA	MR angiography
pASL	pulsed arterial spin labeling
SSFSE	single shot fast spin echo
SWI	susceptibility weighted imaging
US	ultrasound

DISCUSSION

Abdominopelvic Pathology

Appendicitis

US has conventionally been the first-line imaging choice in the emergency setting to assess for various causes of abdominal/pelvic pain in pediatric patients, including evaluation for acute appendicitis [5]. Although US is a great imaging option in pediatric patients, in large part due to its portability, low cost, and lack of ionizing radiation and sedation, it also has the disadvantage of being operator-dependent and can be limited by body habitus and in patients with large amounts of bowel gas [6]. Additionally, US can be limited in detecting alternative diagnoses for the patient's pain, which are usually more apparent on cross-sectional imaging examinations like MRI. Multiple studies have demonstrated that unenhanced, nonsedated MRI is comparable to CT in the diagnosis of acute appendicitis, both highly sensitive and specific, and has shown better sensitivity and specificity compared to US [7–10]. Recent evolution in MRI technology has allowed for the development of rapid, free-breathing, noncontrast sequences that can be effectively utilized in the pediatric population to evaluate both for appendicitis and alternative diagnoses [6]. MRI examinations ordered to evaluate for appendicitis in the pediatric population detected alternative diagnoses in 37.2% of patients in one study and in 18% to 19% of patients in another [6–8]. Examples of potential alternative diagnoses that may be discovered by rapid MRI for appendicitis include infectious or inflammatory enterocolitis, intraperitoneal focal fat infarction, pyelonephritis, ovarian torsion, pancreatitis, osteomyelitis or joint effusion, and biliary pathology among others. An example of omental infarct or intraperitoneal fat infarction is demonstrated in Fig. 1.

At our institution, the rapid MRI appendicitis protocol consists of axial, coronal, and sagittal T2 HASTE (single-shot turbo spin-echo) sequences, axial T2 fat-saturated HASTE sequence, and the option to add an axial diffusion-weighted imaging (DWI) sequence. The examination is performed without contrast or sedation, typically on a 3 T magnet, and extends from the upper abdomen near the gallbladder level through the lower pelvis or pubic symphysis. In total, the scan typically takes less than 15 minutes. A review of the literature demonstrates that other institutions have adopted similar protocols. An institution in Ireland describes their protocol as consisting of axial and coronal T2 single shot fast spin echo (SSFSE) with and without fat saturation, as well as axial DWI [11]. An article from Cincinnati Children's Hospital describes their protocol as consisting of free-breathing coronal T2 SSFSE, axial T2 SSFSE, and axial T2 fat-saturated SSFSE sequences [10].

The diagnostic criteria of appendicitis by MRI are similar to those by US and CT. On MRI, one should evaluate for a dilated appendix (greater than 6 mm in outer diameter), appendiceal wall thickening, and periappendiceal fluid or edema/inflammation (often well visualized on the fat saturated sequences). The abnormal appendix will often be fluid-filled as well [1,6]. The presence of appendicoliths, which will appear as hypointense filling defects within the appendix lumen on all sequences, should also be documented. MRI is useful to assess for signs of perforation, including discontinuity of the appendix wall, free air, a decompressed appendix in the setting of significant periappendiceal inflammation, and the presence of an abscess [1]. DWI sequences are particularly helpful to assess for intra-abdominal abscesses, and at our institution, we have a dedicated MR appendicitis abscess protocol performed in patients where there is concern for abscess related to either perforated appendicitis or following appendectomy, which automatically includes the DWI sequence and extends the field of view (FOV) to include the whole abdomen. An abscess collection will demonstrate restriction diffusion (either layering, peripheral, or central), which will manifest as high signal on the DWI and corresponding low signal on the apparent diffusion coefficient (ADC) map. An example of perforated acute appendicitis with abscess is shown in Fig. 2.

Adnexal or ovarian torsion

In recent years, there has been increased utilization of rapid MRI for the detection of adnexal torsion. Pelvic adnexal torsion is a general term related to twisting of the ovary or fallopian tube on its ligamentous support system, which can lead to vascular compromise of the torsed adnexal structures [12–14]. Prompt detection

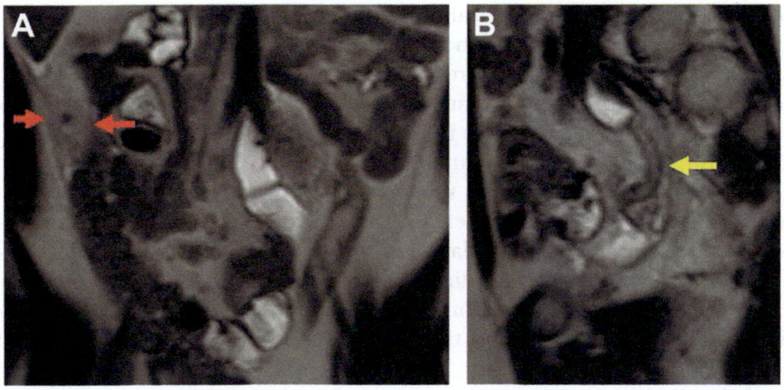

FIG. 1 A 7 year old patient with right lower quadrant pain for several days. (**A**) Coronal T2 HASTE demonstrates focal area of fatty inflammation and stranding centered along the right abdomen fat adjacent to the ascending colon annotated by the *red arrows* with trace reactive fluid by the inferior liver margin. (**B**) Sagittal T2 HASTE demonstrates a normal appendix in the pelvis marked by the *yellow arrow*.

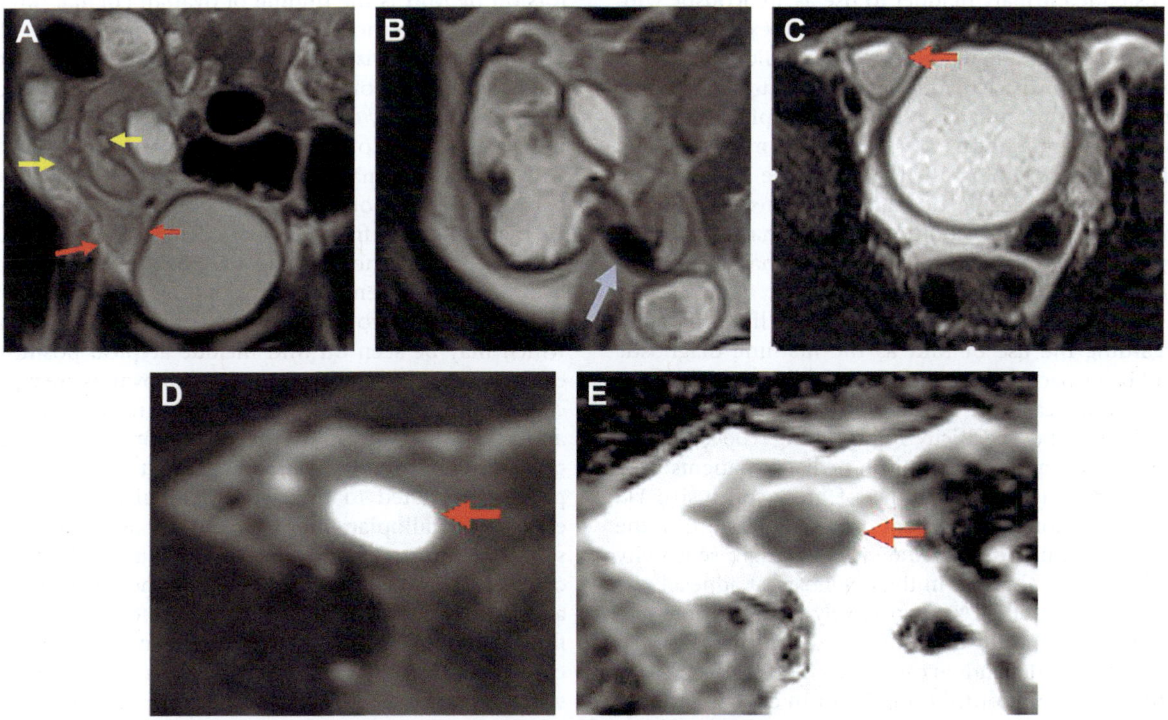

FIG. 2 A 9 year old patient with vomiting and abdominal pain for several days, with findings of acute perforated appendicitis. (**A** and **B**) Coronal T2 HASTE demonstrating dilated fluid-filled appendix with mural irregularity related to perforation denoted by the *yellow arrows*, and hypointense appendicolith in proximal lumen (*blue arrow*), as well as adjacent inflammation. Axial T2 FS (**C**) demonstrating small abscess with fluid-debris level (*red arrow*) in right lower quadrant. Inferiorly the abscess is larger and demonstrates restricted diffusion (*red arrows*) with high DWI signal (**D**) and low ADC signal (**E**), as well as free fluid in the pelvis.

and early initiation of surgical intervention is critical in preventing possible complications such as ovarian or tubal loss, dysfunction, and infertility [12]. Torsion of normal adnexa occurs more frequently in the pediatric population compared to adults, thought to relate to the relative mobility and tortuosity of the adnexa structures in younger patients, though may also develop in the presence of an adnexal mass or cyst [14]. Patients may present with nonspecific symptoms, particularly in the pediatric population, which poses clinical diagnostic challenges and further underlies the importance of being able to efficiently and accurately diagnosis this condition by imaging [14].

Traditionally, transabdominal pelvic US has been the first-line diagnostic modality in female pediatric patients presenting to the ED with concern for adnexal torsion; however, some institutions, including our own, have begun to transition to using MRI as the first-line imaging study for the detection of this condition. Pelvic US in pediatric patients to assess for ovarian torsion may be potentially delayed due to the need for a distended urinary bladder to use as an acoustic window for adequate evaluation of the adnexal structures. Additionally, patients may require fluid boluses to distend the urinary bladder, which can take a variable amount of time and often requires the placement of a peripheral intravenous (IV), and there may be added discomfort for the patient during the examination related to the degree of bladder distension required for the study [15]. Additionally, US may be limited by overlying bowel gas, patient body habitus, and is highly operator-dependent.

Though there is currently relatively little literature regarding the use of MRI as the first-line diagnostic tool in suspected ovarian torsion for the pediatric population, at least one recent study demonstrated high sensitivity and specificity approaching 100% for the diagnosis of adnexal torsion in pediatric patients used as second-line in the setting of an inconclusive US [16]. Additionally, a recent meta-analysis from the adult literature demonstrated both high sensitivity and specificity of MRI in the diagnosis of adnexal torsion of 81% and 91%, respectively [17]. Of note, the diagnostic capability of MRI in the detection of adnexal torsion is not dependent on urinary bladder distension, which is often a contributing factor in delaying the US examination in these pediatric patients. A recent study from a tertiary children's hospital demonstrated a statistically significant difference in scan time between the median MRI scan time (11.4 minutes) and the median historical US scan time (24.1 minutes) in patients with concern for ovarian torsion [15]. In addition, by utilizing MRI as a first-line modality in the diagnosis of adnexal torsion, it is possible to potentially obviate the need for patients to undergo multiple imaging examinations (eg, inconclusive or nondiagnostic US followed by MRI).

The rapid MRI protocol for adnexal torsion at our institution is the same as our protocol for acute appendicitis and includes a 3 plane T2 HASTE (single-shot turbo spin-echo) and an axial fat-saturated T2 HASTE from the level of the upper abdomen near the gallbladder through the lower pelvis, with a scan time between 10 and 15 minutes, usually performed on a 3 T magnet. The examination is performed without contrast and without sedation. A protocol recently published by another tertiary pediatric hospital includes a coronal T2 single shot fast spin echo (SSFE), axial T2W MultiVANE (PROPELLER/BLADE), and an axial T2W sequence with fat saturation [15]. The protocol established by these institutions is also performed without contrast and without sedation.

One main diagnostic feature in recognizing ovarian torsion by MRI is the finding of ovarian edema, often seen as asymmetric ovarian enlargement [12–14,18]. The torsed ovary is usually 3 to 4 times larger than the normal range or 3 times larger than the contralateral normal ovary, often measuring greater than 5 cm in size [14]. Additional findings that may be associated with ovarian edema in the setting of torsion include peripheralization of the ovarian follicles and central T2 hyperintensity from stromal edema [14,18]. Occasionally, ovarian hemorrhage may be seen, identified by a T2W hypointense rim surrounding the perifollicular region [1]. Secondary features of adnexal torsion, which may be seen on MRI include atypical position or situs of the abnormal ovary (normal ovaries are typically seen lateral and slightly posterior to the uterus), and deviation of the uterus toward the torsed ovary secondary to tension on the broad ligament [12]. A whirlpool sign related to the twisted vascular pedicle or edematous fallopian tube, often seen as a rounded soft tissue structure between the uterus and torsed ovary, is considered pathognomonic, though it is not always visualized [12,13,18]. Adnexal or pelvic free fluid and inflammation can also be seen in the setting of adnexal torsion [14]. Adnexal masses are associated with an increased risk for torsion and are readily identified by MRI. One study performed in the pediatric population found that 54% of the positive torsion cases reviewed at their institution were associated with adnexal masses or cysts [14]. Most of these lesions are follicular or paratubal cysts, though benign neoplasms, such as mature teratomas, can also be associated with torsion in approximately 19% of cases [14]. Although a cyst or mass of any size can be associated with torsion, those greater than 5 cm in size are thought to be predisposing risk factors for developing torsion [12]. Figs. 3 and 4 show examples of ovarian torsion identified by rapid MRI.

It is important to remember to consider the possibility of isolated tubal or paraovarian cyst torsion in all patients being evaluated for ovarian torsion. Paraovarian cysts are located in the broad ligament and paratubal cysts are usually attached to the mesosalpinx via a stalk, though the distinction is often made based on location at surgery and not by imaging [12]. Various factors place a patient at risk for tubal torsion, including a paratubal cyst, hydro or hematosalpinx, and tortuous course of the fallopian tube [12]. On MRI, the ovaries will typically appear normal, and there will usually by a cystic mass in the pelvis (often midline in location), which demonstrates an associated whirlpool or beak sign related to abrupt narrowing of the dilated tube. An example of isolated tubal torsion is seen in Fig. 5.

At our institution, following multidisciplinary discussions with our pediatric surgery colleagues and review of the literature, we have come up with a few guidelines to aid our radiologists in the interpretation of MRI examinations ordered to assess for ovarian torsion. If the ovaries measure less than 20 mL in volume and are symmetric in size, we will state there is no MRI concern for ovarian torsion. Conversely, if the ovarian volume measures greater than 20 mL, there is significant size asymmetry, or any other concerning features are seen, we will interpret the examination as concerning for torsion. For studies that have an adnexal lesion on the side of the patient's pain measuring 3 cm or greater, without other secondary findings, we will interpret those examinations as equivocal for adnexal torsion.

Brain pathology

MRI has long been recognized as a preferred method of imaging to detect a variety of intracranial pathologies due to its excellent soft-tissue contrast and high-resolution profile, allowing for optimal evaluation of the brain parenchyma and intracranial compartment. The use of MRI in the pediatric emergency setting was historically limited due to lengthy scan times compared to CT, which made MRI prone to motion degradation and often required the use of sedatives [19]. With technical advances in MRI leading to reduced scan times and the advent of multiple rapid technique protocols, there has been an increased usage of MRI through the ED to assess for intracranial pathology.

One of the initial adaptations for the use of emergent brain MRI in pediatric patients has been to assess for ventriculoperitoneal shunt malfunction in patients with shunted hydrocephalus. Multiple studies have demonstrated the effectiveness of assessing for shunt malformation by MRI, which allows for accurate determination of ventricular size, morphology, shunt position, and the extra-axial spaces [20–23]. Additionally, these studies proved that the examination could be performed successfully without sedation, with typical median scan lengths between 3 and 4 minutes [20,23]. The protocol for the rapid MRI ventricle examination at our institution is similar to those of other institutions, and utilizes axial, coronal, and sagittal T2 HASTE or SSFSE sequences. MRI has essentially replaced CT in the evaluation of patients with shunted hydrocephalus, both in the emergent setting and for routine outpatient surveillance. One major benefit of MRI over CT in this patient population, which often requires multiple or frequent imaging surveillance, is that MRI provides no ionizing radiation exposure or risk for developing radiation-induced cancers [21,22]. Fig. 6 shows an

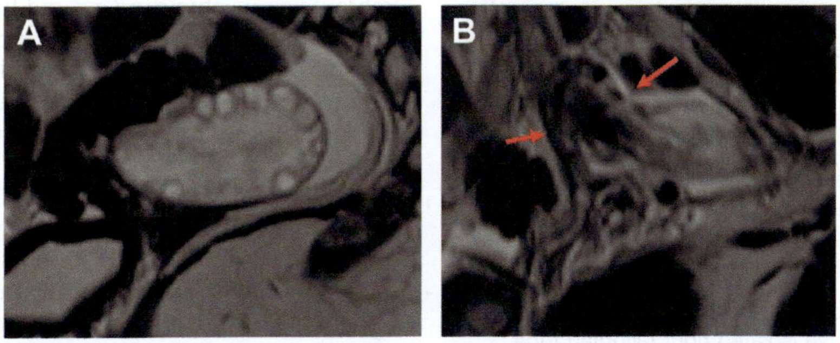

FIG. 3 A 12 year old patient with left pelvic pain found to have left ovarian torsion. (**A**) Sagittal T2 HASTE showing enlarged left ovary with central T2 hyperintense stromal edema and peripheralized follicles, (**B**) demonstrating the twisted vascular pedicle or whirlpool sign (*red arrows*).

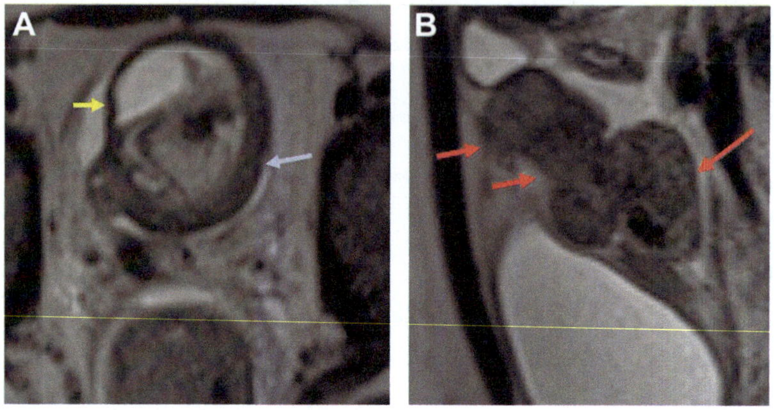

FIG. 4 A 9 year old patient with right lower quadrant pain found to have right ovarian and fallopian tube torsion due to a teratoma. Axial T2 HASTE (**A**) and Sagittal T2 HASTE (**B**) images demonstrating an enlarged right ovary (*blue arrow*) with associated complex cystic mass (*yellow arrow*) and dilated twisted fallopian tube (*red arrow*). Edema and small amount of fluid is seen in the pelvis.

example of a positive MRI ventricle study in the setting of shunt malfunction.

In addition to the shift toward ultrafast or rapid MRI from head CT in assessing patients with ventriculoperitoneal catheters, there has also been increased implementation of other rapid brain techniques in ED settings in recent years. Multiple studies have described the use of rapid protocol techniques as the initial screening examination over CT to evaluate pediatric patients presenting with neurologic symptoms, including those presenting with concern for stroke, migraines, seizures, headache, altered mentation, and vomiting [1,24–28]. In one study, they found a reduction in head CT orders through the ED by 20%, without any missed or undetected pathology by the rapid MRI examinations on patient follow-up [24]. One study noted longer time to imaging and a longer length of stay in the ED in patients who receive rapid brain MRI compared to those who receive a head CT, which partially relates to the longer length of an MR scan and need for patient screening prior to MRI [24]. Although there will be some inevitable delay in obtaining a rapid brain MRI compared to noncontrast head CT, the benefit of better parenchymal assessment that allows the ability to make various important neurologic diagnoses, as well as the lack of ionizing radiation, is an important factor to consider [1,24].

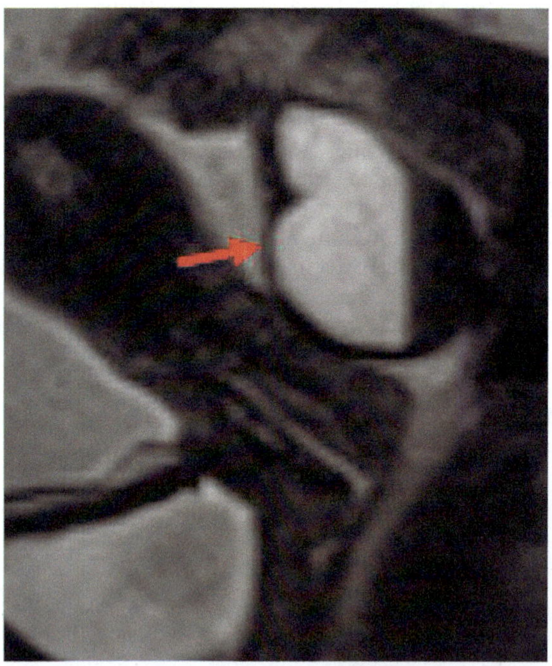

FIG. 5 An 11 year old patient with right lower quadrant/pelvic pain found to have isolated right fallopian tube torsion. Sagittal T2 HASTE showing the dilated fluid-filled fallopian tube within the pelvis posterior to the uterus (*red arrow*), with fluid-hematocrit level.

Rapid brain MRI sequences have proven effective as a screening tool for a variety of intracranial pathologies in various studies [24–26]. MRI is particularly helpful in determining the presence or absence of acute infarct or ischemic stroke, particularly compared to CT that is often not sensitive for the detection of early stroke. The most common risk factors for pediatric stroke secondary to arterial infarct are arteriopathies and congenital

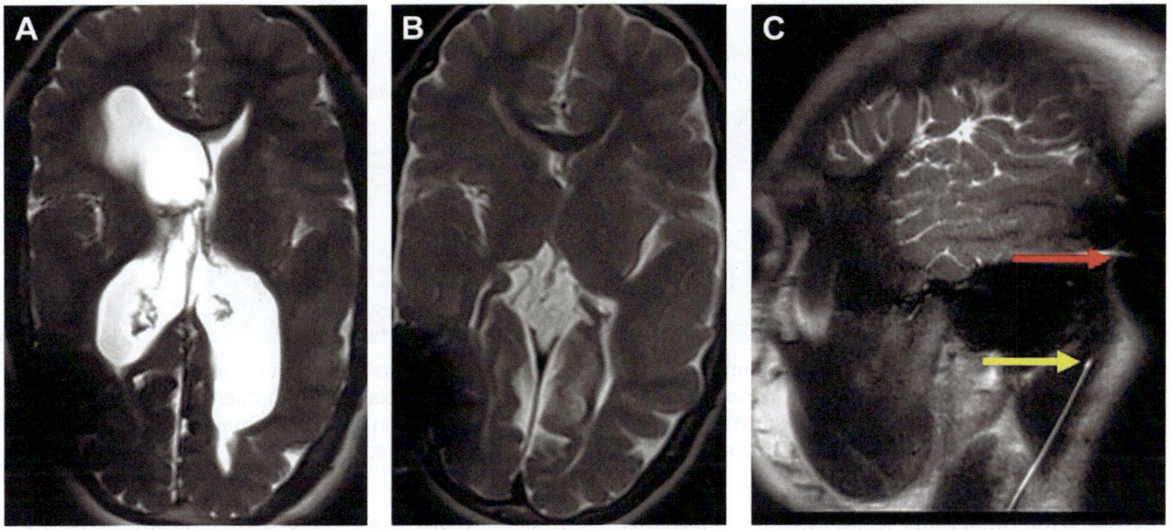

FIG. 6 A 14 year old patient with history of shunted hydrocephalus presenting with emesis and concern for ventriculoperitoneal (VP) shunt malfunction. Axial T2 HASTE sequences demonstrate significantly increased size of the now dilated lateral ventricles (**A**) compared to the comparison study from 2 years prior (**B**) where the lateral ventricles were decompressed. Sagittal T2 HASTE (**C**) demonstrates disconnection of the proximal component of the shunt catheter (*yellow arrow*) from the reservoir (*red arrow*), serving as the cause for shunt dysfunction.

heart disease [1]. DWI sequences are highly sensitive and specific for the detection of ischemia, with one study demonstrating 100% sensitivity by rapid MRI in these patients [1,25]. Evaluation with T2-weighted and fluid attenuated inversion recovery (FLAIR) sequences can help determine the age of the infarct, susceptibility weighted imaging (SWI) can assist in the detection of microhemorrhage, and MR angiography (MRA) can evaluate for arteriopathy or large vessel occlusion [1]. In pediatric patients, there is a high-prevalence of stroke-like conditions or mimics such as hemiplegic migraine, seizures, demyelinating disease, inflammatory conditions, and tumors [1]. Rapid MRI brain protocols are incredibly valuable in both

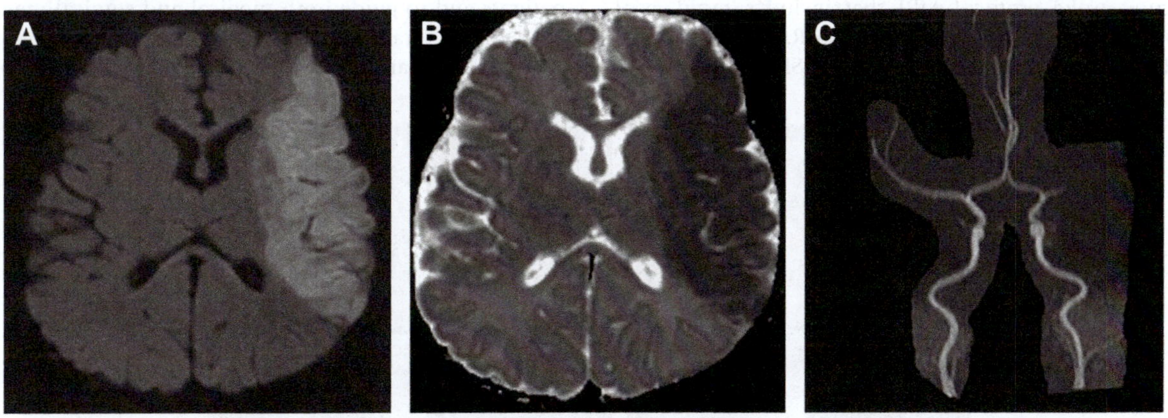

FIG. 7 A 3 month old patient with hypoplastic left heart syndrome status after Norwood palliation and Glenn procedure with right hemiparesis. Axial DWI (**A**) shows large area of restricted diffusion/high signal in the left MCA territory with associated low signal on the ADC map (**B**). Maximum intensity projection (MIP) reformatted image from the time of flight (TOF) MRA (**C**) demonstrates abrupt cutoff of the left MCA related to vessel occlusion.

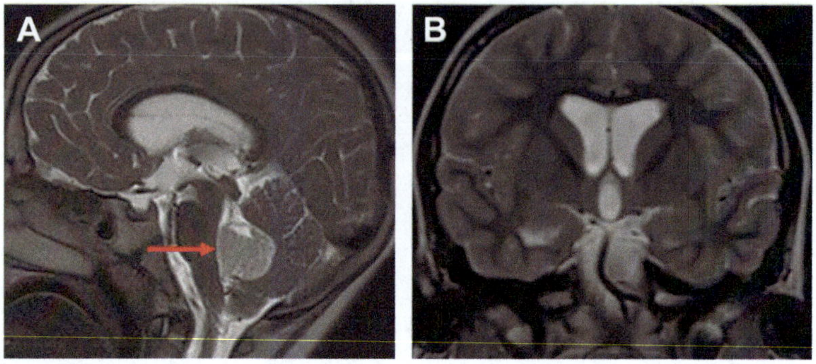

FIG. 8 A 7 year old patient with 2 months of vomiting and dizziness found to have a posterior fossa mass on screening rapid MRI. Subsequent tumor resection demonstrated medulloblastoma. (**A**) Sagittal T2 HASTE demonstrating mixed solid and cystic mass in the posterior fossa centered in the fourth ventricle (*red arrow*), (**B**) and coronal T2 HASTE demonstrates mild associated obstructive hydrocephalus.

detecting acute infarct and in establishing alternative diagnoses. Figs. 7 and 8 showcase examples of intracranial pathology that may be detected by rapid MRI.

At our institution, there are 2 main rapid protocol noncontrast, nonsedated brain protocols that are used in addition to the MRI ventricles examination. There is a general rapid brain MRI, which is used as a screening tool for pediatric patients presenting with a variety of neurologic symptoms, which includes rapid axial DWI, sagittal T1, coronal T2 turbo spin echo (TSE), axial SWI, axial T2 TSE, and axial 2D FLAIR sequences, with the option to add the 3 plane HASTE sequences from the MRI ventricles protocol. This scan typically takes around 15 minutes to complete. The second rapid noncontrast brain protocol is a dedicated acute stroke protocol MRI that includes rapid axial DWI, coronal T2 TSE, axial 2D FLAIR, axial SWI, axial 2D pulsed arterial spin labeling (pASL), and axial 3D time of flight MRA. This scan typically takes 15 to 20 minutes, and the radiologist has the option to omit the MRA and pASL sequences if there is no evidence for acute ischemia or infarct on DWI.

Musculoskeletal pathology

A recent area of emerging research has centered on the development of rapid MRI examination in the evaluation of pediatric musculoskeletal infections, a previously largely unexplored territory. MRI is critical in the diagnosis of musculoskeletal infections that can present various clinical/diagnostic challenges in the pediatric population [2]. MRI, secondary to its excellent soft tissue and bone assessment, is usually necessary to delineate the extent and nature of infection in pediatric patients and to guide both medical and surgical management [2]. Traditional MRI protocols to evaluate for osteomyelitis can take up to several hours to perform,

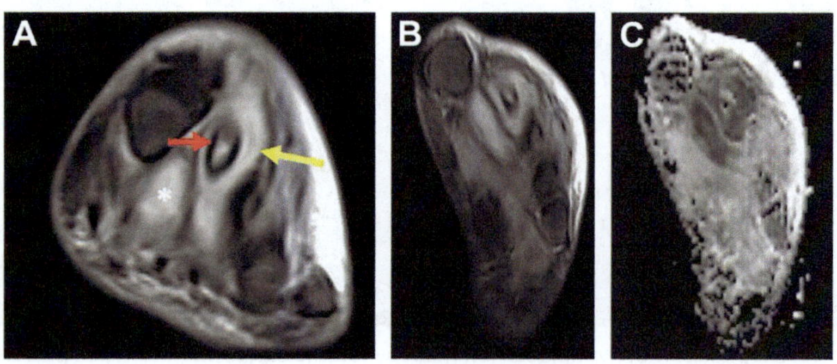

FIG. 9 An 11 year old patient with foot pain and swelling. (**A**) Coronal/short axis T2 demonstrates increased signal in the second metatarsal related to osteomyelitis (*red arrow*) with large surrounding T2 bright subperiosteal abscess (*yellow arrow*) and adjacent soft tissue abscess (*asterisk*) that demonstrate restricted diffusion (**B**) and low ADC (**C**) with T2 bright edema along the dorsal soft tissues.

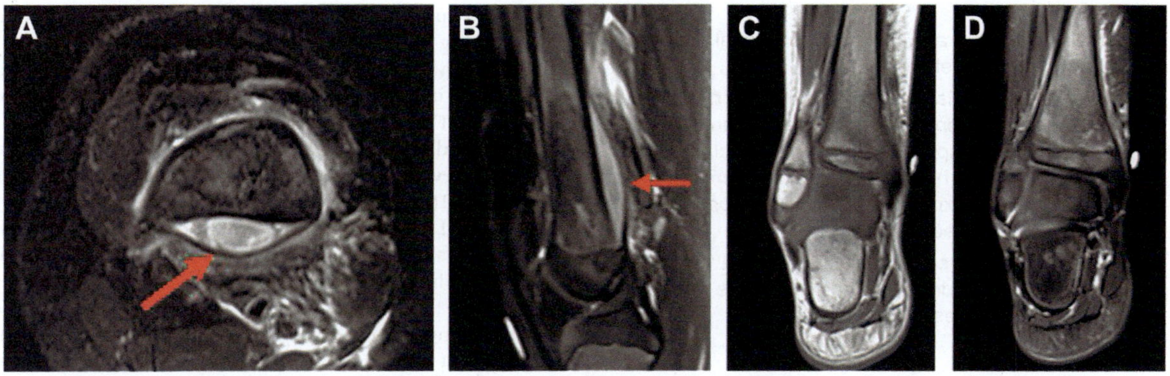

FIG. 10 Examples of musculoskeletal infection. Axial T2 (**A**) and Sagittal T2 (**B**) sequences demonstrate a large subperiosteal abscess along the posterior distal femur (*red arrows*) with soft tissue edema seen about the knee in this patient with distal femoral osteomyelitis. Coronal T1 (**C**) and Coronal T2 (**D**) demonstrate distal left tibial osteomyelitis with high T2 and low T1 signal, as well as surrounding soft tissue edema.

depending on the need for general anesthesia/sedation and are typically performed with and without contrast. A recent study demonstrated that implementation of rapid protocol MRI to assess for acute pediatric musculoskeletal infections eliminated the need for intravenous contrast, minimized anesthesia, improved access to MRI, decreased scan time and time to study interpretation, hospital length of stay, and hospital charges when compared to traditional MRI [29]. Additionally, this study found that rapid protocol MRI to assess for musculoskeletal infection demonstrated high sensitivity in the detection of infection and a low rate of imaging failure [29].

The rapid MRI protocol at our institution includes a larger FOV coronal HASTE sequence (bilateral if possible in younger patients) to localize the area of concern/suspected infection, followed by smaller FOV rapid axial, coronal, and sagittal T2W fat-saturated sequences, coronal T1W sequence, and axial DWI with ADC map tailored to the area of interest. Studies have shown that these rapid abbreviated sequences are sufficient to adequately determine if an infection is present and to assess for complications that might change management or prompt surgical intervention, such as identifying the presence of abscesses and pathologic joint effusions [2,29]. T2-weighted sequences can be used to identify marrow edema, abscesses (intraosseous, intramuscular, soft tissue, and subperiosteal), and joint effusions. Bone marrow changes can be further evaluated on the coronal T1 sequence and can help identify the "penumbra sign" and bony sequestrum, which can be identified in the setting of bone infection [2]. The DWI sequence can be utilized for trouble shooting and serves as a "substitution" for gadolinium contrast, helping to confirm the presence of abscesses and differentiate between osteomyelitis, reactive marrow edema, and necrotic bone [2]. Figs. 9 and 10 demonstrate examples of musculoskeletal infection detected by rapid MRI.

SUMMARY

Rapid protocol noncontrast MRI examinations have been effectively and successfully employed for the assessment of pediatric patients in the emergent setting for acute body, brain, and musculoskeletal imaging indications. Rapid MRI has, thus far, shown to be an incredibly powerful tool in diagnosing and guiding management for various pediatric pathologies encountered in the ED, and further evolution of MR technology and wider acceptance of rapid MRI will likely continue to improve the scan capabilities and expand applications. Limiting the use of contrast and sedation by shifting toward rapid protocol examinations has the potential to help optimize/improve radiology department workflow and could offer hospital cost savings by lowering encounter time.

CLINICS CARE POINTS

- Advancements in MRI technology have allowed for better accessibility of MRI for pediatric patients secondary to decreased scan times and improvement in motion sensitivity.
- Rapid, noncontrast, nonsedated MRI techniques have been successfully employed to various degrees

in pediatric body, brain, and musculoskeletal imaging in the emergency setting.

- Rapid MRI protocols can often replace the need for CT in the assessment of pediatric patients in the ED, particularly with respect to evaluating for acute brain pathologies, which has the potential to decrease ionizing radiation exposure, particularly in patients who may require frequent imaging.
- Diffusion-weighted sequences can act as a "substitute" for contrast administration and can be incredibly helpful in abscess detection.

DISCLOSURE

The authors have nothing to disclose.

REFERENCES

[1] Figueiro Longo MG, Jaimes C, Machado F, et al. Pediatric emergency MRI. Magn Reason Imaging Clin N Am 2022;30:533–52.
[2] Gu JZ, Samet JD. Rapid nonsedated, noncontrast MRI for workup of acute pediatric musculoskeletal infection. Advances in Clinical Radiology 2023;5:107–15.
[3] Kozak BM, Jaimes C, Kirsch J, et al. MRI techniques to decrease imaging times in children. Radiographics 2020;40:485–502.
[4] Gallo-Bernal S, Bedoya MA, Gee MS, et al. Pediatric magnetic resonance imaging: faster is better. Pediatr Radiol 2023;53:1270–84.
[5] Ayyala RS, Dillman JR, Tkach JA, et al. Rapid adominopelvic Mr imaging in the emergency department: establishing a program and addressing the challenges. Pediatr Radiol 2024. https://doi.org/10.1007/s00247-024-06004-5.
[6] Mustaq R, Desoky SM, Morello F, et al. First-line diagnostic evaluation with MRI of children suspected of having acute appendicitis. Radiology 2019;291:170–7.
[7] Dillman JR, Gadepalli S, Sroufe NS, et al. Equivocal pediatric appendicitis: unenhanced MR imaging protocol for nonsedated children—a clinical effectiveness study. Radiology 2016;279(1):216–25.
[8] Moore MM, Kulaylat AN, Hollenbeak CS, et al. Magnetic resonance imaging in pediatric appendicitis: a systematic review. Pediatr Radiol 2016;46(6):928–39.
[9] Ata NA, Trout AT, Dillman JR, et al. Technical and diagnostic performance of rapid MRI for evaluation of appendicitis in a pediatric emergency department. Acad Radiol 2024;31:1102–10.
[10] Ayyala RS, Dillman JR, Tkach JA, et al. Implementation of a program for appendicitis MRI in a pediatric hospital. AJR 2024;222:e2330695.
[11] James K, Duffy P, Kavanagh RG, et al. Fast acquisition abdominal MRI study for the investigation of suspected acute appendicitis in paediatric patients. Insights Into Imaging 2020;11:78.
[12] Strachowski LM, Choi HH, Shum DJ, et al. Pearls and pitfalls in imaging of pelvic adnexal torsion: seven tips to tell it's twisted. Radiographics 2021;41(2):625–40.
[13] Dawood MT, Naik M, Bharwani N, et al. Adnexal torsion: review of radiologic appearances. Radiographics 2021;41(2):609–24.
[14] Sintim-Damoa A, Majmudar AS, Cohen HL, et al. Pediatric ovarian torsion: spectrum of imaging findings. Radiographics 2017;37(6):1892–908.
[15] Epstein KN, Trout AT, Debnath P, et al. Rapid, free breathing non-contrast MRI for first-line imaging evaluation of ovarian torsion in the emergency department. Pediatr Radiol 2024;54:228–35.
[16] Rougier E, Mar W, Della Valle V, et al. Added value of MRI for the diagnosis of adnexal torsion in children and adolescents after inconclusive ultrasound examination. Diagn Interv Imaging 2020;101:747–56.
[17] Watter B, Rimmer M, Rogozinska E, et al. Accuracy of imaging modalities for adnexal torsion: a systematic review and meta-analysis. BJOG 2021;128(1):37–44.
[18] Gomes MM, Cavalcanti LS, Reis RL, et al. Twist and shout: magnetic resonance imaging findings in ovarian torsion. Radiol Bras 2019;52(6):397–402.
[19] Young Ha J, Jin Beak H, Hwa Ryu K, et al. One-minute ultrafast brain MRI with full basic sequences: can it be a promising way forward for pediatric neuroimaging? AJR 2020;215:198–205.
[20] Patel DM, Tubbs RS, Pate G, et al. Fast-sequence MRI studies for surveillance imaging in pediatric hydrocephalus. J Neurosurg Pediatr 2014;13:440–7.
[21] Kim I, Torrey SB, Milla SS, et al. Benefits of brain magnetic resonance imaging over computed tomography in children requiring emergency evaluation of ventriculoperitoneal shunt malfunction: reducing lifetime attributable risk of cancer. Pediatr Emerg Care 2015;31(4):239–42.
[22] Boyle TP, Paldino MJ, Kimia AA, et al. Comparison of rapid cranial MRI to CT for ventricular shunt malfunction. Pediatrics 2014;134(1):e47–354.
[23] Niederhauser BD, McDonald RJ, Eckel LJ, et al. Retrospective review of rapid pediatric brain mr imaging at an academic institution including practice trends and factors affecting scan times. AJNR Am J Neuroradiol 2013;34(9):1836–40.
[24] Ramgopal S, Karim SA, Subramanian S, et al. Rapid brain MRI protocols reduce head computerized tomography use in the pediatric emergency department. BMC Pediatr 2020;20:14.
[25] De Jong G, Kannikeswaran N, DeLaroche A, et al. Rapid sequence MRI protocol in the evaluation of pediatric brain attacks. Pediatr Neurol 2020;107:77–83.
[26] Luque M, Stambo GW. The use of rapid sequence magnetic resonance imaging of the brain as a screening tool for detection of gross intracranial pathology in children presenting to the emergency department with a chief

complaint of persistent of recurrent headaches. Pediatr Emerg Care 2021;37(10):e660–3.
[27] Kessler BA, Goh JL, Pajer HB, et al. Rapid-sequence MRI for evaluation of pediatric traumatic brain injury: a systematic review. J Neurosurg Pediatr 2021;28:278–86.
[28] Young JY, Duhaime AC, Caruso PA, et al. Comparison of non-sedated brain MRI and CT for the detection of acute traumatic injury in children 6 years of age or less. Emerg Radiol 2016;23:325–31.
[29] Chan KS, McBride D, Wild J, et al. A rapid protocol for the evaluation of acute pediatric musculoskeletal infections: eliminating contrast and decreasing anesthesia, scan time, and hospital length of stay and charges. J Bone Joint Surg Am 2024;106:700–7.

Advances in Clinical Radiology 7 (2025) 83–91
ADVANCES IN CLINICAL RADIOLOGY

A Scoping Review of Current Techniques in Posterior Cruciate Ligament Injury Management and Reconstruction

Gabriel Ortiz Celemin, BA[a], Ethan Klepitsch, MD[a], Lucas Buchler, MD[b], Ankur Garg, MD[a], Alison Esteva Sanders, MD[a,*]

[a]Diagnostic Radiology Department, Northwestern University Feinberg School of Medicine, 676 North St Clair Suite 800, Chicago, IL 60611, USA; [b]Department of Orthopaedic Surgery, Northwestern University Feinberg School of Medicine, 676 N. St. Clair Street, Suite 1350, Chicago, IL 60611, USA

KEYWORDS

• Arthroscopy • Posterior cruciate ligament • Double-bundle • Posterior instability

KEY POINTS

- Consensus on superiority of single versus double-bundle posterior cruciate ligament reconstruction does not yet exist; however, there is evidence to support that double bundle is superior at returning posterior tibial translation to near-normal.
- Knee radiographs are important in the preoperative assessment before potential PCL reconstruction. MRI is the preferred modality for assessment of the graft and detection of potential complications.
- Work remains to be done directly comparing PCL remnant-preserving approaches to traditional techniques, but there is a theoretic benefit to preserving this tissue for proprioceptive function.
- The posterior tibial slope is emerging as an important factor affecting graft failure rates following PCL reconstruction.

INTRODUCTION

Posterior cruciate ligament (PCL) injury is a common source of morbidity and mortality, especially for patients presenting with multiligamentous injuries. The decision to undergo PCL reconstruction is nuanced as nonoperative management has historically been favored in cases of isolated PCL injury (Fig. 1). Isolated PCL injury is rare with an estimated occurrence of 1% of total acute knee injuries [1]. More commonly, they present with multiligament involvement with fracture/injury of the posterolateral corner being a poor prognosticator [1]. The clinical features of PCL injury include joint effusion, pain following even low-energy trauma as well as an increased risk of accelerated osteoarthritis (OA) in the long term [1]. With increased posterior instability following the injury, the patellofemoral and medial tibiofemoral articulations are considered particularly vulnerable to the development of OA [1].

The PCL plays a role in stabilizing the healthy knee joint in multiple directions, but especially in preventing posterior tibial translation with posteriorly directed stress [1,2]. Anatomically, the PCL can be divided into the anterolateral bundle (ALB) and the posteromedial bundle (PMB) [1,2]. In the native knee, the ALB is the thicker and stiffer collection of fibers and has

*Corresponding author. *E-mail address:* alison.estevasanders@nm.org

https://doi.org/10.1016/j.yacr.2025.05.007 www.advancesinclinicalradiology.com
2589-8701/25/

ABBREVIATIONS	
ALB	anterolateral bundle
DB-PCLr	double-bundle PCL reconstruction
IKDC	International Knee Documentation Committee
OA	osteoarthritis
PCL	posterior cruciate ligament
PMB	posteromedial bundle
PRP	platelets-rich-plasma
SB-PCLr	single-bundle PCL reconstruction

been thought to undergo the most stress for the knee under load [1,2]. Single-bundle PCL reconstruction replicates the entirety of the PCL with a single allograft, often placed roughly between the 2 insertion points of the ALB and PMB to distribute their respective loads. In contrast, double-bundle PCL reconstruction aims to recreate the 2 anatomic components of the native PCL, most commonly with allografts divided to simulate the ALB and PMB.

In the past decade, a growing body of literature exists describing a shift in PCL reconstructive surgery from single-bundle PCL reconstruction (SB-PCLr), which relies on one group of harvested tendon fibers to replace the damaged PCL toward double-bundle PCL reconstruction (DB-PCLr), which splits the graft into 2 distinct bundles, more closely mimicking native PCL anatomy. As DB-PCLr techniques have been implemented at more surgical centers for some years, enough longitudinal data now exists to consider differences in clinical outcomes between these techniques. Studies using the Lyscholm score, International Knee Documentation Committee (IKDC) Score, Tegner Activity Scale, presence and severity of OA in the injured joint, extent of posterior tibial translation and side-to-side stability and return to sport after a follow-up period will be considered.

PCL reconstruction is a technically challenging endeavor with more inherent risk than anterior cruciate ligament (ACL) reconstruction due to the proximity to neurovascular structures in the posterior compartment of the knee [3]. This article presents advances in the surgical management of PCL injury and insights from recent literature in the radiographic evaluation of the preoperative and postoperative patient across multiple imaging modalities.

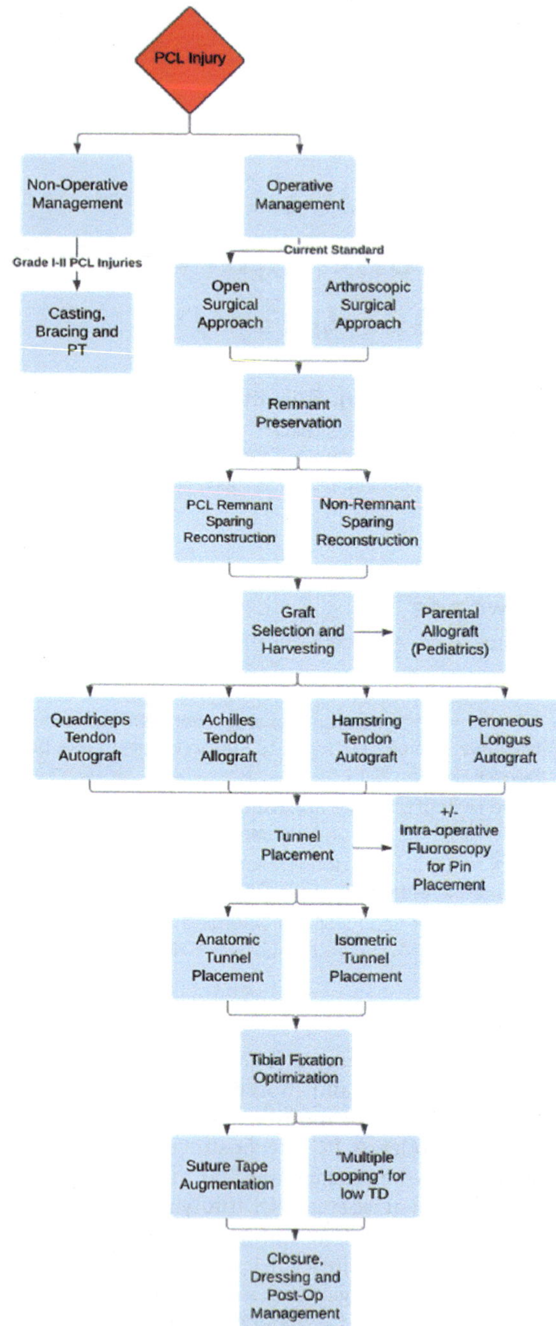

FIG. 1 Flow chart of decision-making branch points in PCL reconstruction options

METHODS

Data for this article was obtained via keyword search of *posterior cruciate ligament reconstruction* OR *double-bundle*

PCL OR *single-bundle PCL* OR *posterior cruciate ligament injury* and filtered for articles published from 2014 to 2025.

The 508 articles produced from this search were screened for appropriateness in the following ways:

- Data from in vivo studies will be highly prioritized except in cases where it describes a novel technique not noted elsewhere
- Data must include an assessment of postoperative outcomes in one of the following ways:
  - Biomechanical stability of the postop joint by clinical assessment and/or stress radiography (especially posterior tibial translation)
  - Functional assessment of postop symptom burden after follow-up period (Lysholm score, IKDC score, Tegner Activity Scale, time to return to sport)
  - Radiographic or clinical presence and severity of OA in the affected joint after a follow-up period

Prior reviews, brief reports, and editorials were also excluded from consideration. From here, the bibliography was further reduced to prioritize highly cited and more recent papers, with studies addressing similar clinical questions grouped for analysis in the discussion section.

DISCUSSION

Several articles have emerged positing new protocols for nearly every operative step of PCL reconstruction. What follows is an overview of the steps of PCL reconstructive surgery.

Posterior cruciate ligament reconstruction protocol

As arthroscopic reconstruction is highly favored and represented by current literature, open surgical approaches will be omitted. After proper positioning, preparation, and draping of the surgical site and induction with anesthesia, a portion of the patient's tendon is harvested for autografting, or a donor allograft is used. The semitendinosus or gracilis tendons are commonly harvested for autografting, as well as recent demonstrations of quadriceps and peroneus longus tendon grafts in the literature; however a paucity of evidence currently exists to suggest clinical superiority in one harvest site [4,5].

Following this, arthroscopic access is obtained, allowing the surgeon to assess the extent of the injuries as well as evaluate and manage associated injuries, as isolated PCL injury is clinically rare [3–5]. From here, the decision may be made to completely debride the remnant PCL fragments to expose their footprint for an entirely non-native reconstruction, or keep the fragments and incorporate them into the reconstruction [6]. Once the surgeon establishes optimal visualization of the relevant anatomic landmarks within the joint space and PCL attachment points, femoral and tibial tunnels are drilled arthroscopically to serve as attachment points for the graft. This may be done under fluoroscopic guidance to confirm optimal placement.

If performing a double-bundle reconstruction, the harvested graft is divided in 2 and prepared with suture, and the 2 pieces are passed through the tunnels corresponding to the anatomic position of the native anterolateral and posteromedial bundles of the PCL [3–5]. A single-bundle reconstruction proceeds similarly; however, only 1 segment of the tendon graft is fixed to the femur and tibia. At this stage, the surgeon may choose to augment the graft reconstruction with suture tape, a technique often referred to as internal bracing [1] (Fig. 2).

To incorporate suture tape using DB-PCLr as an example, the 2 strands of the graft are folded in half to make a 4-strand bundle. Using a suspension device known as an endobutton that will become affixed to the femoral attachment, the graft bundles are looped through along with high-tensile strength braided polyethylene sutures to reinforce the strength of the donor tissue [7]. This construct is then passed into the femoral tunnel and affixed appropriately, providing the theoretic benefit of improved graft longevity and postoperative posterior stability while potentially introducing the risk of overtensioning the graft-suture bundles [7].

Finally, the knee is assessed through a full range of motion to ensure smooth and complete articulation, then the arthroscope and associated tools are removed [3–5]. The portal and harvest sites are then irrigated, closed, and dressed per surgeon preference/institutional protocol.

Double-Bundle PCL Reconstruction Versus single-bundle PCL reconstruction

Within the limitations of the search strategy employed in this study, a paucity of literature addressing direct comparison between SB-PCLr and DB-PCLr and their long-term outcomes continues to exist. Of the 4 comparative studies directly comparing participants receiving SB-PCLr and DB-PCLr, 2 articles reported no clear clinical or functional difference postoperatively after a minimum of 2-year follow-up [8,9]. Of the 2 that reported a difference, it was only evident in the kinematic profile of postoperative knee, assessed with

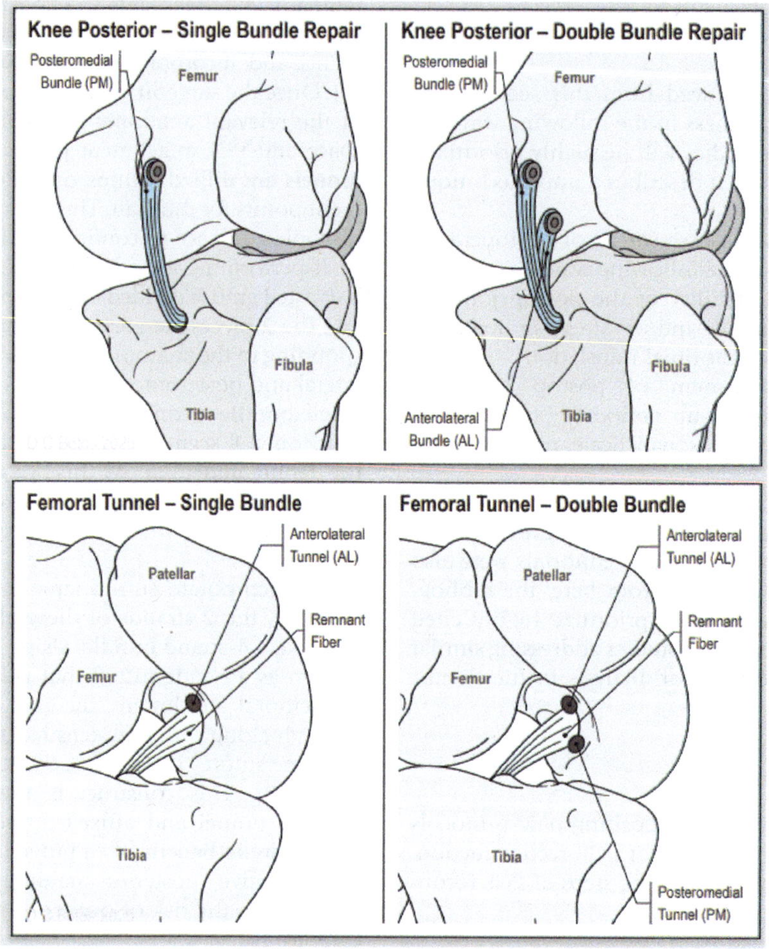

FIG. 2 Anterolateral and posteromedial femoral tunnel locations relative to the remnant PCL attachments for isometric single and DB-PCLr.

measurements of posterior tibial translation and range of motion, but still without a clear clinical difference for the patient between the operations [10,11].

The available literature seems to suggest that whatever possible benefit DB-PCLr has over SB-PCLr is modest and that both modalities are associated with few complications, rates of success comparable with ACL reconstruction, and no documented difference in long-term (10+ year) outcomes including the development of OA in the PCL-deficient knee [8–11].

Preoperative radiographic assessment

Several recommendations to optimize the preoperative assessment have focused on assessment of the tibial morphology and density. Yoon and colleagues published in 2023 regarding the association between posterior tibial slope and 10-year graft failure rates in a 46-patient study and found that a flattened (<5.6°) posterior tibial slope on preoperative imaging predicted a higher likelihood of 10-year graft failure and higher postoperative side-to-side difference on stress radiography. Additionally, the relatively lower bone density of the tibial metaphysis compared to its femoral counterpart has been a well-established challenge to rigid and durable fixation of the reconstructed PCL [12].

The posterior tibial slope can be assessed using lateral radiograph, CT or MRI (Fig. 3). First, to control for malrotation, the posterior femoral condyle overlap should be measured and not greater than 6 mm. Next, the axis of the tibial shaft is drawn as a line that connects the center of 2 circles, placed 5 cm and 15 cm distal to the joint line and touching both the anterior

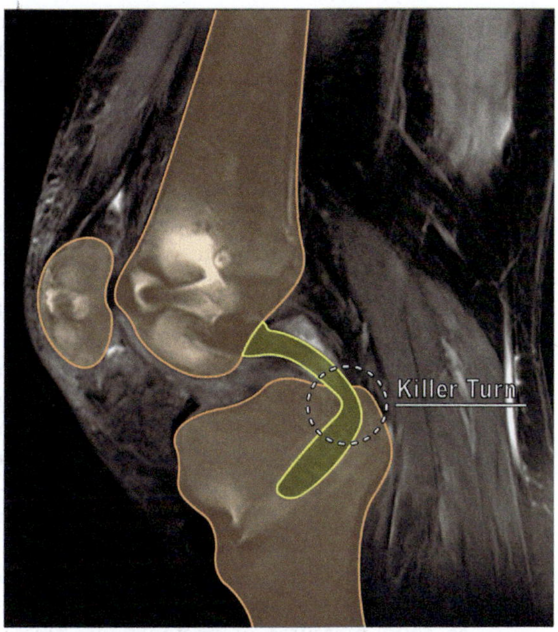

FIG. 3 Killer turn describes the sharp angulation inherent in the proximal anteromedial tibial fixation portion of the repair.

and posterior aspects of the tibial cortex. Next, a tangent line is drawn across the medial tibial plateau. The angle formed between the medial tibial plateau tangent line and the tibial shaft axis is subtracted from 90° to provide the medial posterior tibial slope [13].

Operative technique

Within this basic framework for the steps of this operation, there remains flexibility in what techniques and decisions may be made intraoperatively to complete these steps. While no protocol specifies every surgeon-dependent decision one might encounter during PCL reconstruction, several actionable suggestions have emerged in the last decade of PCL reconstruction literature.

1. Graft selection
    1.1. Recent work regarding the clinical superiority of allograft or autograft tendons in PCL reconstruction was published by Li and colleagues in 2016, reporting no clinically significant difference in patient proprioceptive or functional outcomes at a 5-year follow-up [14]. On assessment of ligamentous laxity, the allograft group was demonstrated to have more laxity than the autograft group. A study published by Sun and colleagues addressing a similar question supports the finding of increased laxity with allograft. The allograft treatment group in this trial had a shorter operative time/incision size and experienced more postoperative leukocytosis/fever without significant differences in functional outcomes [15].
    1.2. A study by Lee and colleagues in 2020 addresses both the safety of hamstring autograft harvest and a key difference in the typical postoperative course between ACL and PCL reconstruction. In a 1:2 matched cohort of patients undergoing ACL reconstruction with hamstring autograft and PCL reconstruction with tibialis anterior allograft, the PCL patients had significant flexor weakness in the operated leg despite receiving a non-native tendon compared to the ACL group [4]. The authors propose one possible mechanism: prolonged immobilization in full extension in the early postoperative period in the PCL recovery group, as opposed to the immediate range of motion (ROM) to 90° in the ACL group [4]. Rhatomy and colleagues compared the peroneus longus tendon with more traditional hamstring graft donor sites and found no significant difference in donor site morbidity or functional outcomes postoperatively [5].
2. Arthroscopic debridement versus PCL remnant preservation
    2.1. In recent years, little has been published directly comparing PCL reconstruction with debridement of the PCL remnant stumps with remnant-preserving approaches. A recent study in *Arthroscopy* noted high rates of return to sport and patient satisfaction as well as satisfactory functional outcomes with a remnant-preserving SB-PCLr [6]. In this study, almost 90% of patients had returned to their sport after 2 years and about 70% reported no pain or limitations to effort [6].
    2.2. A histologic study by Chun and colleagues harvested PCL remnant samples from live patients who underwent PCL allograft with remnant preservation and stained tissue samples to identify neuronal markers. They found evidence to support the presence of mechanoreceptors in PCL remnants, suggesting an added benefit in proprioceptive functional

preservation with remnant-sparing approaches to PCL reconstruction [16].

3. Tunnel Placement and *Killer Turn* Angle Reduction
   3.1. Kernkamp and colleagues conducted a retrospective study of 14 patients with unilateral PCL injury following reconstructive surgery with their healthy knee as a comparator. The patients were imaged with MRI and in multiple planes with fluoroscopy to model their ligament kinematics and evaluate changes in the length of the PCL through 165 potential femoral attachment digitally points. They found that more anatomic attachments reproduced more physiologic changes in ligament length through a range of motion [17].
   3.2. The *killer turn* has been established in PCL literature as a challenge of PCL reconstructive surgery, coined by the American Academy of Orthopedic Surgeons in 1992 to describe the sharp turn inherent in the proximal anteromedial attachment of the tibial fixation portion of the reconstruction, often contributing to increased graft failure and laxity postoperatively (Fig. 4). Vasdev and colleagues propose 1 solution, creating a retrograde socket for graft attachment in the posteromedial aspect of the tibia via an all-inside technique to reduce the killer turn angle [3]. Another solution proposed by Chernchujit and colleagues described as the *arthroscopic transseptal, rod and pulley technique* involved creating tibial transseptal arthroscopic portals for optimal visualization and using a Weissinger rod as a pulley to guide the graft through the tibial tunnel to minimize damage to the graft during passage [18].
   3.3. Tachibana and colleagues detail the natural course of tibiofemoral tunneling following PCL reconstruction up to 1 year of follow-up. Their finding was that every tunnel enlarges up to 6 months of follow-up on CT images, but remains stable at 1 year, with the femoral posteromedial tunnel enlarging to the greatest extent, nearly doubling in diameter on average [19]. The clinical upshot is that initial posterior laxity in the immediate postoperative period may not represent the stability of the graft in the long-term.
   3.4. Osti and colleagues compared and described both radiographs and computed tomography as valid measures of postoperative assessment in femoral and tibial tunnel placement with a high degree of interobserver and intraobserver agreement in angle and positioning [20].
4. Tibial/Femoral Fixation Optimization
   4.1. Noh and colleagues and several others have developed tibial and femoral fixation techniques using *multiple looping*. This involves

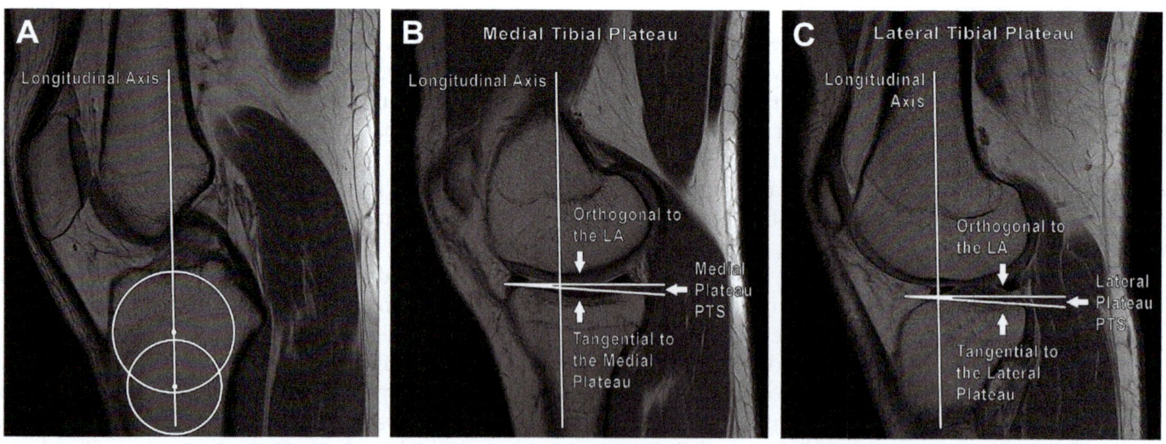

FIG. 4 Posterior tibial slope assessment by MRI. (**A**) Midsagittal slice. (**B**) Medial posterior tibial slope. (**C**) Lateral posterior tibial slope. In assessing medial PTS, the femoral condyle should not exceed 6 mm to control malrotation. The axis of the tibial shaft is located and drawn as described above and made to intersect a tangential line drawn across the medial tibial plateau. The resulting angle is subtracted from 90° to calculate medial posterior tibial slope (PTS).

folding a single-strand graft in half so that it is 2-stranded with a ligament washer at the end to serve as the attachment point for the tether sutures [1]. The group found that functional outcomes by Lysholm Knee score and Tegner Activity Scale reflected patient satisfaction and comparable outcomes with other techniques while theoretically mitigating the risk of graft failure with a fixation technique less dependent on tibial density.

5. Novel Therapeutic Suggestions
   5.1. Messina and colleagues published on the nonoperative management of PCL injury using platelets-rich-plasma (PRP) injection and found that, compared to a group of patients following a standard conservative management protocol, the PRP-treated group was able to begin physiotherapy 2 weeks earlier and completed rehabilitation sooner than the control group [21].

Postoperative radiographic assessment

To effectively interpret postoperative knee imaging in the setting of PCL reconstruction, the radiologist must understand the surgical technique as well as the normal postoperative appearance and complications. Stress radiographs may be obtained in the immediate postoperative period to evaluate tunnel position, fixation material, and joint alignment. In symptomatic patients, MRI is the optimal modality for more in-depth evaluation of the PCL reconstruction [22].

The PCL graft itself should be evaluated with multiple sequences and planes, although an oblique sagittal plane following the course of the graft is ideal. The normal MRI signal characteristics of the graft will vary based on type and age of the graft. Within the first 3 to 4 months after surgery, the avascular graft's signal will be similar to the donor tendon, demonstrating hypointensity on all sequences. Between 4 to 8 months after surgery, remodeling of the graft will be reflected in increased signal on T2WI. During this time, ensuring fiber continuity is important to differentiate normal remodeling from a tear or impingement. At 1 to 2 years, the graft signal should nearly match the native PCL, again hypointense on all sequences. It is also important to note that a variable amount of bone marrow edema is expected adjacent to the tunnels and in the fixation sites for up to 12 months after surgery [23].

Evaluation of single tunnel PCL reconstruction tunnel positioning using cross-sectional imaging has been described by multiple authors and summarized by Alcaľ-Galiano et al. The ideal tunnel locations depend on whether a single bundle or double bundle technique has been employed. In a single bundle technique, the tunnel opening should be located at the anterior half of the native PCL insertion near the AL bundle insertion, at 1 o'clock in the right knee or 11 o'clock in the left knee. This should be approximately 8 to 10 mm from the articular margin [23]. In a double bundle technique, the articular opening sites should be located with one in the anterior third of the native PCL insertion site and the other in the middle to distal third, at 1 o'clock and 3 o'clock in the right knee and at 11 o'clock and 9 o'clock in the left knee [24]. Regardless of technique, the tibial opening in both the inlay and transtibial techniques should be located at the middle of the posterior half of the retrospinal surface, just medial to the articular midline and 8 to 15 mm distal to the articular surface [22].

While some variability in tunnel positioning can be expected, an abnormally placed tunnel is considered one with 75% or more of the articular opening lying outside the anatomic insertion site. The more commonly encountered suboptimal tunnel positions are high and posterior location of the femoral tunnel(s) or increased proximal and/or anterior location of the tibial tunnel. These pitfalls may lead to a vertically oriented graft with limited resistance to posterior tibial translation [23].

Suboptimal tunnel position or the *killer turn* may lead to undue stress on the graft and subsequent graft impingement. On MRI, graft impingement manifests with thickening and increased signal intensity through the intraarticular graft on both T1 and T2 sequences. These signal characteristics will persist or progress over time—an important distinguishing factor between impingement and normal graft remodeling [23].

PCL graft disruption may occur for a variety of reasons at any point post reconstruction. In the setting of increased graft laxity or graft tear, lateral stress radiographs may demonstrate increased posterior tibial translation. MRI will demonstrate more direct signs of graft disruption with full-thickness defect or nonvisualization of the graft with increased T2 signal occupying its expected course [22].

SUMMARY

While a paucity of controlled, randomized trials exists comparing SB-PCLr to DB-PCLr, the current literature reproduces with fair reliability that double-bundle reconstruction is demonstrably superior to single-bundle with respect to reestablishing near-native knee biomechanics. It significantly decreases posterior tibial translation across a range of knee flexion as demonstrated by stress radiography. The clinical significance of these improved biomechanics remains up for debate.

While every operative approach should be tailored to the anatomy and clinical needs of the patient, this article presents a compilation of recent suggestions for operative techniques to guide decision-making in arthroscopic PCL reconstruction. What emerges in the recent literature addressing challenges in PCL reconstruction is increasing consideration for tibial slope as well as for proximal tibial bone density as the substrate for fixation and techniques for augmenting PCLr technique to theoretically extend the lifetime of the reconstruction.

As surgical techniques evolve, radiologists must be able to recognize the normal anatomic locations and appearances of both SB-PCLr and DB-PCLr. Maintaining an understanding of the normal and abnormal MRI signal characteristics of the PCL graft is crucial for the detection of potential complications that may arise following these surgeries.

LIMITATIONS

Given the nature of this article, it lacks the statistical rigor to assess the cumulative size of various treatment effects from the techniques forwarded by the studies presented here. Future publications will work to elucidate the extent of the treatment benefit afforded by emerging approaches to PCL reconstruction.

CLINICS CARE POINTS

- A growing body of literature suggests that double-bundle posterior cruciate ligament reconstruction may more closely replicate native knee biomechanics than a single-bundle technique and may theoretically extend the lifetime of the reconstruction.
- Posterior tibial slope, which can be assessed on radiograph or cross-sectional imaging, is an important preoperative consideration before potential PCL reconstruction. Flattened posterior tibial slope has been associated with higher rates of graft failure.
- Multisequence multiplanar MRI is the preferred modality for evaluation of the PCL reconstruction graft. Understanding the normal and abnormal MRI signal characteristics of the PCL graft is crucial for the detection of potential postoperative complications.
- The *killer turn* refers to the sharp turn required near the tibial fixation portion of the PCL graft, which may predispose to graft impingement.
- In both SB-PCLr and DB-PCLr, the typically encountered suboptimal tunnel positions are excessive high/posterior location of the femoral tunnel(s) and excessively proximal/anterior location of the tibial tunnel. These pitfalls limit the graft's resistance to posterior tibial translation.
- Commonly encountered PCL graft-related complications include impingement, laxity, and disruption.

DISCLOSURES

N/A.

REFERENCES

[1] Noh JH, Yoon KH, Kyung HS, et al. Multiple looping technique for tibial fixation in posterior cruciate ligament reconstruction using free tendon Achilles allograft. Knee Surg Sports Traumatol Arthrosc 2017;25(8): 2640–5.

[2] Ringler MD, Shotts EE, Collins MS, et al. Intra-articular pathology associated with isolated posterior cruciate ligament injury on MRI. Skelet Radiol 2016;45(12): 1695–703.

[3] Vasdev A, Rajgopal A, Gupta H, et al. Arthroscopic all-inside posterior cruciate ligament reconstruction: overcoming the "killer turn ". Arthrosc Tech 2016;5(3): e501–6, Published 2016 May 16.

[4] Lee OS, Lee YS. Changes in hamstring strength after anterior cruciate ligament reconstruction with hamstring autograft and posterior cruciate ligament reconstruction with tibialis allograft. Knee Surg Relat Res 2020;32(1): 27, Published 2020 Jun 5.

[5] Rhatomy S, Abadi MBT, Setyawan R, et al. Posterior cruciate ligament reconstruction with peroneus longus tendon versus hamstring tendon: a comparison of functional outcome and donor site morbidity. Knee Surg Sports Traumatol Arthrosc 2021;29(4):1045–51.

[6] Lee DW, Kim JG, Yang SJ, et al. Return to sports and clinical outcomes after arthroscopic anatomic posterior cruciate ligament reconstruction with remnant preservation. Arthroscopy 2019;35(9):2658–68.e1.

[7] Zhang H, Wang J, Gao Y, et al. Suture tape augmentation improves posterior stability after isolated posterior cruciate ligament reconstruction using hamstring tendon autograft with single-bundle transtibial technique. Arthroscopy 2024;40(7):2045–54.

[8] Deie M, Adachi N, Nakamae A, et al. Evaluation of single-bundle versus double-bundle PCL reconstructions with more than 10-year follow-up. Sci World J 2015;2015: 751465. https://doi.org/10.1155/2015/751465.

[9] Yoon KH, Kim EJ, Kwon YB, et al. Minimum 10-year results of single- versus double-bundle posterior cruciate ligament reconstruction: clinical, radiologic, and survivorship outcomes. Am J Sports Med 2019;47(4): 822–7.

[10] Li Y, Li J, Wang J, et al. Comparison of single-bundle and double-bundle isolated posterior cruciate ligament reconstruction with allograft: a prospective, randomized study. Arthroscopy 2014;30(6):695–700.

[11] Jain V, Goyal A, Mohindra M, et al. A comparative analysis of arthroscopic double-bundle versus single-bundle posterior cruciate ligament reconstruction using hamstring tendon autograft. Arch Orthop Trauma Surg 2016;136-(11):1555–61.

[12] Yoon KH, Lee JH, Kim SG, et al. Effect of posterior tibial slopes on graft survival rates at 10 years after primary single-bundle posterior cruciate ligament reconstruction. Am J Sports Med 2023;51(5):1194–201.

[13] Winkler PW, Wagala NN, Carrozzi S, et al. Low posterior tibial slope is associated with increased risk of PCL graft failure. Knee Surg Sports Traumatol Arthrosc 2022;30-(10):3277–86.

[14] Li J, Kong F, Gao X, et al. ProspECTIVE randomized comparison of knee stability and proprioception for posterior cruciate ligament reconstruction with autograft, hybrid graft, and Γ-IRRADIATED ALLOgraft. Arthroscopy 2016;32(12):2548–55.

[15] Sun X, Zhang J, Qu X, et al. Arthroscopic posterior cruciate ligament reconstruction with allograft versus autograft. Arch Med Sci 2015;11(2):395–401.

[16] Chun KC, Shin CH, Kang HT, et al. Mechanoreceptors in remnant posterior cruciate ligament and achilles tendon allografts after remnant-preserving posterior cruciate ligament reconstruction: hematoxylin-eosin and immunohistochemical assessments. Am J Sports Med 2020; 48(12):3013–20.

[17] Kernkamp WA, Jens AJT, Varady NH, et al. Anatomic is better than isometric posterior cruciate ligament tunnel placement based upon in vivo simulation. Knee Surg Sports Traumatol Arthrosc 2019;27(8):2440–9.

[18] Chernchujit B, Samart S, Na Nakorn P. Remnant-preserving posterior cruciate ligament reconstruction: arthroscopic transseptal, rod and pulley technique. Arthrosc Tech 2017;6(1):e15–20, Published 2017 Jan 2.

[19] Tachibana Y, Tanaka Y, Kinugasa K, et al. Tunnel enlargement correlates with postoperative posterior laxity after double-bundle posterior cruciate ligament reconstruction. Orthop J Sports Med 2021;9(1):23259 67120977834. https://doi.org/10.1177/232596712097 7834:Published 2021 Jan 29.

[20] Osti M, Krawinkel A, Gohm A, et al. The effectiveness of skeletal imaging for quality assessment in posterior cruciate ligament reconstruction: reliability and validity of radiographs and computed tomography. Arch Orthop Trauma Surg 2014;134(12):1731–7.

[21] Messina G, Cataldo P, Mantia F, et al. Platelets-rich-plasma in management of non operative post cruciate ligament injury. Eur J Transl Myol 2023;34(1):11535. https://doi.org/10.4081/ejtm.2023.11535.

[22] Heuck, A., & Woertler, K. (2022, June). Posttreatment imaging of the knee: cruciate ligaments and menisci. In Semin Muscoskel Radiol (Vol. 26, No. 03, pp. 230-241). Thieme Medical Publishers, Inc.

[23] Alcaľ-Galiano A, Baeva M, Ismael M, et al. Imaging of posterior cruciate ligament (PCL) reconstruction: normal postsurgical appearance and complications. Skelet Radiol 2014;43:1659–68.

[24] Noyes FR, Barber-Westin SD. Posterior cruciate ligament revision reconstruction, part 2: results of revision using a 2-strand quadriceps tendon-patellar bone autograft. Am J Sports Med 2005;33(5):655–65.

Advances in Clinical Radiology 7 (2025) 93–101
ADVANCES IN CLINICAL RADIOLOGY

Therapeutic Effectiveness of Lumbar Medial Branch Block and Lumbar Intra-articular Facet Injections, a Review of Current Concepts

Adam Delora, MD[a], Alexander Doubek, DO[b], Vishal Kathardekar, BBA[c], Ian S. Ackers, DO, PhD[d], Kush K. Goyal, MD[e,*]

[a]Cerebrovascular Center, Neurological Institute, Cleveland Clinic, Cleveland, OH 44195, USA; [b]Center for Spine Health, Neurological Institute, Cleveland Clinic, Cleveland, OH 44195, USA; [c]Northeast Ohio Medical University, Rootstown, OH 44272, USA; [d]Department of Physical Medicine & Rehabilitation, Michigan State University and University of Michigan Health - Sparrow, Lansing, MI 48912, USA; [e]Department of Physical Medicine & Rehabilitation, Cleveland Clinic Lerner College of Medicine, Case Western Reserve University, Center for Spine Health, Neurological Institute, Cleveland Clinic, Cleveland, OH 44195, USA

KEYWORDS

• Facet joint injection • Medial branch block • Zygapophyseal joint • Intra-articular facet injection • Corticosteroid • Interventional pain • Radiofrequency ablation • Chronic low back pain

KEY POINTS

- Lumbar facet joint pain is a common cause of low back pain that results in functional impairment that impacts the patient's function and quality of life.
- Diagnosis of lumbar facet joint pain is difficult, with history, physical examination, and imaging being an integral part, but ultimately, many consider medial branch blocks and intra-articular facet injections the gold standard.
- Medial branch blocks and intra-articular facet joint injections are commonly used for diagnosis and prognostication for subsequent procedures, including radiofrequency ablation, but further research needs to be done on their diagnostic and therapeutic utility.

INTRODUCTION

Lumbar facet joint (LFJ) pain is a significant contributor to chronic low back pain (LBP), a condition with a substantial impact on public health. The annual prevalence of LBP in the American population ranges from 15% to 45%, with a lifetime incidence as high as 80%, making it one of the leading causes of years lived with disability [1–3]. A comparative review of the socioeconomic cost of LBP estimates the costs at ~$40 billion or ~$2000 per patient per year in the United States alone, with the prevalence of LBP continuing to increase with the aging population [4]. LBP can result from various causes, among which the LFJs are a common cause. Facetogenic LBP is identified in 15% to 41% of individuals experiencing LBP, highlighting its role as a major cause of disability and reduced quality of life [5]. In patients who underwent provocation lumbar discography or diagnostic facet joint (FJ) or sacroiliac joint blocks, the most common generators of axial LBP included intervertebral disc (internal disc disruption [IDD]), LFJs, sacroiliac joints, along with several other less common causes like insufficiency fractures and fusion

*Corresponding author. *E-mail address:* goyalk@ccf.org

https://doi.org/10.1016/j.yacr.2025.05.008
www.advancesinclinicalradiology.com
2589-8701/25/

ABBREVIATIONS

CT	computed tomography
FJ	facet joint
FJP	facet joint pain
IA	intra-articular
IDD	internal disc disruption
LBP	low back pain
LFJ	lumbar facet joint
MBB	medial branch block
RFN	radiofrequency neurotomy
SIJP	sacroiliac joint pain

hardware–mediated soft tissue pain with an estimated prevalence of facet joint pain (FJP) of 30.6% (95% CI, 24.2% to 37.9%) [6].

FJP can arise from degeneration, inflammation, or trauma, leading to localized and referred pain. Various treatment modalities have been developed to address facetogenic LBP, including conservative approaches, such as physical therapy, and more invasive interventions, like medial branch block (MBB), intra-articular (IA) FJ injections, and denervation. These procedures aim to alleviate pain by targeting the FJ and its associated neural pathways. This article aims to provide an overview of facetogenic back pain and examine the efficacy, advantages, and limitations of MBB and IA FJ injections as therapeutic options for its treatment.

ANATOMY AND PATHOPHYSIOLOGY

LFJs are synovial joints formed by the articulation of the inferior and superior articular process of 2 adjacent lumbar vertebrae (Fig. 1). They are surrounded by a fibrous capsule enclosing the bones and articular cartilage and extend into the periosteum. The capsule consists of an inner layer with a thin, sleevelike synovial membrane made of fibers and another layer of adipose tissue [7,8]. Extending from the joint capsule at the upper and lower poles, the membrane projects between the articular facets to form a fibroadipose meniscoid, which distributes forces evenly across the joint and improves its stability [9]. Similar to other joints, the cartilage of the FJ is aneural. The subchondral bone, synovium, and joint capsule are innervated extensively [10]. LFJs are innervated by the medial branch, a nerve from the dorsal ramus of the spinal nerve. Each joint capsule has 2 medial branch nerves innervating it, one from the same spinal level and another from the level above. The medial branches originate from the dorsal rami and innervate the FJ and the multifidus muscle [11].

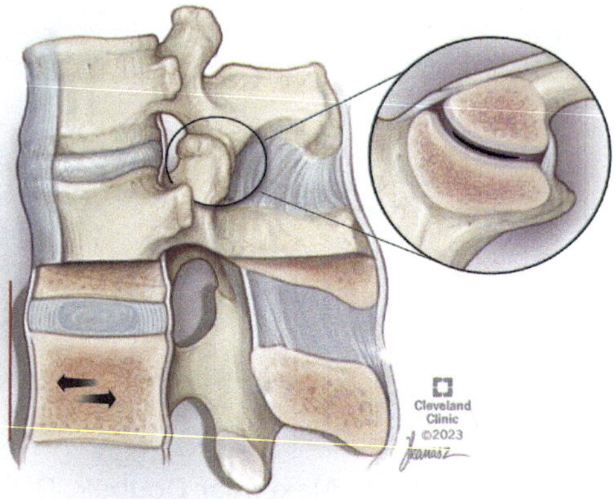

FIG. 1 The FJs with cross-sections of the joint showing the joint and capsule. (*Reprinted with permission*, Cleveland Clinic Foundation © 2025. All Rights Reserved.)

The most common cause of facetogenic LBP is LFJ osteoarthritis or arthropathy. Its degenerative process involves cartilage, subchondral bone, synovium, joint capsule, and periarticular soft tissues (Fig. 2) [12]. One mechanism for LFJ osteoarthritis was elevated subchondral bone resorption and turnover [13]. LFJ osteoarthritis has been found in patients with LBP from ages ranging from 15 all the way through older adults with a mean age of 67, suggesting that LFJ osteoarthritis is highly prevalent among individuals across a wide age range with LBP [14,15]. The causes of osteoarthritis can be multifactorial. Although osteoarthritis is prevalent, a retrospective showed that the cause of axial back pain is more likely to be IDD in younger patients,

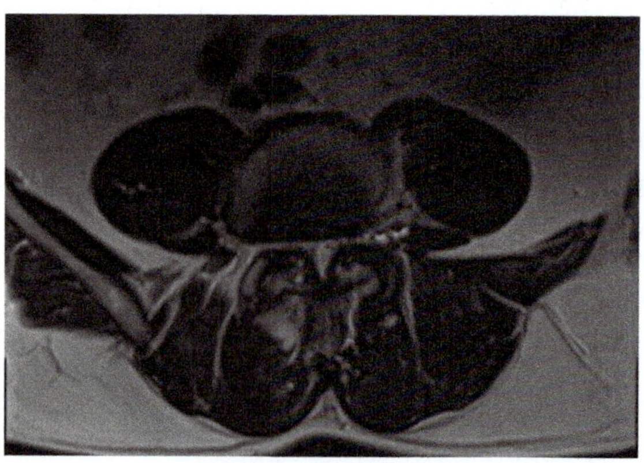

FIG. 2 Facet arthropathy on T2-weighted MRI. Note the increased facet hypertrophy, osteophytes, and subchondral sclerosis.

and FJP and sacroiliac joint pain (SIJP) increase with age [16]. Several studies suggest that degeneration of the intervertebral disc and the 2 LFJs may influence each other or that LFJ degeneration may follow disc degeneration [17,18]. Eubanks and colleagues [19] found that in younger patients, FJ osteoarthritis may occur before disc degeneration, which provided an alternate mechanism compared with other studies that may have indicated that they were linked. Inflammation or trauma to the LFJ is also a cause for facetogenic LBP, and it has been suggested that increased inflammatory cytokines contribute to the pain [20,21].

The medial branch traverses through the fibro-osseous canal created by the mammillary process superiorly, the accessory process inferiorly, the bony groove between the mammillary and accessory processes anteriorly, and the mammillary accessory process posteriorly [7]. The multifidus is the deepest and most medial muscle layer of the paraspinal musculature (Fig. 3) [11]. The lumbar paraspinal musculature is an integral structure in regard to the anatomy and function of the LFJ. The paraspinal musculature provides motion and stabilization of the spine [22]. The paraspinal musculature also provides proprioception primarily through the multifidus [23]. The multifidus also contributes to spinal segmental stability by opposing flexion and providing increased stiffness at the spinal segment [24,25]. The multifidus has the largest cross-sectional area with the shortest fiber length, which allows the multifidus to produce the highest force of all paraspinal musculature. This inherently provides stability rather than motion [24]. Because there is a concern for a possible increase in lumbar spine instability owing to radiofrequency ablation causing denervation of the multifidus muscle, other therapeutic options are of interest to the spine/pain community.

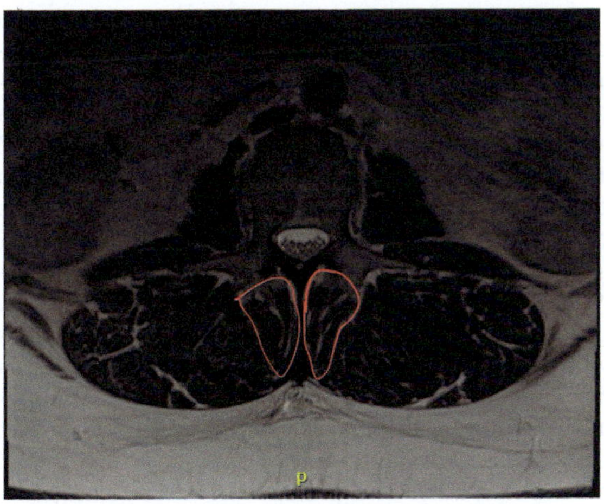

FIG. 3 T2-weighted MRI highlighting the location of multifidus muscles. (*Red circles*) identifying multifidus muscle on MRI.

Certain radiographic features make IA facet injection difficult. More specifically, facet arthropathy at the most posterior aspect of the lumbar facet may lend to difficult or nonaccessible IA facet injection. Therefore, reviewing lumbar MRI and computed tomography (CT) scans is paramount to preprocedure planning. CT scan (if available) will provide a better approximation of accessibility of the posterior aspect of the facet and will allow for better planar to cross-sectional correlation (Fig. 4) than MRI. For younger patients (age <50) where facet arthropathy is not as prevalent compared with age greater than the 50s, it may be possible to offer IA facet injections (see Fig. 2). For example, in young athletes with mechanical and axial back pain, an IA approach may be beneficial. The medial branch technique is the more prevalent technique, as most patients with mechanical and axial back pain are aged greater than 50 [16]. In addition, IA facet injections are particularly useful for aspiration and/or rupture of a synovial cyst [26].

Previous literature, along with a more recent publication, supports a therapeutic effect of lumbar facet steroid with medial branch and IA technique with patients with spondylolisthesis [27]. This study showed no statistically significant difference in pain relief or patient-reported outcomes in patients receiving MBB or IA facet injection with or without spondylolisthesis. Some patients had radiographic dynamic instability with open facet sign on MRI and/or change greater than 3 mm in standing radiograph compared with supine MRI [28].

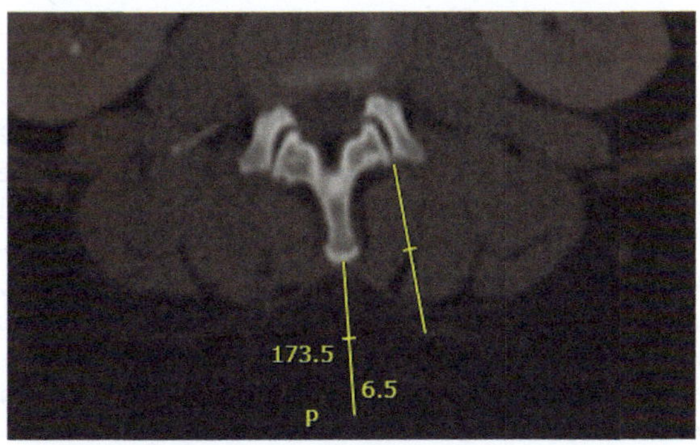

FIG. 4 CT image depicting angle measurement for needle trajectory while performing FJ access. This analysis can be used for cross-sectional to planar correlation to aid in access.

DIAGNOSIS

Diagnosing LFJ pain represents a diagnostic challenge owing to overlap with other causes of LBP. With a poor correlation between imaging and the gold-standard diagnostic blocks, understanding how to use the history and physical examination to guide diagnosis and treatment is paramount. Using discography and diagnostic blocks to diagnose the cause of LBP, a previous retrospective chart review showed the prevalence of IDD, FJP, and SIJP was 42%, 31%, and 18%, respectively [16]. Accurate diagnosis is essential to effective treatment. A thorough history and physical examination can help guide imaging and diagnostic procedures. A retrospective chart review of patients who underwent diagnostic spinal procedures found that significantly fewer patients with IDD (67.3%; $P=.0003$) reported paramedian pain as compared with cases of FJP (95.0%) or SIJP (96.0%), which reported less midline pain. In addition, only 15.4% who reported midline pain had FJP [29]. A multivariate retrospective review looking at the relationship between age, hip/girdle pain, leg pain, and thigh pain found that IDD was much more common in younger patients than FJP or SIJP. As patients age, the presence of thigh pain predicts FJP-mediated pain over SIJP [30]. A study in 1976 that carried out contrast-enhanced LFJ injection under fluoroscopy with an irritant found that the most common pain referral patterns were to the buttock, greater trochanter, and posterior thigh, and it was challenging to differentiate patterns of radiation from the L4-5 or L5-S1 joints [31].

Physical examination maneuvers have sparse evidence for ruling in and out facet-mediated joint pain. The extension rotation test, which is also known as Kemp's Test or facet loading, is a common physical examination maneuver that shows poor sensitivity in most studies but may have some negative predictive value, with negative results helping to rule out FJP, whereas positive results may not be clinically meaningful [32]. Finding a test or historical feature to rule in FJP has proved difficult, with one study looking at the site of back pain, the pattern of referral pain, forward flexion, extension, rotation of the trunk in both directions, rotation with extension, and straight leg test, and none of these maneuvers or historical features were found to be associated with response to the confirmatory block [33]. Subsequent research focused on combinations of historical features and physical examination findings that were able to predict responders. One example is Revel's Criteria, which included age greater than 65, pain relief with recumbent position, and absence of pain with coughing, forward flexion, rising from flexion, extension, and extension/rotation. Five of seven positive variables identified 92% of responders and 80% of nonresponders to injection [34]. A prospective study that used McKenzie-trained physical therapists and single diagnostic injections found that FJP did not have pain when rising from sitting and lacked centralization of pain [35]. A subsequent study with 2 diagnostic blocks and physical therapist evaluation also showed that the absence of pain when rising from sitting correlated with relief and that lack of centralization and positive extension rotation were highly sensitive but not specific. Increasing age also predicted pain relief with diagnostic injections [36]. This study also combined their data to make a pain prediction rule with age greater than 50, improved pain when walking or sitting, paraspinal pain at onset, Modified Somatic Perception Questionnaire score greater than 14, extension rotation test, and absence of centralization during repeated movement testing. They were unable to reproduce the results of Revel's Criteria. Altogether, the history and physical examination tend to have a higher sensitivity and negative predictive value, helping physicians to determine patients whose blocks will likely not result in relief.

According to consensus practice guidelines, response to IA facet injections or MBBs is the gold standard for diagnosing the FJs as the cause of LBP [37]. Using imaging to predict response to diagnostic blockade has proven difficult in multiple imaging modalities. Radiographs can show narrowing of the FJ space, subarticular bone erosions, subchondral cysts, and osteophyte formation, and hypertrophy of the articular process that is better seen on oblique views has been found to have 55% sensitivity and 69% specificity in distinguishing the presence from the absence of FJ osteoarthritis when compared with CT [38]. Although MRI is better at delineating active synovial inflammation, FJ effusions, and other causes of LBP, like IDD, to help rule out FJP, CT is better at evaluating the bony cortex margin [39]. Unfortunately, facet degeneration on CT does not correlate to the presence of LBP. As many as 8% to 14% of patients without back pain have some level of facet degeneration on CT or MRI that increases with age [40,41]. More recent research has looked at different imaging features and imaging modalities and their ability to predict response to the diagnostic block. One such study looked at facet synovitis and facet arthropathy. The presence of facet arthropathy on MRI did not predict response to lumbar facet injections, but the presence of bilateral facet synovitis

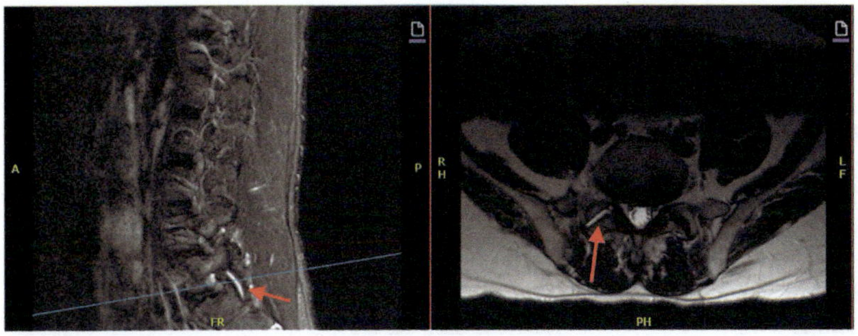

FIG. 5 FJ effusion seen on the right-sided FJ. (left) Sagittal T2-weighted short tau inversion recovery MRI. (*right*) Axial T2-weighted MRI.

characterized by edema and inflammatory changes affecting the FJs, adjacent bone marrow, and surrounding soft tissues seen on fat-saturated T2-weighted imaging had lower pain scores and decreased burden from work and daily activity (Fig. 5) [42]. Further research should be carried out looking at the relationship between facet synovitis and a positive MBB as compared with IA injection with and without steroids. Several studies have looked at the ability of SPECT (single-photon emission computed tomography)-CT to predict a positive response to IA facet injection or MBBs and results have been mixed; consensus guidelines currently do not support its use [37,43–46].

TREATMENT

MBB is a procedure in which the use of anesthesia blocks the transmission of pain signals from the nerves. Although this does not alter the course of underlying pathologic condition, it can provide symptomatic pain relief for people experiencing LBP. It must be performed on at least 2 spinal levels, one at the level of the FJ and the other at the level above, and using a local anesthetic, such as lidocaine or bupivacaine, can be done with or without steroids (Figs. 6 and 7) [47]. Typically, an MBB is performed as a diagnostic block before a radiofrequency neurotomy (RFN) to confirm the source of LBP and predict the success of an RFN [48]. Several studies show varying lengths of relief with these diagnostic injections [49,50]. One study by Cohen and colleagues [51] found no pain relief beyond the diagnostic window when using bupivacaine and corticosteroid. However, these results should be tempered with understanding that the inclusion criteria were based on 3 months or more of axial low back with paraspinal muscle tenderness and not a mechanical examination to confirm facet-mediated pain. A different study by Sadeghian and Motiei-Langroudi [50] demonstrated that LFJ blocks may potentiate effects lasting an average length of 2 months. Another study demonstrating longer-term relief of LBP was conducted by Liu and colleagues [52], which showed that 35% of patients experience prolonged relief beyond the expected timeframe. Those who showed extended pain relief typically had LBP symptoms that lasted less than 6 months (more of an acute onset) as well as unilateral back pain, although the mechanism for the prolonged pain reduction was unclear. Recently, research has shown that MBBs have a greater therapeutic benefit compared with IA injections, according to a review by Manchikanti and colleagues [53]. This could be for several reasons, one being the procedure is technically less difficult than IA injections [54].

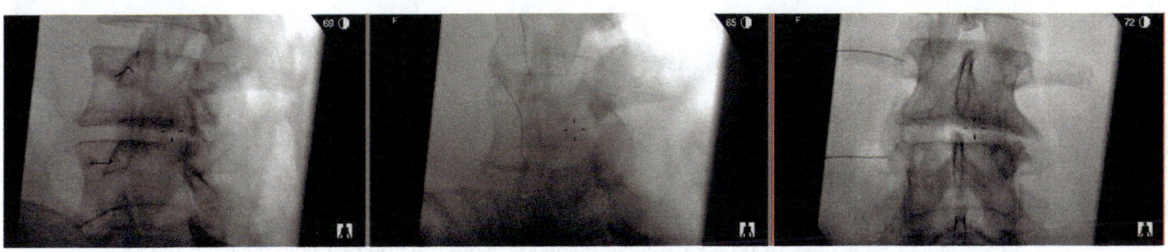

FIG. 6 Optimal lumbar MBB needle placement on fluoroscopy.

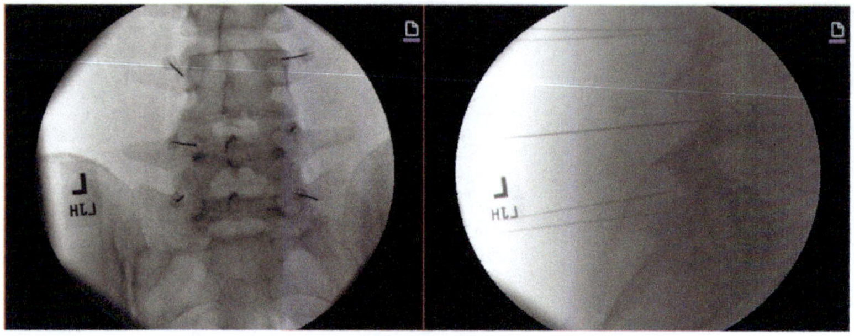

FIG. 7 Suboptimal lumbar MBB needle placement on fluoroscopy.

IA injections may play a key role in the treatment of facetogenic back pain by injecting an anesthetic and a steroid into the joint capsule. This provides pain relief by interrupting the transmission of pain signals both centrally and peripherally and by reducing inflammation in the affected joint (Fig. 8) [55]. IA injections, through several studies, have been shown to be effective in the reduction of facetogenic LBP at various follow-up periods. Fuchs and colleagues [56] found that patients receiving steroid injections had a 56% reduction in pain scores compared with a 40% reduction in pain scores for those receiving a hyaluronate injection at 6 months postinjection. Lakemeier and colleagues [57] randomly assigned patients to either IA steroid injections or radiofrequency denervation, a procedure where the medial branch nerves of the corresponding FJs are ablated at 80°C to 90°C, and found that there were no significant differences in pain relief and functional improvement. Carette and colleagues [58] showed that after 1 month, 42% of patients who received methylprednisolone indicated a marked or very marked improvement in LBP compared with 33% of patients who received a placebo injection, and at 6 months postinjection patients who were treated with the steroid reported less pain and physical disability. Although IA injections do provide pain relief for LBP, it is unclear whether patients can receive long-term relief. Kennedy and colleagues [59,60], in 2 studies, demonstrated that there was no significant difference in the need for RFN in patients who received IA or saline groups at a 1-year follow-up. There is low-grade evidence that IA and MBBs with corticosteroid provide clinically significant therapeutic benefit beyond their diagnostic window, and therefore, their use should be limited to pre-RFN procedures, which is currently consistent with 2020 North American Spine Society (NASS) Low Back Pain Guidelines. Although RFN has become the standard treatment for facetogenic LBP, there are important physiologic ramifications when performing lumbar medial branch RFN. There is mixed evidence that denervation of the medial branches via RFN may cause atrophy of the multifidus [61,62]. A study by Smuck and colleagues [63] measuring the cross-sectional area of the multifidus pre-RFN and post-RFN demonstrated a decrease in the size of multifidus following RFN treatment. The change in the cross-sectional area did not reach statistical significance, although it did show a trend toward size reduction in the posttreatment group ($P = .06$). There was a statistically significant increase in disc

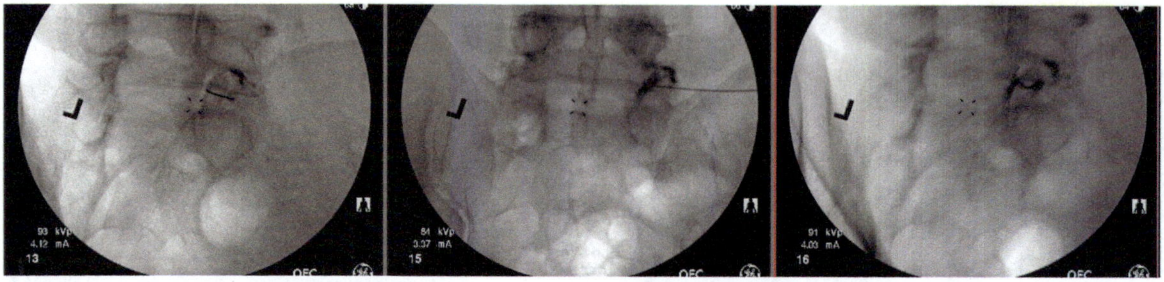

FIG. 8 Successful IA FJ access using fluoroscopic guidance. Note the contrast flow outlining the joint confirming joint access.

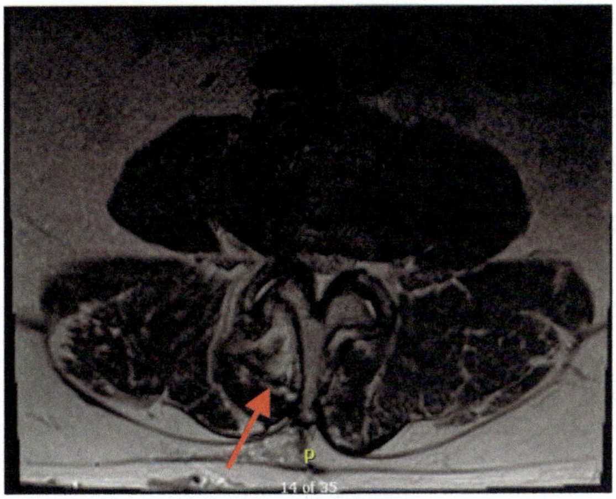

FIG. 9 T2 MRI depicting increased fat atrophy within multifidus. (*Arrow*) demonstrating multifiudus atrophy.

degeneration using the Pfirrmann grading system (Fig. 9). The long-term clinical significance of iatrogenic multifidus atrophy is not fully understood. A retrospective analysis by Caragea and colleagues [64] evaluating the long-term progression of spondylolisthesis following RFN did not demonstrate the acceleration of spondylolisthesis. However, patients with post-RFN lumbar fusion were excluded from this study.

SUMMARY

LFJ pain represents a significant contribution to chronic LBP, a condition that substantially impacts quality of life and public health. As highlighted, the pathophysiology of facetogenic LBP is complex, involving degenerative, inflammatory, and traumatic processes that necessitate targeted treatment approaches. MBB and IA FJ injections are widely used interventions that aim to alleviate pain by addressing the FJ and its associated neural pathways. MBB is particularly valued for its diagnostic utility in identifying facetogenic pain and predicting the success of subsequent RFN. Although some studies have demonstrated short-term pain relief with MBB for mechanical back pain, evidence suggests limited therapeutic benefit beyond the diagnostic window in many cases when inclusion criteria are based primarily on paraspinal muscle tenderness. Conversely, IA injections have been shown to reduce inflammation and provide symptomatic relief in select patient populations. However, similar to MBB, their long-term efficacy remains uncertain, with mixed results regarding sustained pain relief and functional improvement. Despite their potential benefits, both MBB and IA injections are primarily considered diagnostic tools, as supported by the 2020 NASS Low Back Pain Guidelines. The declining use of these interventions over recent years underscores the need for further research to better define their role in managing facetogenic LBP and to explore alternative or adjunctive treatments that may offer more enduring outcomes.

Ultimately, although MBB and IA injections are valuable components of a multifaceted approach to managing facetogenic LBP, ongoing studies are essential to clarify their efficacy, refine patient selection criteria, and optimize treatment protocols to improve clinical outcomes.

CLINICS CARE POINTS

- Intra-articular facet injections are particularly useful for aspiration and/or rupture of lumbar facet synovial cyst.
- Reviewing lumbar MRI and computed tomographic scans is paramount to preprocedure planning. A computed tomographic CT scan can provide a better approximation of accessibility of the posterior aspect of the facet.
- Lumbar facet arthropathy, especially when associated with spondylolisthesis, can affect placement of spinal needles for medial branch technique.
- Treatment of facet arthropathy includes intra-articular facet injection, lumbar medial branch block with corticosteroid, and lumbar facet medial branch radiofrequency ablation with varying degrees of evidence for therapeutic benefit.

DISCLOSURE

None.

REFERENCES

[1] Shraim M, Cifuentes M, Willetts JL, et al. Length of disability and medical costs in low back pain: do state workers' compensation policies make a difference? J Occup Environ Med 2015;57(12):1275–83.

[2] Ehrlich GE. Low back pain. Bull World Health Organ 2003;81(9):671–6.

[3] Andersson GB. Epidemiological features of chronic low-back pain. Lancet 1999;354(9178):581–5.

[4] Chang D, Lui A, Matsoyan A, et al. Comparative review of the socioeconomic burden of lower back pain in the United States and globally. Neurospine 2024;21(2):487–501.

[5] Curtis L, Shah N, Padalia D. Facet joint disease. In: StatPearls. Treasure Island (FL): StatPearls Publishing; 2025.

[6] DePalma MJ, Ketchum JM, Ruchala M, et al. Prevalence of disc, facet joint or sacroiliac joint pain in low back pain patients utilizing an algorithmic approach: GP100. Spine Journal Meeting Abstracts 2010;242.

[7] Kapetanakis S, Gkantsinikoudis N. Anatomy of lumbar facet joint: a comprehensive review. Folia Morphol (Warsz) 2021;80(4):799–805.

[8] Yamashita T, Minaki Y, Ozaktay AC, et al. A morphological study of the fibrous capsule of the human lumbar facet joint. Spine (Phila Pa 1976) 1996; 21(5):538–43.

[9] Bogduk N, Engel R. The menisci of the lumbar zygapophyseal joints. A review of their anatomy and clinical significance. Spine (Phila Pa 1976) 1984;9(5): 454–60.

[10] O'Leary SA, Paschos NK, Link JM, et al. Facet joints of the spine: structure-function relationships, problems and treatments, and the potential for regeneration. Annu Rev Biomed Eng 2018;20:145–70.

[11] Bogduk N, Wilson AS, Tynan W. The human lumbar dorsal rami. J Anat 1982;134(Pt 2):383–97.

[12] Du R, Xu G, Bai X, et al. Facet joint syndrome: pathophysiology, diagnosis, and treatment. J Pain Res 2022; 15:3689–710.

[13] Netzer C, Distel P, Wolfram U, et al. Comparative analysis of bone structural parameters reveals subchondral cortical plate resorption and increased trabecular bone remodeling in human facet joint osteoarthritis. Int J Mol Sci 2018;19(3):845.

[14] Li J, Muehleman C, Abe Y, et al. Prevalence of facet joint degeneration in association with intervertebral joint degeneration in a sample of organ donors. J Orthop Res 2011;29(8):1267–74.

[15] Suri P, Hunter DJ, Rainville J, et al. Presence and extent of severe facet joint osteoarthritis are associated with back pain in older adults. Osteoarthr Cartil 2013; 21(9):1199–206.

[16] DePalma MJ, Ketchum JM, Saullo T. What is the source of chronic low back pain and does age play a role? Pain Med 2011;12(2):224–33.

[17] Bashkuev M, Reitmaier S, Schmidt H. Relationship between intervertebral disc and facet joint degeneration: a probabilistic finite element model study. J Biomech 2020;102:109518.

[18] Goda Y, Sakai T, Harada T, et al. Degenerative changes of the facet joints in adults with lumbar spondylolysis. Clin Spine Surg 2017;30(6):E738–42.

[19] Eubanks JD, Lee MJ, Cassinelli E, et al. Does lumbar facet arthrosis precede disc degeneration? A postmortem study. Clin Orthop Relat Res 2007;464:184–9.

[20] Kim JS, Ali MH, Wydra F, et al. Characterization of degenerative human facet joints and facet joint capsular tissues. Osteoarthr Cartil 2015;23(12):2242–51.

[21] Igarashi A, Kikuchi S, Konno S, et al. Inflammatory cytokines released from the facet joint tissue in degenerative lumbar spinal disorders. Spine (Phila Pa 1976) 2004; 29(19):2091–5.

[22] Gellhorn AC, Katz JN, Suri P. Osteoarthritis of the spine: the facet joints. Nat Rev Rheumatol 2013;9(4):216–24.

[23] Bastide G, Zadeh J, Lefèbvre D. Are the "little muscles" what we think they are? Surg Radiol Anat 1989;11(4): 255–6.

[24] Macintosh JE, Bogduk N. The biomechanics of the lumbar multifidus. Clin Biomech (Bristol) 1986;1(4):205–13.

[25] Panjabi M, Abumi K, Duranceau J, et al. Spinal stability and intersegmental muscle forces. A biomechanical model. Spine (Phila Pa 1976) 1989;14(2):194–200.

[26] Kuriakose B, Bashir D, Saremi A, et al. Effectiveness of lumbar facet synovial cyst aspiration and/or rupture. Adv Clin Radiol 2024;6(1):99–106.

[27] Ackers IS, Witzke JA, Saremi A, et al. Therapeutic effectiveness of lumbar medial branch block and lumbar intra-articular facet injections: a propensity-matched cohort study. Cureus 2025;17(3):e79962.

[28] Saremi A, Goyal KK, Benzel EC, et al. Evolution of lumbar degenerative spondylolisthesis with key radiographic features. Spine J 2024;24(6):989–1000.

[29] Depalma MJ, Ketchum JM, Trussell BS, et al. Does the location of low back pain predict its source? Pharm Manag PM R 2011;3(1):33–9.

[30] Laplante BL, Ketchum JM, Saullo TR, et al. Multivariable analysis of the relationship between pain referral patterns and the source of chronic low back pain. Pain Physician 2012;15(2):171–8.

[31] Mooney V, Robertson J. The facet syndrome. Clin Orthop Relat Res 1976;115:149–56.

[32] Stuber K, Lerede C, Kristmanson K, et al. The diagnostic accuracy of the Kemp's test: a systematic review. J Can Chiropr Assoc 2014;58(3):258–67.

[33] Schwarzer AC, Derby R, Aprill CN, et al. Pain from the lumbar zygapophysial joints: a test of two models. J Spinal Disord 1994;7(4):331–6.

[34] Revel M, Poiraudeau S, Auleley GR, et al. Capacity of the clinical picture to characterize low back pain relieved by facet joint anesthesia. Proposed criteria to identify patients with painful facet joints. Spine (Phila Pa 1976) 1998;23(18):1972–6 [discussion: 1977].

[35] Young S, Aprill C, Laslett M. Correlation of clinical examination characteristics with three sources of chronic low back pain. Spine J 2003;3(6):460–5.

[36] Laslett M, McDonald B, Aprill CN, et al. Clinical predictors of screening lumbar zygapophyseal joint blocks: development of clinical prediction rules. Spine J 2006; 6(4):370–9.

[37] Cohen SP, Bhaskar A, Bhatia A, et al. Consensus practice guidelines on interventions for lumbar facet joint pain from a multispecialty, international working group. Reg Anesth Pain Med 2020;45(6):424–67.

[38] Pathria M, Sartoris DJ, Resnick D. Osteoarthritis of the facet joints: accuracy of oblique radiographic assessment. Radiology 1987;164(1):227–30.

[39] Kalichman L, Hunter DJ. Lumbar facet joint osteoarthritis: a review. Semin Arthritis Rheum 2007;37(2): 69–80.

[40] Wiesel SW, Tsourmas N, Feffer HL, et al. A study of computer-assisted tomography. I. The incidence of positive CAT scans in an asymptomatic group of patients. Spine (Phila Pa 1976) 1984;9(6):549–51.

[41] Jensen MC, Brant-Zawadzki MN, Obuchowski N, et al. Magnetic resonance imaging of the lumbar spine in people without back pain. N Engl J Med 1994;331(2): 69–73.

[42] Green MS, Hal MV, Onimus M, et al. Association between MRI findings of facet arthropathy and synovitis with health-related outcome and pain scores following therapeutic lumbar facet injections. Anesthesiol Res Pract 2024;2024(1):7889539.

[43] Scholten P, Sheikh M, Atchison J, et al. Correlating SPECT-CT activity in lumbar facet joints with response to lumbar medial branch and L5 dorsal ramus blocks. Interventional Pain Medicine 2024;3(1):100387.

[44] Ackerman WE, Ahmad M. Pain relief with intraarticular or medial branch nerve blocks in patients with positive lumbar facet joint SPECT imaging: a 12-week outcome study. South Med J 2008;101(9):931–4.

[45] Tender GC, Davidson C, Shields J, et al. Primary pain generator identification by CT-SPECT in patients with degenerative spinal disease. Neurosurg Focus 2019; 47(6):E18.

[46] Freiermuth D, Kretzschmar M, Bilecen D, et al. Correlation of 99m Tc-DPD SPECT/CT scan findings and diagnostic blockades of lumbar medial branches in patients with unspecific low back pain in a randomized-controlled trial. Pain Med 2015;16(10):1916–22.

[47] Won HS, Yang M, Kim YD. Facet joint injections for management of low back pain: a clinically focused review. Anesth Pain Med (Seoul) 2020;15(1):8–18.

[48] Wong MJ, Rajarathinam M. Ultrasound-guided axial facet joint interventions for chronic spinal pain: a narrative review. Can J Pain 2023;7(2):2193617.

[49] Kershen LM, Nacey NC, Patrie JT, et al. Fluoroscopically guided facet injections: comparison of intra-articular and periarticular steroid and anesthetic injection on immediate and short-term pain relief. AJNR Am J Neuroradiol 2018;39(11):2161–5.

[50] Sadeghian H, Motiei-Langroudi R. Sonography guided lumbar nerve and facet blocks: the first report of clinical outcome from Iran. Radiography (Lond) 2018;24(1): 52–6.

[51] Cohen SP, Doshi TL, Constantinescu OC, et al. Effectiveness of lumbar facet joint blocks and predictive value before radiofrequency denervation: the facet treatment study (FACTS), a randomized, controlled clinical trial. Anesthesiology 2018;129(3):517–35.

[52] Liu M, Shaparin N, Nair S, et al. Chronic low back pain: the therapeutic benefits of diagnostic medial branch nerve blocks. Pain Physician 2021;24(4):E521–8.

[53] Manchikanti L, Hirsch JA, Falco FJ, et al. Management of lumbar zygapophysial (facet) joint pain. World J Orthop 2016;7(5):315–37.

[54] Perolat R, Kastler A, Nicot B, et al. Facet joint syndrome: from diagnosis to interventional management. Insights Imaging 2018;9(5):773–89.

[55] Baroncini A, Maffulli N, Eschweiler J, et al. Management of facet joints osteoarthritis associated with chronic low back pain: a systematic review. Surgeon 2021;19(6): e512–8.

[56] Fuchs S, Erbe T, Fischer H-L, et al. Intraarticular hyaluronic acid versus glucocorticoid injections for nonradicular pain in the lumbar spine. J Vasc Interv Radiol 2005;16(11):1493–8.

[57] Lakemeier S, Lind M, Schultz W, et al. A comparison of intraarticular lumbar facet joint steroid injections and lumbar facet joint radiofrequency denervation in the treatment of low back pain: a randomized, controlled, double-blind trial. Anesth Analg 2013;117(1):228–35.

[58] Carette S, Marcoux S, Truchon R, et al. A controlled trial of corticosteroid injections into facet joints for chronic low back pain. N Engl J Med 1991;325(14):1002–7.

[59] Kennedy DJ, Huynh L, Wong J, et al. Corticosteroid injections into lumbar facet joints: a prospective, randomized, double-blind placebo-controlled trial. Am J Phys Med Rehabil 2018;97(10):741–6.

[60] Kennedy DJ, Fraiser R, Zheng P, et al. Intra-articular steroids vs saline for lumbar Z-joint pain: a prospective, randomized, double-blind placebo-controlled trial. Pain Med 2019;20(2):246–51.

[61] Dreyfuss P, Stout A, Aprill C, et al. The significance of multifidus atrophy after successful radiofrequency neurotomy for low back pain. Pharm Manag PM R 2009; 1(8):719–22.

[62] Guven AE, Evangelisti G, Burkhard MD, et al. Asymmetrical atrophy of the paraspinal muscles in patients undergoing unilateral lumbar medial branch radiofrequency neurotomy. Pain 2024;165(9):2130–4.

[63] Smuck M, Crisostomo RA, Demirjian R, et al. Morphologic changes in the lumbar spine after lumbar medial branch radiofrequency neurotomy: a quantitative radiological study. Spine J 2015;15(6):1415–21.

[64] Caragea M, Le A, Curtis T, et al. Does medial branch radiofrequency neurotomy accelerate degenerative lumbar spondylolisthesis compared to natural progression? A cross-sectional cohort study. Interv Pain Med 2023; 2(4):100289.

Advances in Clinical Radiology 7 (2025) 103–128
ADVANCES IN CLINICAL RADIOLOGY

Updates and Advances in Neuroimaging of Neonatal Encephalopathy

Vivek Pai, MD[a,b,1], Ting Guo, PhD[c,1], Manohar Shroff, MD, FRCPC[a,b,*]
[a]Division of Neuroradiology, Department of Diagnostic and Interventional Radiology, The Hospital for Sick Children, 170 Elizabeth Street, Toronto, Onatrio M5G 1E8, Canada; [b]Department of Medical Imaging, University of Toronto, 263 McCaul Street, 4th Floor, Toronto, Onatrio M5T 1W7, Canada; [c]Department of Neurosciences and Mental Health, The Hospital for Sick Children Research Institute, Toronto, Canada

KEYWORDS
• Neonatal encephalopathy • Hypoxic-ishemic encephalopathy • MRI

KEY POINTS

- Neonatal encephalopathy is most commonly caused by hypoxic-ischemic encephalopathy (HIE), though other causes (eg, infections, metabolic derangements/disorders, trauma, and congenital disorders) may be encountered.
- Timing the MRI after treatment of therapeutic hypothermia is crucial in accurately estimating the extent of brain injury and providing appropriate prognosis in patients with HIE.
- Posthemorrhagic ventricular dilatation is a delayed manifestation of intraventricular haemorrhage in preterm neonates with serial head ultrasound being an important imaging tool for diagnosis and follow-up assessment.

INTRODUCTION

Neonatal encephalopathy (NE) encompasses a broad continuum of disorders causing altered neurologic function in neonates [1]. According to the World Health Organization, NE is one of the top 10 causes of lost years of life [1]. Nearly half of the cases diagnosed with NE are due to hypoxic-ischemic encephalopathy (HIE), that is, impaired brain function caused by insufficient cerebral oxygenation and blood flow [1,2]. Other common causes of NE include infections, metabolic derangements/disorders, trauma, and congenital disorders. Irrespective of the cause, NE typically manifests with decreased level of consciousness, reduced reactivity, reduced spontaneous activity, abnormal tone, poor suck and/or diminution of primitive reflexes [3]. It is important to note that NE may be acute or chronic; the etiologies of these are distinct, but clinical overlap may exist, making diagnosis and management challenging [3]. Thanks to its excellent inherent spatial and contrast resolution, devoid of radiation, MRI is the imaging modality of choice in the evaluation of a patient with NE [3]. Using conventional imaging techniques, MRI accurately defines lesional extent, estimates the time of insult, and helps identify the cause of NE (HIE and beyond) [4]. With the advent of newer imaging techniques, MRI promises even better diagnostic capabilities in NE [4]. In this article we discuss the common causes of NE with an imaging review and provide an overview of the new and emerging techniques in the diagnosis of NE.

[1] First authors.

*Corresponding author. Division of Neuroradiology, Department of Diagnostic and Interventional Radiology, The Hospital for Sick Children, 170 Elizabeth Street, Toronto, Onatrio M5G 1E8, Canada. *E-mail address:* Manohar.shroff@sickkids.ca

https://doi.org/10.1016/j.yacr.2025.05.009 www.advancesinclinicalradiology.com
2589-8701/25/

ABBREVIATIONS

ADC	apparent diffusion coefficient
AHW	anterior horn width
ASL	arterial spin labeling
AUC	area under curve
BGT	basal ganglia–thalamus
CI	confidence interval
CMV	cytomegalovirus
CNS	central nervous system
CSF	cerebrospinal fluid
cUS	cranial ultrasound
DKI	diffusion kurtosis imaging
DL	deep learning
dMRI	diffusion MRI
DTI	diffusion tensor imaging
DWI	diffusion-weighted imaging
EEG	electroencephalogram
Epo	erythropoietin
fNIRS	functional near-infrared spectroscopy
fUS	functional ultrasound
GABA	gamma-aminobutyric acid
GM	germinal matrix
HIE	hypoxic-ischemic encephalopathy
ISO	isotropic volume fraction
IVH	intraventricular hemorrhage
MCA	middle cerebral artery
MK	mean kurtosis
MRA	magnetic resonance angiography
MRS	magnetic resonance spectroscopy
NAA	*N*-acetylaspartate
NDI	neurite density index
NE	neonatal encephalopathy
NH	neonatal hypoglycemia
NODDI	neurite orientation dispersion and density imaging
ODI	orientation dispersion index
PAIS	perinatal arterial ischemic stroke
PLICs	posterior limbs of the internal capsules
PVHD	posthemorrhagic ventricular dilatation
PVHI	periventricular hemorrhagic infarction
RK	radial kurtosis
ROI	region-of-interest
rs-fMRI	resting-state fMRI
SNR	signal-to-noise ratio
SWI	susceptibility-weighted imaging
TH	therapeutic hypothermia
TOBY	total body hypothermia for neonatal encephalopathy
TOF	time-of-flight
WM	white matter

HYPOXIC-ISCHEMIC ENCEPHALOPATHY

HIE is a consequence of altered or loss of normal cerebral autoregulation due to a combination of inadequate cerebral blood flow (ie, ischemia) and impaired oxygen delivery to the brain (ie, hypoxia) [5]. Perinatal asphyxia is the most important cause of neonatal HIE [6]. In the setting of HIE, the combination of reduced cerebral blood flow, hypoxemia, hypercarbia, and hypotension trigger a cascade of deleterious neurologic events (inflammatory mediators and excitatory neurotransmitter release, free radical formation, calcium accumulation, lipid peroxidation, and breakdown of the blood-brain barrier) culminating in permanent neuronal death [6]. The incidence of neonatal HIE is estimated at 2.5 per 1000 nonanomalous term live births and approximately 7 per 1000 preterm births [5]. Albeit advances in detection and marked improvement in obstetric/perinatal care, HIE still accounts for almost 23% of world's neonatal deaths and remains a major contributor (up to 25%) of permanent neurologic deficits (cerebral palsy, mental retardation, and seizures) among survivors [5,7].

Rationale of MRI and Therapeutic Hypothermia

The diagnosis of HIE is often complex and mandates a multidisciplinary approach. Neonates with clinically suspected HIE typically have a low Apgar score (ie, 0–3 in 5 mins) along with metabolic acidosis (cord blood pH <7.1), need for resuscitation, abnormal neurology (coma and hypotonia), and/or multiorgan dysfunction [5,6]. Within the initial 24 hours of life, neonates present with apnea and seizures along with abnormal electroencephalographic recording [6]. MRI is by far the most sensitive and specific imaging technique available for the diagnosis of neonatal HIE. Diffusion-weighted imaging (DWI) obtained between 24 hours and 8 days of life allows detection of cytotoxic edema, even in the absence of an imaging correlate on conventional T1-weighted images and T2-weighted images [6]. Additionally, MRI plays a crucial role in prognostication of long-term outcomes. However, accurate timing of MRI examination in neonates with HIE is of critical importance to accurately ascertain the extent of injury. This is especially pertinent with the advent of therapeutic hypothermia (TH) as the mainstay in the management and neuroprotection of neonates with HIE [8]. TH reduces secondary energy failure after an acute ischemic event [9]. Results from a Cochrane Review suggest that TH at 33 to 34 °C for a period of 72 hours (of life) reduces the incidence of death or significant neurodevelopmental disability among survivors at the age of 18 or 24 months [8,10]. In the Total Body Hypothermia for Neonatal Encephalopathy (TOBY) trial (n = 131), TH was associated with a reduction in lesions in the basal ganglia or thalamus (odds ratio 0·36, 95% confidence interval [CI] 0·15–0·84; $P = 0{\cdot}02$), white matter (0·30, 0·12–0·77; $P = 0{\cdot}01$), and abnormal posterior limb of the internal capsule (0·38, 0·17–0·85; $P = 0{\cdot}02$) [11]. Studies also suggest that among neonates undergoing TH, an MRI performed between days 2 and 4 optimally identifies lesions on DWI; these are seen after day 10 of life on T1-and T2-weighted sequences [12].

Emerging Therapies in Neonatal Hypoxic-Ischemic Encephalopathy

The rationale for neuroprotective strategies is to mitigate the central nervous system (CNS) effects of secondary energy failure [13]. The main mode of action of therapies in experimental/animal models of HIE is to slow down pathophysiology of HIE including decreasing the oxidative stress, antagonizing the release of excitatory neurotransmitters, immunomodulation, and reduce apoptosis [13]. Some of these agents underwent clinical trials (eg, Erythropoietin, darbepoietin, stem cells, melatonin, Monosialogangliosides, Xenon, allopurinol, topiramate, magnesium sulfate) while others are in preclinical studies (eg, Endocannabinoids, Argon, and Azithromycin) [13]. Erythropoietin (Epo) and Epo receptors have been noted to be upregulated following a hypoxic ischemic injury; Epo has been observed to provide an antioxidant as well as anti-inflammatory effect while reducing excitotoxic injury [13]. Although the administration of multiple doses of Epo (1000 U/kg) was related to less MRI brain injury in phase II [14], it did not lower the risk of death or neurodevelopmental impairment in phase III of the HEAL trial [15].

MRI Patterns and Appearances of Hypoxic-Ischemic Encephalopathy

At MRI, the appearances of HIE-related brain injury vary with the duration and severity of the asphyxia, with pronounced differences between term and preterm neonates. Among term neonates encountering a mild to moderate reduction in blood flow or partial hypoxia over a prolonged duration, shunting from the anterior and posterior circulations takes place to maintain perfusion within vital structures (ie, basal ganglia, brain stem, and cerebellum) [7]. The resultant brain injury demonstrates a watershed predominant distribution in the cerebrum [5]. It is worth noting that the vascular supply of the brain changes with fetal maturation. In preterm neonates, ventriculopetal penetrating arteries provide blood supply to the periventricular regions, extending inwards from the brain surface [5]. Hence hypoperfusion in preterm neonates leads to injury to the periventricular white matter injury [5]. In term neonates, ventriculofugal blood vessels are also developed, which radiate into the brain from the lateral ventricles; hence the intervascular border zone moves to a parasagittal location [5]. Imaging of term neonates with partial prolonged hypoxia demonstrates a peripheral pattern with involvement of the deep and subcortical white matter with or without cortical involvement [16]. In the acute phase, areas of involvement show cortical-subcortical restricted diffusion, which evolves over days to weeks with eventual cortical thinning and diminution of the underlying white matter (Fig. 1) [7]. In the chronic phase, a ulegyric configuration of the involved cortices (thinning of the base/stem of the cortices with relative sparing of the crests). This has been attributed to a *watershed within watershed* phenomenon that renders the base of the cortex more susceptible to hypoxia relative to the crest [17].

In the setting of acute sentinel event (profound hypotension, hypoxia, or cardio-pulmonary arrest of short duration), shunting of blood to pivotal structures is inadequate and hence, injury typically affects the more metabolically active regions (ie, ventrolateral thalami, posterior putamina, perirolandic regions, corticospinal tracts, and hippocampal formations; termed as the Basal Ganglia–Thalamus [BGT] Pattern) [7,18]. Identification of this pattern of injury is best assessed on DWI within the first 24 hours of life with progressive increase in the conspicuity of the diffusion restriction and signal abnormality over the next few days (Fig. 2). However, DWI would yield false negative results approximately 1 week after the event as diffusion restriction is known to pseudonormalize with increased diffusivity over time [7]. On T1-weighted images, neonates with BGT pattern of injury demonstrate no or minimal change in the signal intensity within the first 2 to 3 days. Over days 3 to 7, abnormal areas of hyperintensity are noted along with loss of the expected hyperintensity within the posterior limbs of the internal capsules (PLICs) (absent posterior limb sign) [19]. On T2-weighted images, signal abnormality may not be obvious within the first day of life; over the first 2 to 3 days and later, the normal hypointense foci of the posterolateral putamina, PLICs, and ventrolateral thalami may be indistinct [7]. Long-term outcomes of neonates with the BGT pattern of injury are poor, with most presenting with dyskinetic cerebral palsy [18].

Although not common, neonates who experience a profound, prolonged hypoxic-ischemic episode with catastrophic reduction in cerebral perfusion, present

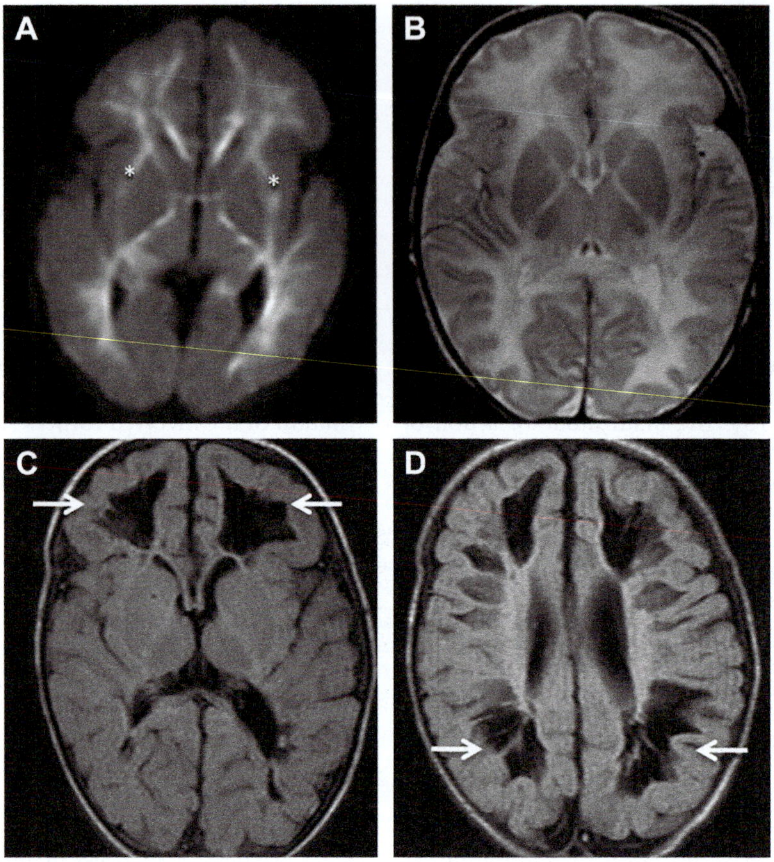

FIG. 1 Imaging appearances of partial prolonged HIE in a term neonate born after prolonged labor. Axial DWI (**A**) and axial T2 (**B**) images reveal extensive restricted diffusion (*asterisk* in **A**) and corresponding hyperintense signal abnormality, respectively, involving the cerebral WM symmetrically, sparing the deep gray nuclei and the cortices. Follow-up FLAIR images (*C*, *D*) obtained 1 month later reveal evolution of the signal abnormality with extensive cystic encephalomalacia (*solid arrows* in **C, D**) associated with volume loss.

with diffuse, widespread injury to the central vital structures as well as the cerebral cortex and white matter (encompassing the basal ganglia-thalamus and peripheral patterns of injury) [7]. On DWI, the involved cerebral hemispheres show uniform restricted diffusion (*white cerebrum sign*) (Fig. 3) [7]. An abnormal increase of the T1-weighted signals within the basal ganglia and the ventrolateral thalami may also be noted; however, this is a subjective finding, especially given that these structures do demonstrate some degree of intrinsic T1 hyperintensity [20]. Hence, care must be taken to interpret the abnormal T1 hyperintensity in conjunction with other clinico-radiological findings [5,20]. It is noteworthy that while these imaging patterns are typical and conceptual, in our clinical experience, overlapping atypical patterns and/or asymmetric extent of involvement of the brain are not uncommon. The knowledge of complicated labor, laboratory workup, and clinical course from labor to the initial MRI scan are critical in narrowing down a diagnosis of HIE.

Classification of Brain Injury in Neonatal Hypoxic-Ischemic Encephalopathy

Several classification systems have been developed to grade and score MRI abnormalities encountered in the clinical setting of HIE. Among them, Barkovich [21], Rutherford [22,23], National Institute of Child Health and Human—Neonatal Research Network [24,25], Washington University in St. Louis (WashU) [26,27], and Weeke [28] have been more widely used

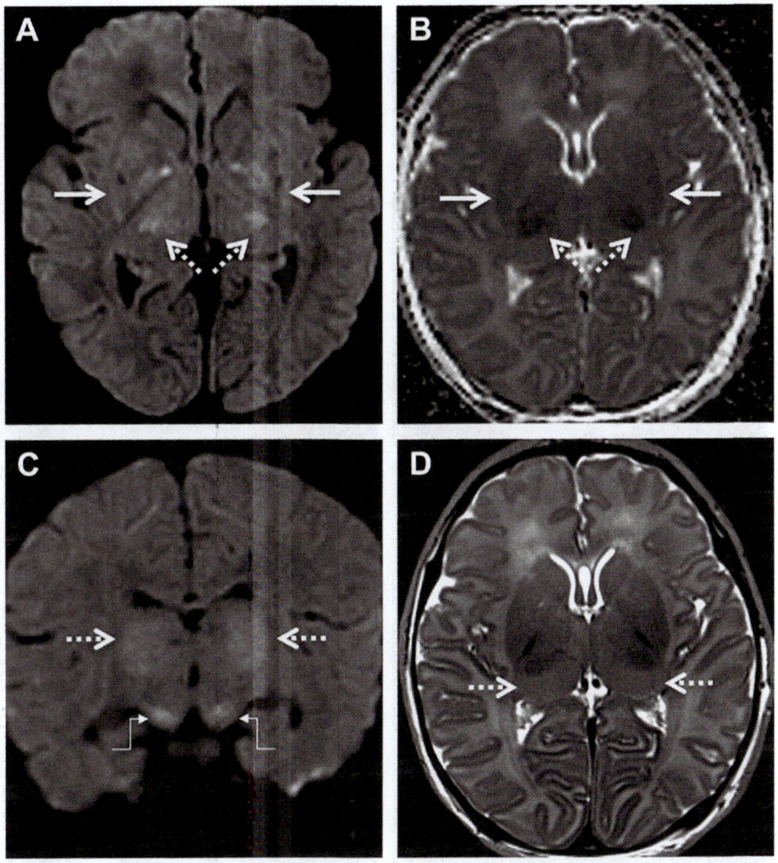

FIG. 2 MRI appearances of profound HIE in a 4-day-old term neonate with shoulder dystocia at the time of delivery. The neonate was born unresponsive with an Apgar score of 0/2/3 and required resuscitation for 3 minutes followed by intubation. Axial DWI (**A**) and ADC (**B**) images reveal symmetric restricted diffusion involving the lentiform nuclei (*solid arrows*) and the dorsolateral thalami (*dotted arrows*). Coronal DWI (**C**) demonstrates the involvement of the thalami (*dotted arrows*) along with symmetric involvement of the cerebral peduncles (*stepped arrows*). Axial T2 (**D**) reveals hyperintense swelling of the involved thalami (*dotted arrows*).

(Table 1). Most of these use T1-and T2-weighted sequences analyzed on scans obtained 2 weeks post birth [29]. As the most recent system, the Weeke system considers T1, T2, and DWI to objectively score signal abnormalities in a wide variety of anatomic areas [29]. The regions evaluated include the deep structures (BGT, posterior limb of the internal capsule, brainstem, hippocampus, and perirolandic cortices), white matter/cortex (cortex, periventricular white matter, optic radiations, and corpus callosum), and cerebellum [29]. Involvement of each anatomic structure is scored based on extent: focal (score of 1) or extensive (score of 2) and laterality: unilateral (score of 1) or bilateral (score of 2) [29]. Intracranial hemorrhage, punctate white matter lesions, and cerebral sinovenous thrombosis are also taken into account. The maximum score is summed up to 57 or 55 with or without magnetic resonance spectroscopy (MRS) results in the BGT [29]. In a recently published consensus based on Canadian experience, MR spectroscopy has been excluded in view of untested reproducibility across different centers as well as concerns surrounding accuracy and reliability [29]. A summary of these classification systems is provided in Table 1.

OTHER CAUSES OF NEONATAL ENCEPHALOPATHY

Germinal Matrix Hemorrhage

The germinal matrix (GM) is gelatinous, metabolically active, cellular structure along the subependymal region of the ventricles [30,31]. It represents the initial

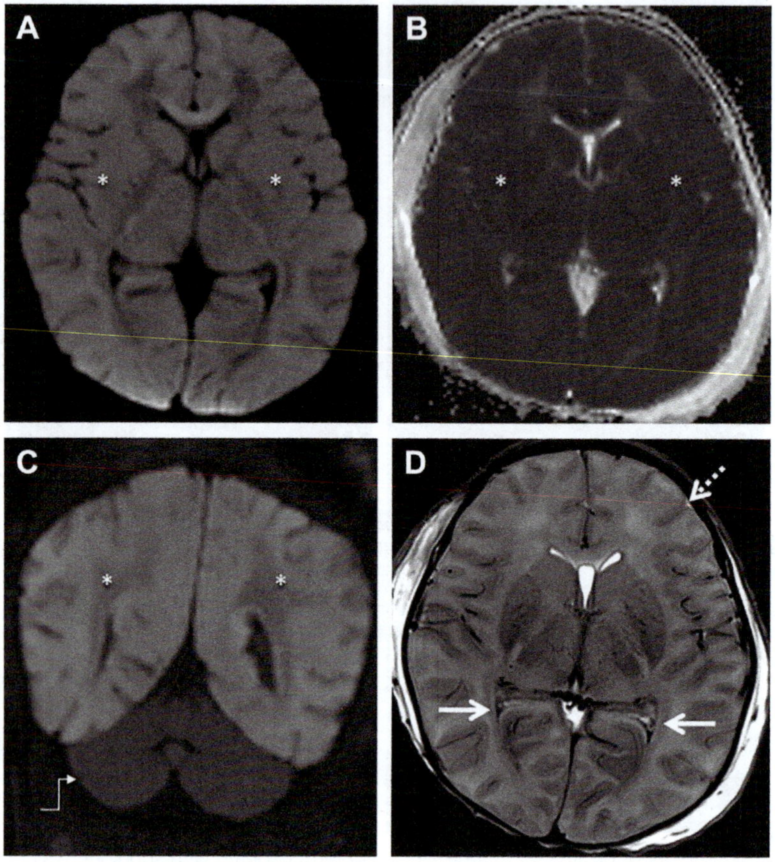

FIG. 3 MRI appearances of global HIE in a term baby neonate. The delivery was complicated by prelabor rupture of membranes (PROM) for 3 days followed by fetal decelerations mandating emergency C-section. Axial DWI (**A**) and ADC (**B**) reveals confluent restricted diffusion (*asterisk* in **A, B**) extensively involving both the cerebral hemispheres. Coronal DWI (**C**) redemonstrates the diffuse cerebral involvement (*asterisk*) and helps identify the relative sparing of the posterior fossa structures (only the cerebellum [*stepped arrow*] is shown in this image). Axial T2 (**D**) shows the diffuse swelling of the cerebral parenchyma with effacement of the sulcal spaces (*dotted arrows*) and the ventricles (*solid arrows*).

site for neuronal and glial cell differentiation, before they migrate to remote sites within the brain [30,31]. Vascularization of the germinal matrix begins by the 7th or 8th week of gestation and persists through the third trimester. It is worthwhile noting that these vessels are not supported by astrocytic processes or adventia and are not protected by autoregulation [30,31]. Preterm neonates are prone to severe systemic and autonomic complications, which causes the capillaries within the GM to rupture leading to localized or diffuse intraventricular hemorrhage [30,31].

The most commonly used system for GM hemorrhage contains 4 categories: Grade 1: hemorrhage localized to the subependymal GM; Grade 2: intraventricular hemorrhage (IVH) occupying lesser than 50% of the lateral ventricle, without ventricular dilation, and Grade 3: IVH occupying greater than 50% of the lateral ventricles with or without ventricular dilation. The previous Grade 4, now described as periventricular hemorrhagic infarction (PVHI; occurring due to impaired medullary venous drainage rather than a parenchymal extension of IVH), represents IVH along with hemorrhage in the adjacent parenchyma (Fig. 4) [32]. T2* imaging/susceptibility weighted imaging is extremely sensitive in - identifying GM hemorrhage [32]. However, of greater concern is the development of posthemorrhagic ventricular dilatation (PHVD), which refers to progressive ventricular dilatation due to GM hemorrhage occurring

TABLE 1
Common Scoring Systems for Neonatal Brain Injury in Infants with Neonatal Encephalopathy

Scoring System	Birth GA	Timing of MRI	MRI Modalities	ROIs	Methods & Scores	Neurodevelopmental Outcomes: Timing of Assessment	Neurodevelopmental Outcomes: Assessment Tests	Patterns Predict Adverse Outcome	Trials Applied
Barkovich et al, [21] 1998	> 36 wk	1–17 d Mean: 7d	• T1-WI • 1st & 2nd echo T2-WI • Gadolinium-enhanced T1-WI	• BGT/Perirolandic cortex, • W (Parasagittal or Borderzone) • Cerebral cortex	• BGT: 0–4 • W: 0–5 • BGT/watershed: 0–4 • Summation (BGT + W): 0–9 • Enhancement: 0–4	3 mo (n = 53) 12 mo (n = 32)	3M & 12M – Neuromotor: normal, abnormal, and unclear 12M – BSID-II: NDI	BG/W 1st-echo T2-WI in the 2nd week	
Rutherford [22,23]	37–42 wks [22]	• <10 d (94%) • 11–17 d (6%)	• T1-WI • T2-WI	• PLIC [22]	• PLIC: abnormal, equivocal, and normal [22]	• 12 mo (n = 72) [22]	Griffiths developmental scales	• Absence of normal PLIC signal [22]	TOBY [23,114,115] CoolCap [116]
	36 wk [23]	<6 wk [23]	• T1-WI • T2-WI	• BGT, WM, PLIC [23]	• BGT/WM/PLIC: I-V [23]	• 12 or 18 mo (n = 48) [23]	Griffiths developmental scales	• Pattern I and II [23]	
NICHD NRN [24,25]	Cooled: 39.1±1.5 wk Control: 38.6±1.6 wk	• 15±12 d (n = 97) • <7 d (n = 39) 24	• T1-WI • T2-WI	• BGT • ALIC, PLIC • Watershed • Cerebral hemispheres	0: normal 1A: minimal cerebral lesions 1B: extensive cerebral lesions 2A: BGT/ALIC/PLIC/W 2B: BGT/ALIC/PLIC/W & cerebral lesions 3: cerebral devastation	• 18–22 mo (n = 136) [24] • 6–7 y (n = 124) [25]	• 18–22 M: BSID-II, GMFCS, hearing & vision assessment [24] • 6-7Y: WPPSI-III or WISC-IV, NEPSY, GMFCS [25]	• 18–22M: 3 & 2B [24] • 6-7Y: 3 & 2B [25]	NICHD-NRN Trials [117,118]
WashU [26,27]	36–41 wk (n = 59)	6.2±4.1 d (0–17 d)	• T1-WI • T2-WI • DWI	• BGT: ○ Caudate ○ Lentiform ○ Thalamus ○ PLIC • WM • Cortex • Cerebellum • Brainstem	GS (global score): 48–186 • Mild: 49–59 • Moderate: 60–80 • Severe [3]: 81 Each score ′ 2 hemispheres ′ 3 modalities • WM, Cx, Cb: 1–4 • BGT: (1–4) ′ 4 subregions • BS: 1–3	No outcome			HEAL [15]

(continued on next page)

TABLE 1
(continued)

Scoring System	Birth GA	Timing of MRI	MRI Modalities	ROIs	Methods & Scores	Neurodevelopmental Outcomes: Timing of Assessment	Neurodevelopmental Outcomes: Assessment Tests	Patterns Predict Adverse Outcome	Trials Applied
	38.5±1.6 wk (n = 57)	4±2 d (n = 50) 10±2 d (n = 54)	• T1-WI • T2-WI • DWI	• BGT: ○ Caudate ○ Lentiform ○ Thalamus ○ PLIC • WM • Cortex • Cerebellum • Brainstem	• Total score 0–138 • Grade: ○ Mild: 1–11 ○ Moderate: 12–32 ○ Severe: 33–138 Each score ′ 2 hemispheres′ 3 modalities • WM, Cx, Cb: 0–3 • BGT: (0–3) ′ 4 sub-regions • BS: 0–2	18–24 mo	BSID-III	Total score cut-off: 10.5–11.5 Subcortical (BGT & PLIC) score	
Weeke et al, [28] 2018	39.9±1.6 wk (n = 97) 40.3±1.4 wk (n = 76)	Median [IQR] 6 [5–7] days 6 [5–8] days	• T1-WI • T2-WI • DWI • MRS	• DGM (0–23): ○ BG, Thal, BS, PLIC, Perirolandic Cx ○ HC (ext: 0–1, lat: 0–2) • WM/Cx (0–21): ○ Cx, WM, OR, pWMI, PH ○ CC (ext: 0–1, lat: 0) • Cerebellum (0–8): ○ Cb, CbH • Additional (0–3): ○ IVH, SDH, SVT • *MRS (0–2): NAA, Lactate*	• Total: 55 or 57 with MRS Ext + Lat + Additional + MRS • Extent (ext): ○ Focal <50%: 1 ○ Extensive ^{3}50%: 2 • Laterality (lat) ○ Unilateral 1; bilateral 2 • Additional: ○ Present 1 • MRS: 1 for reduced NAA, 1 for increased lactate	• 2 y ○ 24.1±0.4 M ○ 25.9±1.7 • School age ○ 5.9±0.3 y (n = 53) ○ 7.5±0.8 y (n = 46)	• 2 y: BSID-III, GMFCS • School age ○ WPPSI-III-NL ○ WISC-IV-SE & GMFCS	DGM score Cutoff – *no MRS*: • 2y 9.5 • School age 11.5	

Abbreviations: ALIC, anterior limb of the internal capsule; BG, basal ganglia; BS, brainstem; BSID, bayley scales of infant and toddler development; Cb, cerebellum; CbH, cerebellar hemorrhage; CC, corpus callosum; Cx, cortex; GE, gradient echo; GMFCS, gross motor function classification system; HC, hippocampus; NEPSY, developmental neuropsychological assessment; OR, *optic radiation; pWMI, punctate white matter injury; SDH, subdural hemorrhage; SE, spin echo; SVT, sinovenous thrombosis; Thal, thalamus;* W, *Watershed;* WISC, wechsler intelligence scale for children; WPPSI, Wechsler Preschool and Primary Scale of Intelligence.

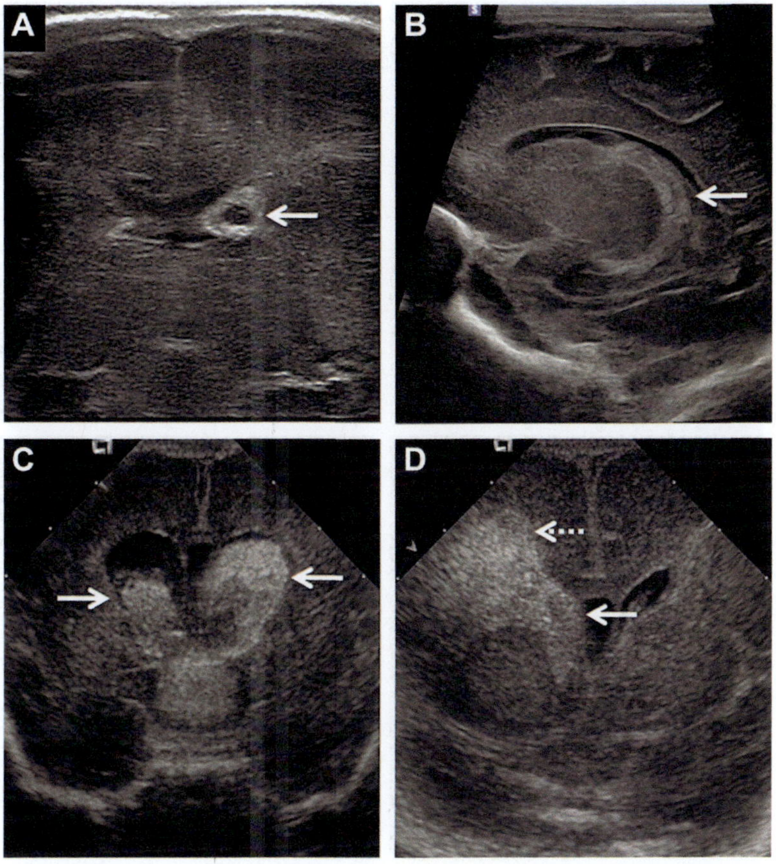

FIG. 4 Ultrasound appearances of the different grades of IVH in preterm neonates (**A–D**). Grade 1 IVH (**A**) seen as an echogenic focal hemorrhage (*solid arrow*) localized to the subependymal germinal matrix. Grade 2 IVH (**B**) evidenced by the echogenic IVH (*solid arrow*) layering posteriorly, occupying lesser than 50% of the lateral ventricle with normal ventricular caliber. Grade 3 (**C**) IVH (*solid arrows*) occupying greater than 50% of the lateral ventricles with ventricular dilation (note hemorrhage occupying greater than 50% of the lateral ventricles without ventricular dilatation is also considered grade 3 IVH). PVHI (**D**) seen as an ill-defined area of echogenicity (*dotted arrow*) in the periventricular white matter on the background of IVH (*solid arrow*). (*Images courtesy of* Dr Oscar M. Navarro, The Hospital for Sick Children, Toronto, Canada.)

within 7 to 10 days of the IVH (Fig. 5) [30]. Poor cerebrospinal fluid (CSF) resorption secondary to hemorrhage-induced irreversible deposition of collagenous connective tissue (altering ventricular compliance) and release of transforming growth factor (causing upregulation of fibroblast production) are the main contributors to PHVD [30]. Prompt identification of PHVD is crucial as it takes place before clinical onset of increased intracranial pressure. Hence serial surveillance imaging—is warranted, with cranial ultrasound (cUS) playing an indispensable role. Transfonatelle cUS offers a convenient, low-cost, portable, noninvasive modality both for screening and following up neonates with IVH, particularly those who are hemodynamically unstable for transfer to a radiology department [6]. The *ventricular index* (distance between the midline and the lateral border of the lateral ventricle obtained in the coronal plane at the level of the foramina of Monro) and the *anterior horn width*(AHW: widest diagonal width of the anterior horn in the coronal plane anterior to the thalamic notch) are the most common indices obtained and compared to previously published reference values (Fig. 6) [32].

Perinatal Arterial Ischemic Stroke

With an approximate incidence of 1:2300 to 1:5000 births, perinatal stroke forms an important contributor to long-term morbidity [33,34]. Perinatal ischemic

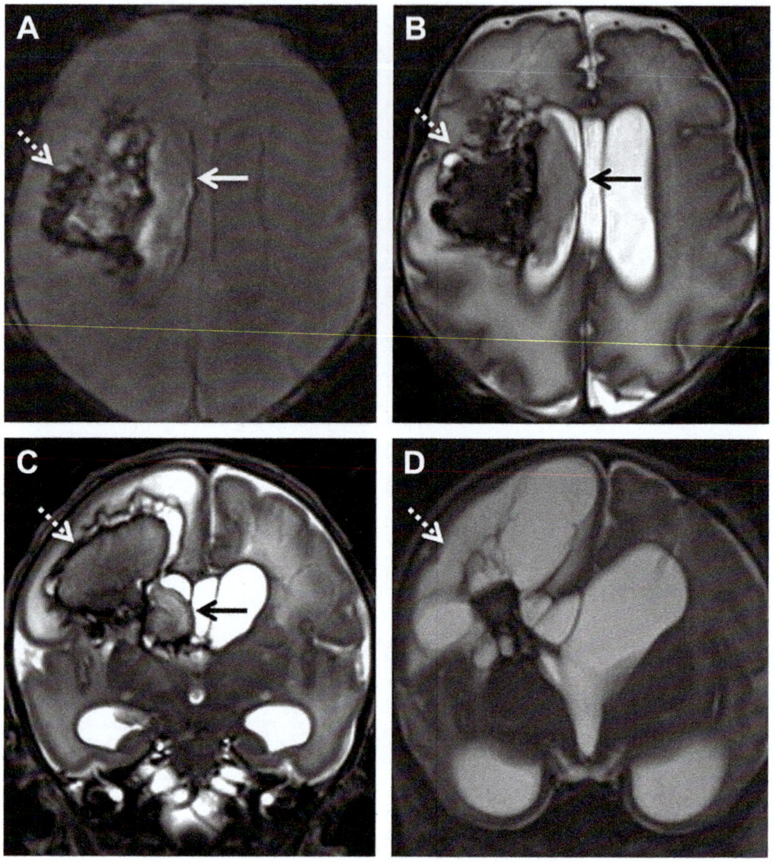

FIG. 5 MRI appearances of PVHI and its evolution in a preterm neonate born at 31 weeks of gestation. Axial SWI (**A**), axial T2 (**B**) and coronal T2 (**C**) reveal moderate ventriculomegaly with confluent hemorrhagic products within the right lateral ventricle (*solid arrows* in **A–C**) and in the right fronto-parietal deep white matter (*dotted arrows*), the latter in keeping with PVHI. Coronal T2 (**D**) follow-up obtained 3 weeks later reveals temporal evolution of the PVHI seen in the form of a large area of porencephaly (*dotted arrow*) along with severe increase in the size of the lateral ventricles and the third ventricle representing PHVD.

stroke is defined as *a group of heterogeneous conditions in which there is focal disruption of cerebral blood flow secondary to arterial or cerebral venous thrombosis or embolization, between 20 weeks gestational age and the 28th postnatal day, confirmed by neuroimaging or neuropathologic studies* [34]. As per the National Institute of Neurologic Disorders and Stroke, perinatal stroke can be divided into ischemic (arterial or venous) stroke and hemorrhagic stroke [34]. Arterial ischemic stroke constitutes the majority (80%) of ischemic strokes in the perinatal period; however, venous infarcts are thought to be underreported with up to 43% of all cases of pediatric cerebral sinovenous thrombosis occurring during the neonatal period [34]. In this section we focus our discussion on perinatal arterial ischemic stroke (PAIS).

PAIS is another major contributor to long-term neurologic morbidity (eg, cerebral palsy, epilepsy, and cognitive impairment) [35]. Symptomatic PAIS has an incidence of approximately 1 in 4000 term live born infants [35]. The clinical presentation of PAIS in term neonates includes seizures (80%–92% of cases) after a rather uneventful birth, usually with normal Apgar scores and cord pH values [35]. The timing of clinical presentation of PAIS is often after the first 2 hours of birth with some as late as the 3rd or 4th day of life [35]. Seizures are usually, but not invariably, contralateral to the site of infarction, and are commonly clonic in nature [35]. Occasionally, the clinical presentation can be more subtle such as apnea, dyskinesis, poor feeding, hypotonia, and

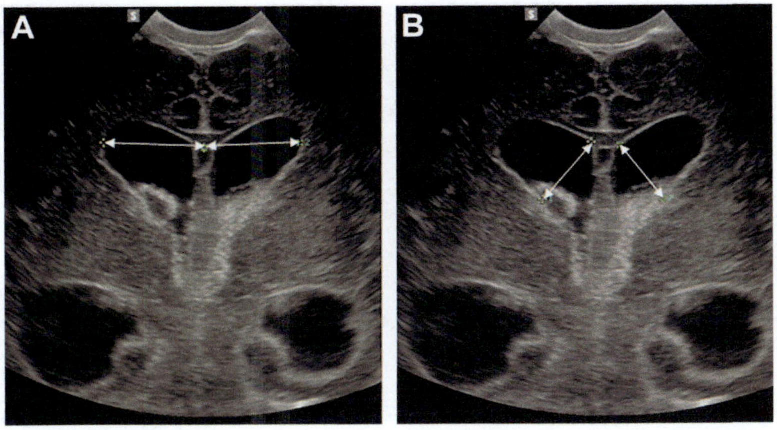

FIG. 6 Coronal ultrasound images in a patient with PHVD demonstrating methods to measure the ventricular index (*arrows* in **A**) and AHW (*arrows* in **B**). (*Images courtesy of* Dr Oscar M. Navarro, The Hospital for Sick Children, Toronto, Canada.)

irritability [35]. Risk factors for PAIS are not certain, but HIE is comorbidity [33]. Nevertheless, the risk of PAIS is highest in the peripartum period, thought to be related to the activation of coagulation cascades during normal birth [34]. Thromboembolism risk factors (fetal or neonatal, maternal, and placental factors) are found in 42%–78% of patients with PAIS with congenital heart disease being another independent risk factor [34]. From a pathophysiological standpoint, PAIS and HIE are similar processes with the former being a result of focal reduction in blood supply while the latter is a more global process [36]. In both PAIS and HIE, the involved brain progresses through phases of primary cell death, secondary energy failure (with subsequent programmed cell death pathways), and a tertiary phase of remodeling and neurodegeneration [36]. In some cases, both PAIS and HIE may coexist with similar intrapartum risk factors [36].

In terms of territorial distribution, most PAIS occur in the middle cerebral artery (MCA) territory, with a left sided predominance (3–4 times more common than the right) [34]. This is because the left internal carotid artery is more directly aligned with the direction of blood flow within the ascending aorta [34]. MRI is the mainstay in the diagnosis of PAIS, with DWI being the workhorse [33]. Acute arterial infarcts show restricted diffusion within minutes of insult [33]. The diffusion abnormality progresses over days, with the nadir of apparent diffusion coefficient (ADC) hypointensity occurring on day 3 of the insult [33]. Eventually, diffusion signals begin to decrease, undergoing pseudonormalization within 4 to 21 days after the acute event [33]. Apart from detection of the PAIS, DWI also plays an important role in identifying network injury (i.e., Wallerian degeneration representing secondary axonal effects of cell injury in tracts and nuclei connected to the primary site of arterial insult) [37]. It is thought to occur due to the initial transmission of excitotoxic injury followed by cell death secondary to the lack of trophic support [37]. Commonly affected tracts and nuclei include the corticospinal tract, commissures, optic radiations, and the thalamus, the latter demonstrating regional differences depending on the primary site of involvement [37]. Notably, involvement of the middle part of the cerebral peduncle (course of the corticospinal tract) is described as an important prognostic site for cerebral palsy [37].

Other sequences such as T2* gradient echo or susceptibility-weighted imaging (SWI) (to rule out hemorrhagic transformation), a T1-weighted sequence (for asymmetry of myelination) and a T2-weighted sequence (for evaluation of mass effect) play an ancillary role in the diagnosis of PAIS [33]. Magnetic resonance angiography (*MRA*) using a three-dimensional time-of-flight (TOF) technique is critical to identify the site and extent of occlusion [33]. Embolic occlusion of the mainstem MCA is seen only in about 10 to 20% of cases, presumably due to breakdown of the embolus by the time imaging is obtained (Fig. 7). In our experience, the feeding mainstem artery and cortical arborization distal to the site of occlusion is usually paradoxically increased compared to the contralateral unaffected side, a phenomenon known as luxury perfusion (Fig. 8).

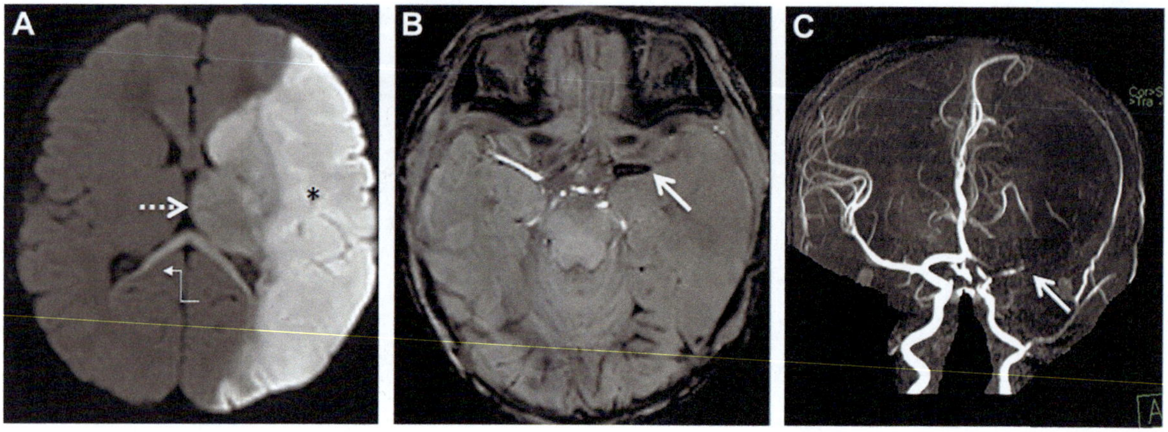

FIG. 7 Left MCA territory infarct in a 2-day-old term neonate presenting with seizures. There were no antenatal complications and delivery was uneventful (Apgars: 9/9/9). Axial DWI (**A**) reveals a large left MCA territory infarct (*asterisk*) with pre-Wallerian degeneration involving the left thalamus (*dotted arrow*) and the splenium of the corpus callosum (*stepped arrow*). Axial SWI (**B**) image reveals a focal thrombus (*solid arrow*) within the left M1-MCA. TOF MR Angiography (TOF-MRA); (**C**) reveals loss of flow signals along the left MCA mainstem (*solid arrow*) with loss of distal arborization.

Metabolic Disorders: Hypoglycemia

Metabolic disorders encompass a wide range of disorders and collectively are an important cause of neonatal encephalopathy. Inborn errors of metabolism are a heterogeneous group of conditions characterized by the deficiency in production, synthesis, metabolism, storage, or transport of biochemical compounds [38]. They are broadly classified into 4 major groups based on the mechanism of clinical presentation: (1) intoxication disorders (ie, accumulation of toxic metabolic products proximal to the metabolic block; eg, aminoacidopathies/organic acidemias), (2) energy production disorders (deficiency in energy production or utilization; eg, mitochondriopathies), (3) disorders of the biosynthesis and breakdown of complex molecules (eg, lysosomal or peroxisomal disorders.), and (4)

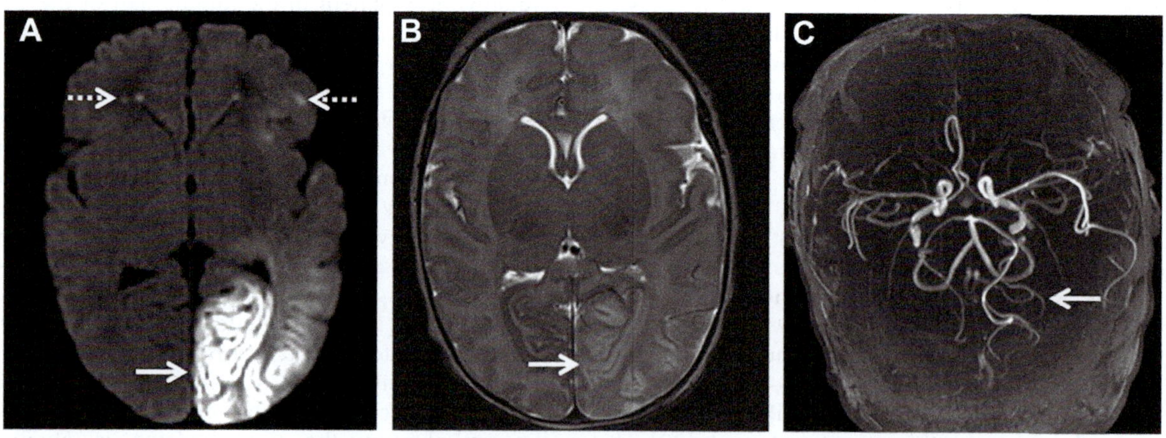

FIG. 8 Imaging appearances of luxury perfusion in a 3-day old term neonate presenting with jerky movement of right leg. Axial DWI (**A**) reveals a wedge-shaped left posterior cerebral artery territory infarct (*solid arrow*) with scattered punctate foci of white matter injury (*dotted arrows*) in the frontal lobes bilaterally. Axial T2 (**B**) reveals corresponding hyperintensity, with loss of grey-white matter differentiation (*solid arrow*) within the involved left occipital lobe. MIP-TOF-MRA (TOF-MRA; **C**) reveals asymmetric enlargement of the left PCA (*solid arrow*) in keeping with luxury perfusion.

neurotransmitter defects (usually affecting monoamine synthesis or gamma-aminobutyric acid (GABA) metabolism; eg, pyridoxine dependency) [38]. On the other hand, neonatal hypoglycemia (NH) is the most common metabolic condition causing encephalopathy in newborns [39,40]. NH has an incidence of approximately 1 to 6 per 1000 live term births; however, some authors believe that its incidence is often underestimated as relevant symptomatology such as (stupor, jitteriness, and seizures) are often lacking or inconspicuous in most affected neonates, making NH go undetected until clinical seizures develop [39,40].

NH (<46 mg/dL) is estimated to occur in about 5% to 15% of normal term neonates and can lead to long-term visual impairment, epilepsy, and cognitive deficits [39]. However, some authors suggest that absolute glucose values are often not useful, as multiple factors (eg, cerebral blood flow, duration of hypoglycemia, and exacerbating factors [hypoxia and hyperbilirubinemia]) impact the degree and extent of brain injury [40]. MRI plays an important role in the diagnosis of NH. In a study by Wong and colleagues, MRI findings were found to have a positive predictive value of 82% and negative predictive value of 78%, with clinical hypoglycemia being associated with a 17.6-fold higher odds of MRI identification ($P<.001$) [39]. The typical imaging features of symptomatic NH include signal abnormalities (restricted diffusion with corresponding T2-hyperintensity) involving the cerebral hemispheres with a parieto-occipital cortical-subcortical predominance [38]. Cortical involvement is usually along the superficial layers, supporting the concept that the release of excitatory amino acids from synaptic endings within the CSF enhances neuronal death, as opposed to the involvement of deeper cortical layers in HIE [38]. Additionally, the hippocampal formations, basal ganglia, and peri-Rolandic cortices are often spared in NH (vs HIE) [38]. Fig. 9.

Recent studies using continuous glucose monitoring for 72 hours in neonates $\geq$ 36 weeks gestation with NE showed some interesting results [41,42]. Higher maximum glucose levels on the first day of life were associated with widespread changes in mean diffusivity on MRI acquired around day 5 of life [41]. Maximum glucose during first 2 days of life predicted neonatal basal ganglia thalamus (area under curve [AUC] = 0.811) and watershed (AUC = 0.858) injury, and a glucose threshold of greater than 10.1 mmol/L was related to higher internalizing behavior score (P=.029), lower neuromotor score (P=.035), and higher odds for cerebral palsy (P=.014) at 19 months [42].

Infection

Neonatal (and fetal) CNS infections differ significantly from CNS infections in other demographics. The damage is usually more severe and widespread in the developing brain with outcomes depending on the gestational age at which the infection was contracted, the maternal immune status, and the neurotropic properties of the infectious agent [43]. Typically, CNS infections occurring during the initial 2 trimesters manifest as congenital malformations, whereas those occurring in the third trimester or immediately following birth demonstrate destructive lesions in the brain [44]. Another key feature of the immature

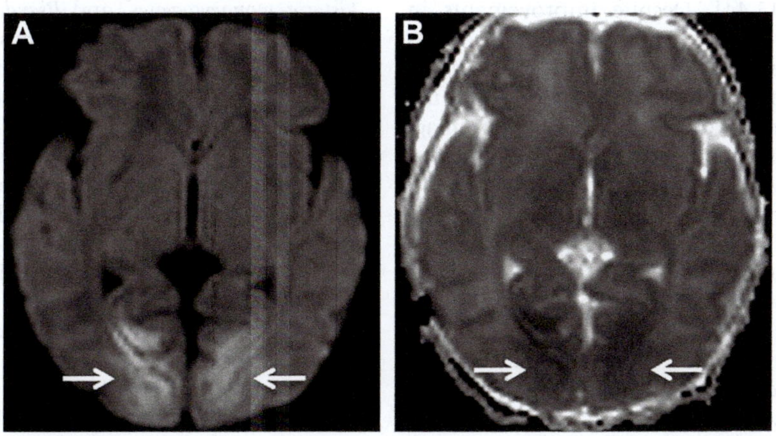

FIG. 9 Imaging appearances of neonatal hypoglycemia in a 3-day-old patient presenting with seizures. Axial DWI (**A**) and ADC (**B**) reveal symmetric restricted diffusion (*solid arrow*) involving the mesial occipital lobes.

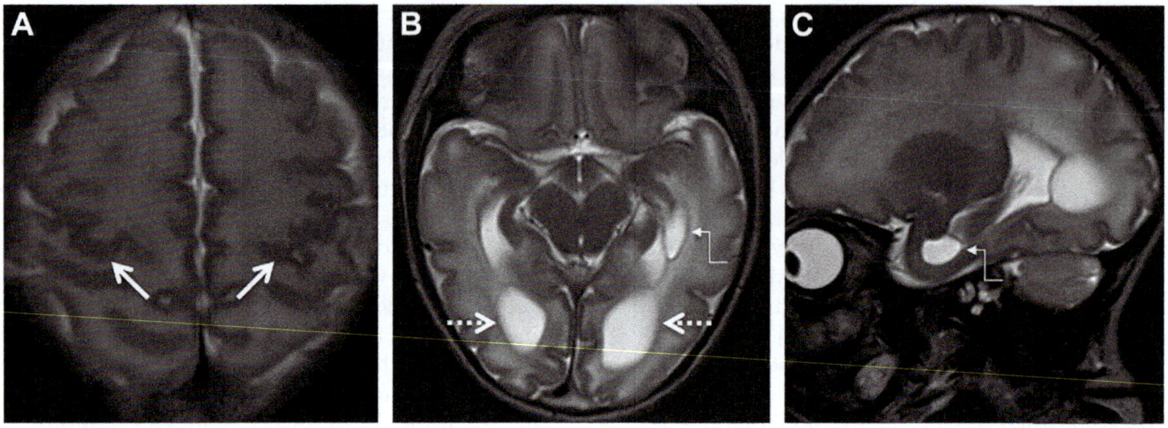

FIG. 10 Imaging appearances of a 3-day-old neonate born at 35 weeks of gestation presenting with encephalopathy, apnea, microcephalic, and dysmorphic facial features. Axial T2 (**A**) reveal subtle polymicrogyria (*solid arrows*) involving the perirolandic cortices. Axial (**B**) and sagittal (**C**) reveal large cysts along the occipital horns on both sides (*dotted arrows* in **B**) and the left temporal horn (*stepped arrow* in **B**, **C**).

brain is the difference in its response to infection; response to injury is not via astroglial reaction, rather the immune response repairs damage and removes abnormal cells while compensating for destroyed tissue. In other words, the immune-mediated inflammatory response, which leads to the damage produced by viral infection among older patients, is absent or less pronounced among neonates (and fetuses) [45].

The term TORCH (acronym denoting infection with Toxoplasma gondii, Rubella, Cytomegalovirus [CMV], and Herpes viruses [mainly herpes simplex virus]) is an important cause of congenital and perinatal infections [43,44]. Despite improvements in the methods of diagnosis and prevention, these agents are still encountered [44]. Maternofetal transmission usually occurs via a transplacental route or across the birth canal at the time of delivery [44]. On neuroimaging, most of these infections demonstrate a wide overlap [44]. CNS toxoplamosis infection leads to microcephalus, parenchymal calcification, ependymitis, and aqueduct stenosis (leading to hydrocephalus), often devoid of cortical malformations [44]. Rubella usually presents with ventriculomegaly, multifocal areas of white matter T2 hyperintensity (frontal predominant), cyst formations, parenchymal calcifications, cataracts, and inner ears anomolies [44]. CMV typically presents with microcephaly, malformations of cortical development, cerebellar hypoplasia, and white matter lesions, with or without temporal lobe or polar abnormalities (enlarged temporal horns, temporal polar cysts) [44] (Fig. 10). Neonatal herpes simplex virus infection typically presents with areas of reduced cortical diffusion and parenchymal hemorrhage often with meningeal enhancement [44]. However, the spectrum of maternofetal transmission of infectious agents has expanded over the years with the addition of several agents such as lymphocytic choriomeningitis virus, parechovirus, varicella-zoster virus, and Zika virus [44].

In neonates, a plethora of gram positive and negative organisms such as Streptococcus agalactiae (group B streptococcus), *Escherichia coli*, *Staphylococcus* species, *Listeria monocytogenes*, and *Pseudomonas* species have been implicated in the pathophysiology of meningitis and sepsis [46]. Of these, group B *Streptococcus* is the most common organism isolated in neonates with meningitis [46]. Initial signs of bacterial meningitis in neonates are often subtle (eg, low-grade fever, poor feeding/suck, and somnolence) eventually progressing to vomiting, lethargy, and seizures; meningeal signs are often absent [44]. Systemic manifestations such as shock and disseminated intravascular coagulopathy may also present. On imaging cUS may reveal echogenic widened sulcal spaces and hyperemia [44]. In the early stages of neonatal meningitis, CT and MRI may be unremarkable; however, in advanced cases, hydrocephalus with or without purulent layering within the ventricles as well as ependymal and/or leptomeningeal enhancement are common [44]. Thrombosis (arterial or venous), ischemic damage to the brain, abscess formation, and empyema may also be shown [44].

ADVANCES IN IMAGING

Prompt detection of perinatal brain injury is of paramount importance in encephalopathic neonates to initiate appropriate pharmacologic and/or cooling therapies, which hold promise in aiding the maturing brain in its early self-repair mechanisms, thereby salvaging neurons following the insult [47]. While conventional MRI techniques are more sensitive in identifying the extent of brain injury, relative to other modalities (ie, cUS and CT), they are limited to only gross anatomic assessment and do not offer nuanced in vivo analysis of microstructure and biochemistry [47]. In this section we discuss the role of advanced imaging modalities in the diagnosis and treatment of neonatal encephalopathy.

Small Footprint MRI Systems

For optimal MRI quality, a high signal-to-noise ratio (SNR) is a prerequisite. Hence 2 major criteria need to be fulfilled, that is, use of an appropriately sized head coil (SNR is inversely proportional to the coil radius [CR] to the exponent 5 over 2 [$CR^{5/2}$]), and use of high field strength (1.5T/3T; SNR is directly proportional to the B0) [48]. In terms of machine hardware, we have seen a resurgence of low-field, small foot-print MRI systems in neonatal imaging [49,50]. With reduced siting requirements, these systems can now be installed as point-of-care units near or in the NICU, improving access to imaging and reducing transport (hence eliminating the need to change lines and reducing exposure to infections) as well as reducing wait times [49,50]. The considerable reduction in the size of the MRI system also improves physical and visual access to the neonate as compared to an adult-sized scanner [49]. In addition, it provides an excellent option for imaging the sickest and most unstable NICU patients who are supported by devices (eg, nitric oxide administration) who are difficult to transport out of the NICU and traditionally cannot enter into a 1.5T or 3T MRI room [49].

Magnetic Resonance Spectroscopy

MRS is a noninvasive technique that provides information about metabolic processes (energy metabolism), neuronal integrity, and cell proliferation and degradation including necrosis [51]. Based on the concept of chemical shift (ie, differences of proton precession in different nuclear environments based on the surrounding electron cloud), MRS provides a distinct *readout* compared to routine MRI, that is, a spectrum instead of a cross-sectional image [51,52]. This MR spectrum comprises of resonances (or peaks) of metabolites (in significantly smaller quantities compared to water and fat) and shows a graph representing the signal intensity as a function of frequency (expressed as parts per million) [51,52]. Spectra may be obtained from 1 specific region of interest in the brain (single-voxel MRS) or from multiple regions [52]. In vivo 1H MRS, the most frequently used MRS technique in clinical practice, focuses on carbon-bound protons within the 1 to 5 ppm range of the chemical shift scale and depicts metabolites present at high enough concentrations [53]. These include the neuronal metabolite *N*-acetylaspartate (NAA), choline-containing compounds (glycerophosphocholine and phosphocholine), neurotransmitters glutamate and γ-aminobutyric acid, creatine, myo-inositol, and lactate (Lac) [53].

The common metabolites expected on MRS in a healthy neonate brain include NAA (synthesized in brain mitochondria, with a peak at 2.02 ppm), followed by creatine at 3.03 (and 3.94) ppm [51]. NAA is an important marker for intact neurons (also thought to be an integral part of myelinization), while creatine is thought to represent energy metabolism [51]. Choline is another important peak (observed at 3.22 ppm) representing membrane, phospholipid, and myelin metabolism [51]. At birth, choline is the predominant peak; however, with brain maturation, the levels of NAA and creatine steadily rise within the first 3 months of life with choline persisting as the dominant peak, only to eventually decline thereafter [51]. At 6 months of age, NAA is the most prominent detectable marker on MRS [51].

Importantly, in a healthy individual, irrespective of age, lactate (terminal metabolite of glycolysis) is below the detectability of MRS [51,53]. In the setting of inadequacy of mitochondrial respiration, with energy supply being dependent on glycolysis, an increase in lactate is noted reflecting inefficient energy production [51,53]. In neonates with HIE, lactate levels rise almost immediately and demonstrates a characteristic doublet peak at 1.3 ppm on MRS obtained with a short or long echo time (TE 35ms, and 288 msec, respectively), but inverts on MRS acquired using an intermediate echo time (TE 144 msec) (Fig. 11) [7]. Elevated lactate-creatinine and lactate-choline ratios were found to indicate poor long-term neurologic outcomes [7]. Furthermore, increased NAA concentration and Lactate/NAA ratios and decreased NAA/creatine ratios in thalamus and parietal white matter (WM) were significantly associated with

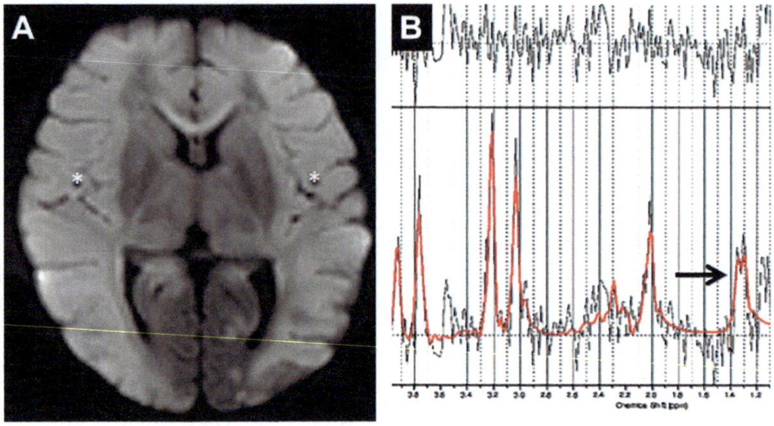

FIG. 11 Lactate peak on MRS in a term born neonate with global HIE. Axial DWI (**A**) reveals confluent restricted diffusion (*asterisk*) extensively involving both the cerebral hemispheres. MRS (TE 288 msec; **B**) reveals a large lactate peak (*solid arrow*) resonating at 1.3 ppm.

worse neurodevelopmental outcomes and increased risk of having cerebral palsy [54,55]. Another important consideration in patients with HIE is understanding the evolution of lactate levels; lactate levels typically decrease or return to normal within 24 hours after birth (pseudonormalization) followed by a rise between 24 and 48 hours (known as secondary energy failure) with a peak at 5 days [7]. Additionally, lactate peaks may be normally seen in preterm neonates and within the CSF, making it imperative to not interpret MRS peaks in isolation [7]. Beyond HIE, MRS also plays a crucial role in specific inherited metabolic disorders, including but not limited to, mitochondrial disorders (elevated lactate peaks), pyruvate and succinate dehydrogenase complex deficiencies (presence of pyruvate, succinate, lactate, and/or alanine), organic acidopathies (branched chain amino acids), nonketotic hyperglycinemia (elevated glycine), Canavan disease (elevated N-acetylaspartate [NAA]), and creatine transporter deficiency (absent or very low creatine levels) (Figs. 12 and 13) [53].

It is important to note that the utilization of MRS, despite its promise to demonstrate metabolite changes and guide diagnosis, is highly variable in different practice settings, with standardization across centers being a

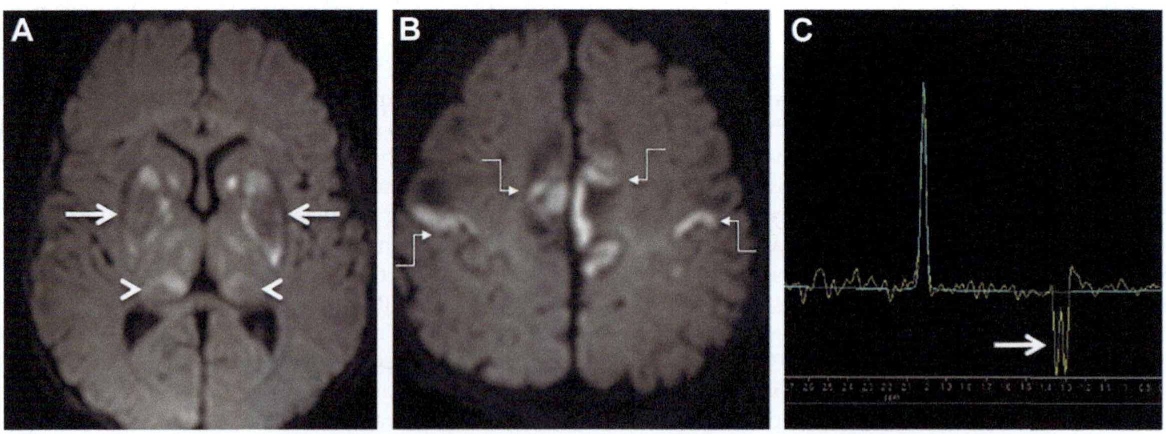

FIG. 12 Lactate peak on MRS in a 2-week-old patient with Leigh syndrome. Axial DWI (**A, B**) reveals symmetric restricted diffusion involving the lentiform nuclei (*solid arrows* in **A**) and medial thalami (*arrowheads* in **A**) as well as along the frontal cortices (*stepped arrows* in **B**). MRS (TE 144 msec; **C**) reveals a large, inverted lactate peak (*solid arrow*).

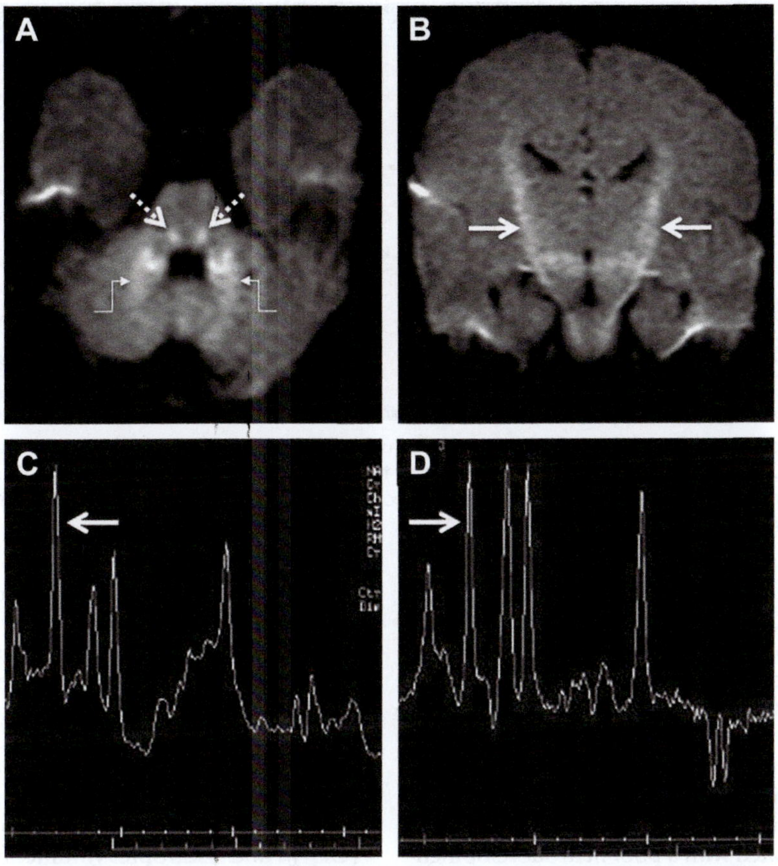

FIG. 13 Role of MRS in a neonate with nonketotic hyperglycinemia presenting with encephalopathy. Axial (**A**) and coronal (**B**) DWI reveal symmetric restricted diffusion involving the early myelinating structures (middle cerebellar peduncles [*stepped arrows* in **A**], dorsal pons [*dotted arrows* in **A**], corticospinal tracts [*solid arrows* in **B**]) without associated swelling. MRS obtained at TE 30 msec (**C**) and 144 msec (**D**) reveals a prominent peak at 3.5 ppm (*solid arrows*). It is important to note that myoinositol and glycine are observed at approximately 3.5 ppm; however, myoinositol only resonates at a short TE, but not on intermediate and long TEs. Hence the persistence of a peak at around 3.5 ppm on TE 144 msec and 288 msec indicates a glycine peak.

major challenge due to issues with background noise, the qualitative nature of data, and variable performance on different MRI systems/vendors [29].

Arterial Spin Labeling

Arterial spin labeling (ASL) is an unenhanced, noninvasive perfusion technique, which employs endogenous blood water as a diffusible tracer agent [56,57]. Protons within arterial blood are magnetically labeled with an RF inversion pulse applied below the imaging volume (ie, in the neck vessels) [56,57]. Based on the technique of labeling, ASL can be divided into continuous (application of long flow-induced inversion pulse) ASL, pulsed ASL (short inversion pulse applied to a large volume of the neck vessels), and pseudocontinuous ASL (using a train of short RF pulses thereby mimicking effects of continuous ASL) [56]. Of these, the latter is commonly employed in clinical practice due to the higher SNR and less labeling artifacts [56,57]. A crucial initial step in ASL is obtaining a control image (ie, without labeling); the 2 datasets are subtracted to provide a perfusion-weighted image [56,57]. Multiple repeat acquisitions are often needed to improve SNR in ASL [56]. Additionally, ASL is more challenging in neonates due to the low baseline cerebral blood flow relative to children and adults, making

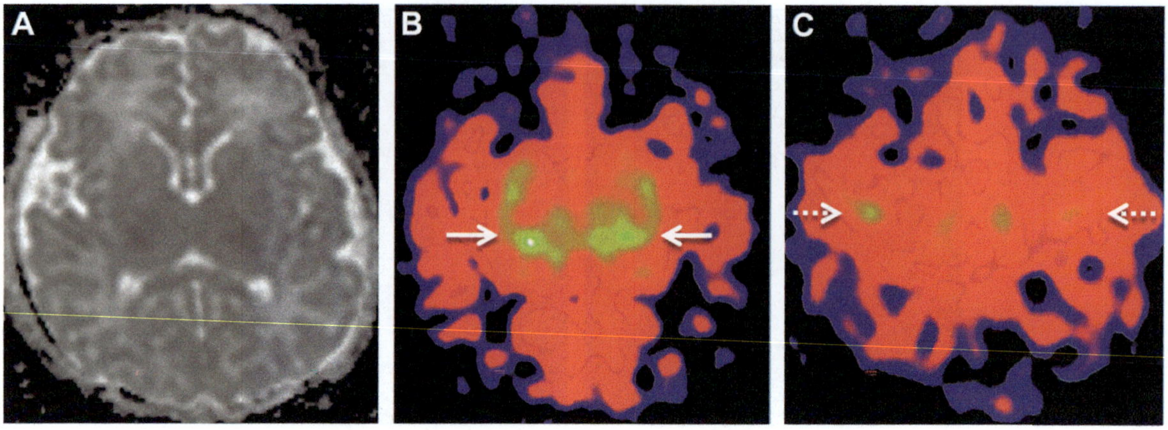

FIG. 14 Normal appearance of ASL in a neonate. Axial ADC (**A**) reveals no evidence of focal signal drop. Axial ASL (**B, C**) reveals mildly elevated perfusion in the deep gray nuclei (*solid arrows* in **B**) and in the sensorimotor cortices (*dotted arrows* in **C**). (*Image courtesy of* Dr Mai-Lan Ho, University of Missouri, Columbia, Missouri, United States of America.)

optimum postlabeling delay for better contrast-to-noise ratio difficult [56]. Despite this, studies have shown some promise of ASL in asphyxiated newborns [58]. In asphyxiated term neonates, ASL obtained during the first week of life showed an initial hypoperfusion followed by a hyperperfusion phase, which correlated with the subsequent development of brain injury, despite institution of TH [59]. Additionally, a higher ASL perfusion value in neonates with HIE ($n = 28$) was associated with a poor neurodevelopmental outcome at 9 or 18 months of age [60] (Figs. 14 and 15).

Magnetic Resonance Thermometry

Based on the shift in the water resonance peak in MRS and changes in the diffusion coefficient, MR thermometry allows direct measurement of brain temperature during TH, and provides important information to assess the effectiveness of TH and estimate the severity of brain injury [61–64]. However, due to the relatively low-spatial and temporal resolution, challenges in acquisition and reconstruction, and other practical issues for infants requiring ventilation support or electroencephalogram (EEG) monitoring, MR thermometry has so far only been used as a research tool.

Multishell Diffusion MRI

Multishell diffusion MRI (dMRI) data characterize the water diffusion signal with multilevels of diffusion-weighting. In addition to allowing assessment of brain tissue abnormalities with traditional diffusion tensor imaging (DTI) metrics using manual region-of-interest (ROI)-based labeling and tract-based spatial statistics, multishell dMRI data can be analyzed using multicompartment diffusion models, such as the neurite orientation dispersion and density imaging (NODDI) models, and diffusion kurtosis imaging (DKI) to provide a more sensitive measure of brain microstructure and brain structural connectivity [65–68].

NODDI calculates 3 main parameters, neurite density index (NDI), orientation dispersion index (ODI), and isotropic volume fraction (ISO) [69]. NDI reflects density of axons and dendrites in tissue, ODI indicates structural complexity by measuring the angular variability or fanning of neurites, and ISO quantifies free water content (eg, from edema). Compared to conventional DTI, NODDI metrics allow more specific biological interpretations of the measured tissue, improved sensitivity to subtle microstructural changes, and better assessment of gray matter maturation (Fig. 16) [70].

In addition to DTI metrics (fractional anisotropy [FA], mean diffusivity [MD], etc), DKI capturing the kurtosis of water diffusion (deviation from Gaussian behavior) also provides kurtosis metrics including mean kurtosis (MK), axial kurtosis, and radial kurtosis (RK) [71,72]. DKI permits more accurate depiction of microstructural damage and distinction of areas with different degrees of injury. Although DKI is less specific about microstructural components than NODDI, it makes fewer assumptions about tissue models and is easier to implement clinically.

Despite the increased interests in NODDI and DKI, there have been very few publications in neonatal

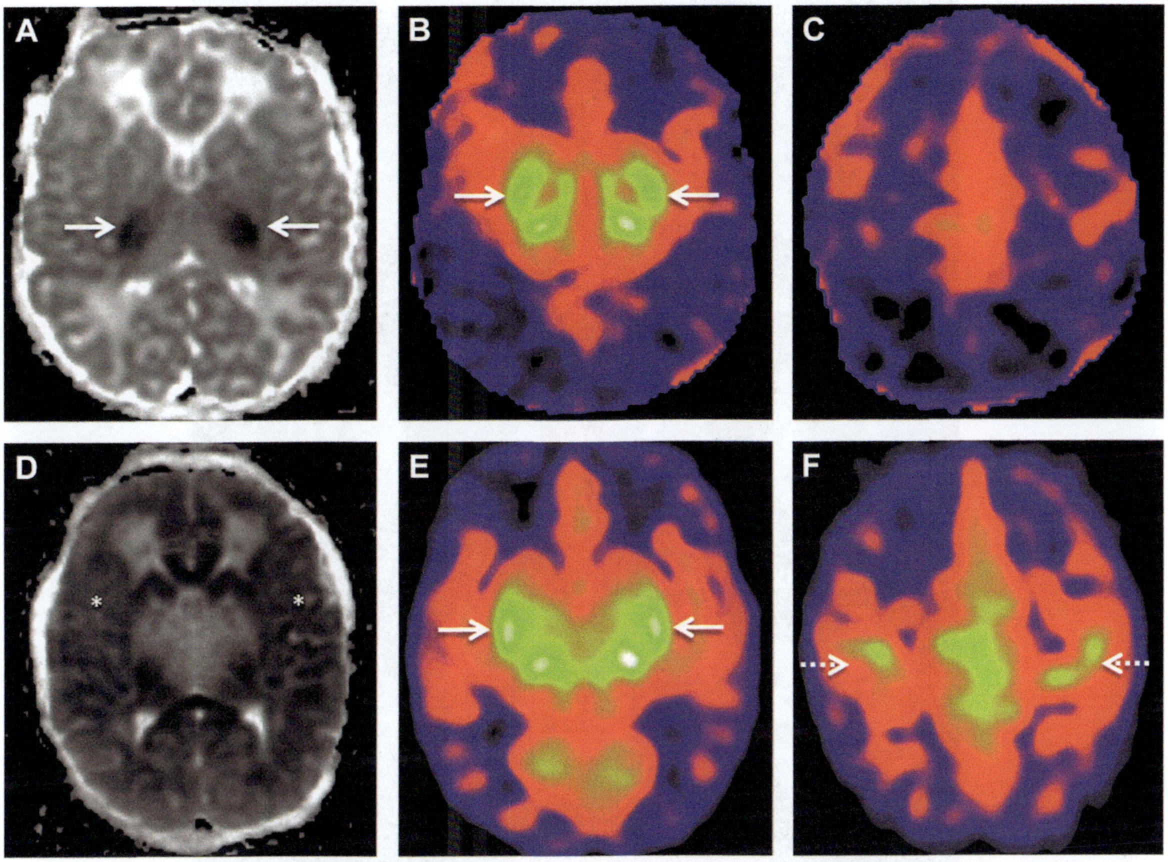

FIG. 15 Hyperperfusion injury in 2 different neonates. Patient 1 (**A–C**) with a history of delivery complicated by placental abruption. Axial ADC (**A**) reveals symmetric restricted diffusion (*solid arrows*) involving the dorsolateral thalami and the posterior limbs of the internal capsules. ASL (**B, C**) reveals corresponding hyperperfusion injury involving the deep gray nuclei (*solid arrows* in **B**) on the background of hypoperfusion in the rest of the brain parenchyma. Patient 2 (**D–F**) also with a history of delivery complicated by placental abruption. Axial ADC (**D**) reveals diffuse, symmetric restricted diffusion involving both the cerebral hemispheres (*asterisk*) in keeping with global HIE. ASL (**B, C**) reveals symmetric hyperperfusion injury involving the deep gray nuclei (*solid arrows* in **E**) and the perirolandic regions (*dotted arrows* in **F**). (*Image courtesy of* Dr Mai-Lan Ho, University of Missouri, Columbia, Missouri, United States of America.)

populations. In preterm infants, NDI was positively related to FA in cingulum, fornix, corticospinal tract, and optic radiations, but not inferior longitudinal fasciculus, and NDI positively correlated with PMA at scan [73]. Neonatal brain abnormality assessed with Kidokoro score predicted reduced FA and increased ODI in widespread WM tracts at 7 years in children born very preterm [74,75]. MK in both WM and deep gray nuclei was associated with PMA at scan [76]. Another study of 59 infants and children 0 to 4.6 years showed that MK depicted continued WM microstructural changes in the 2nd year of life, but FA plateaus at around 5 months. Furthermore, MK allowed more sensitive characterization of gray matter maturation that was not detected by DTI metrics, suggesting its great potential in studying the developing brain [70]. Most recently, MK in the PLIC and thalamus was found to be different in preterm infants with versus without low-grade IVH, and that MK in the genu and thalamus, and RK in the cerebellum were associated with lower neonatal behavioral neurologic assessment scores at 40 weeks in the group with IVH [77]. As of yet, the literature does not seem to include studies using NODDI or DKI in human infants

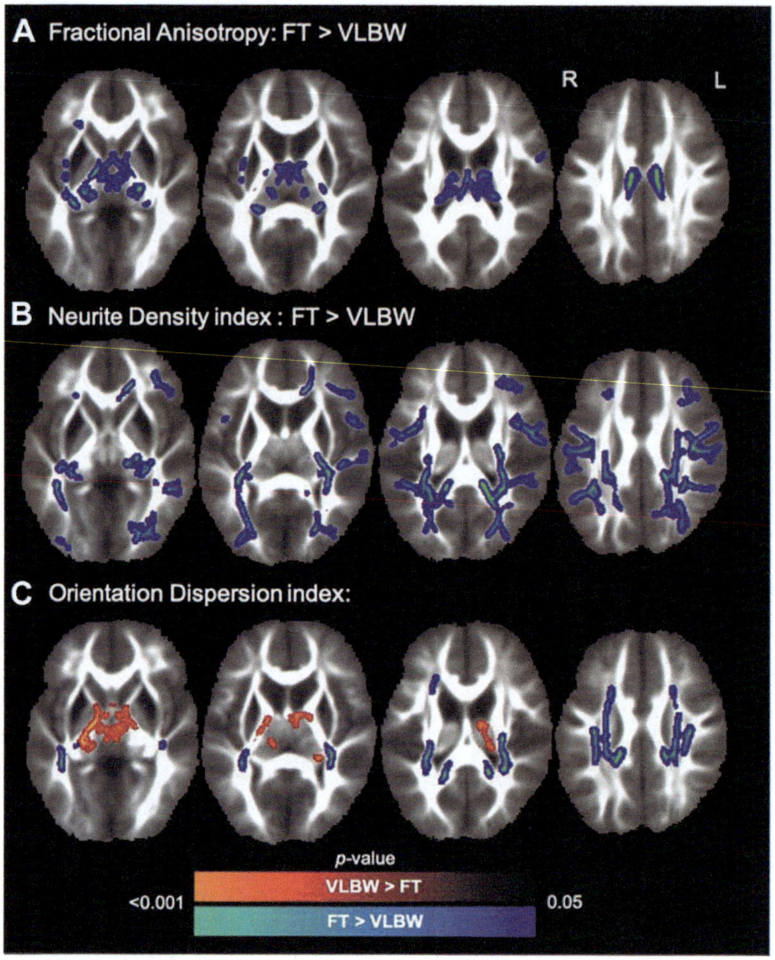

FIG. 16 FA and NODDI between group. (**A**) The blue areas are in keeping with regions in which FA was significantly lower in very low birth weight (VLBW) neonates compared to full term (FT) children. (**B**) Voxels with significantly lower NDI in VLBW children are indicated in blue. (**C**) Voxels in red depict regions with increased ODI in VLBW children including the corpus callosum and posterior limb of the internal capsule. Blue areas are regions with reduced ODI in VLBW children including the superior and posterior corona radiata and the superior longitudinal fasciculus. Significance was held at pcorr lesser than 0.05. Color bars indicate p-values. (*Reproduced* under CC BY-NC-ND license with due permission from the Dr. Julie Sato, The Hospital for Sick Children, Toronto, Canada [69].)

with NE or HIE. However, animal studies have demonstrated higher ODI and ISO in multiple brain regions in severe HIE rats compared mild HIE rats [78], and that the injured area delineated by MK corresponded to more severe pathologic findings by light microscopy in piglets [79].

Structural connectivity

Comprehensive investigation of brain networks through assessing structural connectivity between brain regions is important [80]. It allows understanding of the specific pathways involved in performing various functions and provides insight into developmental brain plasticity—the ability to reorganize or *rewire* brain networks to perform different functions after neonatal brain injury [81]. Decreased brain network integration and segregation are associated with increased neuromotor deficit scores in 6-month-old infants with perinatal HIE [82]. In school-age children with neonatal HIE, alterations in brain connectivity were observed, and reduced structural brain connectivity was associated, with poorer motor and cognitive outcomes [83,84].

Assessing connectivity in large neonatal HIE cohorts across the spectrum of brain injury patterns and severity may identify new MRI predictors of outcomes.

Resting-State Functional MRI (rs-fMRI)

Rs-FMRI measures temporal correlation of spontaneous, low-frequency, blood oxygen level-dependent signal alterations across the brain to map organized networks at the *resting state*, for example, default mode, sensorimotor, visual, and salience networks [85,86]. Functional connectivity of the brain can be investigated using seed-based correlation, independent component analysis, graph theory analysis, and regional homogeneity [85,87–90]. Although rs-fMRI has been widely applied to other populations, only a few studies in infants and children with NE have been published. Research found reduced functional connectivity in infants with HIE compared to healthy controls and greater reductions in connectivity in infants with severe HIE [91,92]. Connectivities in multiple regions are different in infants with mild HIE compared to infants with moderate/severe HIE [93]. The degree of functional connectivity abnormality in the first month was related to neonatal clinical factors and outcome at 6 months [94]. The rs-fMRI holds promise for detecting functional connectivity disruptions, assessing the effects of risk factors and therapies, understanding the development of functional networks in normal maturation and in recovery/plasticity after brain injury, and in identifying biomarkers for outcomes in infants with NE [80,91,93–97].

Functional Near-Infrared Spectroscopy and Functional Ultrasound

Functional near-infrared spectroscopy (fNIRS) uses near-infrared light (650–1000 nm) to measure changes in cerebral hemoglobin oxygenation and deoxygenation [98]. It allows bedside assessment of resting-state functional connectivity in infants. Reduced long-range functional connectivity and higher local network efficiency were found in infants with HIE compared to those in healthy controls [99]. A recent study in 19 infants with HIE demonstrated comparable resting-state functional connectivity generated by fNIRS and fMRI, with greater clustering coefficients, network efficiency, and modularity in HIE infants than in healthy controls, suggesting potential use of these features as biomarkers [100]. However, fNIRS has limited spatial resolution and is currently more suitable for measuring cortical activities.

Functional ultrasound (fUS) is another novel noninvasive bedside imaging technique that permits measurement of resting-state functional connectivity. fUS allows for sensitive detection of significantly decreased thalamo-cortical networks in very preterm neonates as compared to healthy term newborns [101]. Its high SNR, spatiotemporal resolution (250 mm, 1 s time scale), and capability to simultaneously image both cortical and subcortical structures make fUS a feasible and useful tool to monitor dynamic changes in functional networks and identify abnormal connectivity patterns in vivo for HIE infants.

Harmonization

Interscanner and intercentre differences used to be a challenge for multicentre neuroimaging studies. However, recent advancement in computational models permit preservation of biological variability and removal of unwanted intersite variability. ComBat, a popular batch-effect correction tool, allows for harmonization not only—of FA and MD maps but also—of fMRI-derived connectivity measures [102–104]. Meyers and colleagues presented a semiautomatic pipeline, Diffusion Imaging of Neonates by Group Organization, and demonstrated its feasibility—in harmonizing multicentre diffusion tensor tractography in infants with congenital heart disease [105]. These advanced computational methods paved the way for large multicentre studies of functional and structural imaging in infants with NE.

Deep Learning

Machine learning-based techniques, especially deep learning (DL)-based techniques can leverage comprehensive data from clinical, multimodal MRI, and socioeconomic factors and hold great promise for more accurate prediction of neurodevelopmental outcomes [106–108]. A deep learning approach has been developed to incorporate both clinical and neuroimaging features to predict motor outcome at 12 to 24 months in infants with HIE [106]. Using only 3 features, lentiform nucleus injury on T1 imaging, gestational age, and cord parenchymal hemorrhage, the DL approach achieved 85% accuracy in outcome prediction [106]. With the availability of more enriched data from the Developing Human Connectome Project [80], Baby Connectome Project [109,110], Fetal-Neonate Brain Development [111,112], and Healthy Brain and Child Development study [113], and continuing advancement in DL-based analytical approaches, we can afford the opportunities of better neurodevelopmental outcome prediction across the spectrum of brain injury severities to allow novel treatment targets and timely customized interventions for improved outcomes in infants with NE.

SUMMARY

The clinical management of a patient with NE entails detailed investigation to identify the underlying etiology. While HIE is the most common cause of NE, it is crucial to identify other clinical mimics causing NE, which entail diametrically different management strategies and prognoses. Despite thorough physical examination and laboratory investigations, MRI plays a crucial role in the diagnosis of NE. With advances in MRI techniques, computing methods, and clinical trials to substantiate their role in investigating NE, reliable identification of microstructural damage and prediction of functional outcomes of patients with NE are achievable. Finally, judicious use of conventional and advanced MRI techniques with standardized protocols for imaging and reporting is needed to not only improve diagnostic output but also ensure uniformity across centers for data collation and future research.

FUNDING

None.

ACKNOWLEDGMENTS

We wish to acknowledge the image contributions by Dr Oscar Navarro, The Hospital for Sick Children, Toronto, Canada; Dr Julie Sato, The Hospital for Sick Children, Toronto, Canada; Dr Mai-Lan Ho, University of Missouri, Columbia, Missouri, United States of America.

DISCLOSURE

The authors have nothing to disclose.

REFERENCES

[1] McIntyre S, Nelson KB, Mulkey SB, et al. Neonatal encephalopathy: focus on epidemiology and underexplored aspects of etiology. Semin Fetal Neonatal Med 2021;26:101265.

[2] Kurinczuk JJ, White-Koning M, Badawi N. Epidemiology of neonatal encephalopathy and hypoxic-ischaemic encephalopathy. Early Hum Dev 2010;86:329–38.

[3] Sandoval Karamian AG, Mercimek-Andrews S, Mohammad K, et al. Neonatal encephalopathy: etiologies other than hypoxic-ischemic encephalopathy. Semin Fetal Neonatal Med 2021;26:101272.

[4] Barkovich AJ. MR imaging of the neonatal brain. Neuroimaging Clin N Am 2006;16:117-35, viii-ix.

[5] Varghese B, Xavier R, Manoj VC, et al. Magnetic resonance imaging spectrum of perinatal hypoxic-ischemic brain injury. Indian J Radiol Imaging 2016;26:316–27.

[6] Chao CP, Zaleski CG, Patton AC. Neonatal hypoxic-ischemic encephalopathy: multimodality imaging findings. Radiographics 2006;26(Suppl 1):S159–72.

[7] Ghei SK, Zan E, Nathan JE, et al. MR imaging of hypoxic-ischemic injury in term neonates: pearls and pitfalls. Radiographics 2014;34:1047–61.

[8] Park J, Park SH, Kim C, et al. Growth and developmental outcomes of infants with hypoxic ischemic encephalopathy. Sci Rep 2023;13:23100.

[9] Bonifacio SL, Glass HC, Vanderpluym J, et al. Perinatal events and early magnetic resonance imaging in therapeutic hypothermia. J Pediatr 2011;158:360–5.

[10] Jacobs SE, Berg M, Hunt R, et al. Cooling for newborns with hypoxic ischaemic encephalopathy. Cochrane Database Syst Rev 2013;2013:CD003311.

[11] Rutherford M, Ramenghi LA, Edwards AD, et al. Assessment of brain tissue injury after moderate hypothermia in neonates with hypoxic-ischaemic encephalopathy: a nested substudy of a randomised controlled trial. Lancet Neurol 2010;9:39–45.

[12] Charon V, Proisy M, Ferre JC, et al. Comparison of early and late MRI in neonatal hypoxic-ischemic encephalopathy using three assessment methods. Pediatr Radiol 2015;45:1988–2000.

[13] Nair J, Kumar VHS. Current and emerging therapies in the management of hypoxic ischemic encephalopathy in neonates. Children 2018;5.

[14] Wu YW, Mathur AM, Chang T, et al. High-dose Erythropoietin and hypothermia for hypoxic-ischemic encephalopathy: a phase II trial. Pediatrics 2016;137.

[15] Wu YW, Comstock BA, Gonzalez FF, et al. Trial of Erythropoietin for hypoxic-ischemic encephalopathy in newborns. N Engl J Med 2022;387:148–59.

[16] Izbudak I, Grant PE. MR imaging of the term and preterm neonate with diffuse brain injury. Magn Reson Imaging Clin N Am 2011;19:709–31, vii.

[17] Chacko A, Andronikou S, Mian A, et al. Cortical ischaemic patterns in term partial-prolonged hypoxic-ischaemic injury-the inter-arterial watershed demonstrated through atrophy, ulegyria and signal change on delayed MRI scans in children with cerebral palsy. Insights Imaging 2020;11:53.

[18] de Vries LS, Groenendaal F. Patterns of neonatal hypoxic-ischaemic brain injury. Neuroradiology 2010;52:555–66.

[19] Barkovich AJ, Westmark K, Partridge C, et al. Perinatal asphyxia: MR findings in the first 10 days. AJNR American Journal of Neuroradiology 1995;16:427–38.

[20] Heinz ER, Provenzale JM. Imaging findings in neonatal hypoxia: a practical review. AJR Am J Roentgenol 2009;192:41–7.

[21] Barkovich AJ, Hajnal BL, Vigneron D, et al. Prediction of neuromotor outcome in perinatal asphyxia: evaluation of MR scoring systems. Ajnr American Journal of Neuroradiology 1998;19:143–9.

[22] Rutherford MA, Pennock JM, Counsell SJ, et al. Abnormal magnetic resonance signal in the internal capsule predicts poor neurodevelopmental outcome in infants with hypoxic-ischemic encephalopathy. Pediatrics 1998;102:323–8.
[23] Okereafor A, Allsop J, Counsell SJ, et al. Patterns of brain injury in neonates exposed to perinatal sentinel events. Pediatrics 2008;121:906–14.
[24] Shankaran S, Barnes PD, Hintz SR, et al, Eunice Kennedy Shriver National Institute of Child H, Human Development Neonatal Research N. Brain injury following trial of hypothermia for neonatal hypoxic-ischaemic encephalopathy. Arch Dis Child Fetal Neonatal Ed 2012;97: F398–404.
[25] Shankaran S, McDonald SA, Laptook AR, et al, Eunice Kennedy Shriver National Institute of Child H, Human Development Neonatal Research N. Neonatal magnetic resonance imaging pattern of brain injury as a biomarker of childhood outcomes following a trial of hypothermia for neonatal hypoxic-ischemic encephalopathy. J Pediatr 2015;167:987–93.e3.
[26] Trivedi SB, Vesoulis ZA, Rao R, et al. A validated clinical MRI injury scoring system in neonatal hypoxic-ischemic encephalopathy. Pediatr Radiol 2017;47:1491–9.
[27] Bednarek N, Mathur A, Inder T, et al. Impact of therapeutic hypothermia on MRI diffusion changes in neonatal encephalopathy. Neurology 2012;78:1420–7.
[28] Weeke LC, Groenendaal F, Mudigonda K, et al. A novel magnetic resonance imaging score predicts neurodevelopmental outcome after perinatal asphyxia and therapeutic hypothermia. J Pediatr 2018;192: 33–40.e2.
[29] Mohammad K, Reddy Gurram Venkata SK, Wintermark P, et al, Newborn Brain Health Working Group of the Canadian Neonatal N. Consensus approach for standardization of the timing of brain magnetic resonance imaging and classification of brain injury in neonates with neonatal encephalopathy/hypoxic-ischemic encephalopathy: a Canadian perspective. Pediatr Neurol 2025;166: 16–31.
[30] Egesa WI, Odoch S, Odong RJ, et al. Germinal matrix-intraventricular hemorrhage: a tale of preterm infants. Int J Pediatr 2021;2021:6622598.
[31] Cherian S, Whitelaw A, Thoresen M, et al. The pathogenesis of neonatal post-hemorrhagic hydrocephalus. Brain Pathol 2004;14:305–11.
[32] You SK. Neuroimaging of germinal matrix and intraventricular hemorrhage in premature infants. J Korean Neurosurg Soc 2023;66:239–46.
[33] Lee S, Mirsky DM, Beslow LA, et al. Pathways for neuroimaging of neonatal stroke. Pediatr Neurol 2017;69: 37–48.
[34] Lai LM, Sato TS, Kandemirli SG, et al. Neuroimaging of neonatal stroke: venous focus. Radiographics 2024;44: e230117.
[35] Dudink J, Mercuri E, Al-Nakib L, et al. Evolution of unilateral perinatal arterial ischemic stroke on conventional and diffusion-weighted MR imaging. AJNR Am J Neuroradiol 2009;30:998–1004.
[36] Gonzalez FF, Monsell SE, Cornet MC, et al. Perinatal arterial ischemic stroke diagnosed in infants receiving therapeutic hypothermia for hypoxic-ischemic encephalopathy. Pediatr Res 2024;97(3):1140–6.
[37] Lequin MH, Dudink J, Tong KA, et al. Magnetic resonance imaging in neonatal stroke. Semin Fetal Neonatal Med 2009;14:299–310.
[38] Poretti A, Blaser SI, Lequin MH, et al. Neonatal neuroimaging findings in inborn errors of metabolism. J Magn Reson Imaging 2013;37:294–312.
[39] Wong DS, Poskitt KJ, Chau V, et al. Brain injury patterns in hypoglycemia in neonatal encephalopathy. AJNR Am J Neuroradiol 2013;34:1456–61.
[40] Volpe JJ. Neurology of the newborn. 5th edition. Philadelphia: W. B. Saunders Company; 2008.
[41] Tam EWY, Kamino D, Shatil AS, et al. Hyperglycemia associated with acute brain injury in neonatal encephalopathy. Neuroimage Clin 2021;32:102835.
[42] Kamino D, Widjaja E, Brant R, et al. Severity and duration of dysglycemia and brain injury among patients with neonatal encephalopathy. eClinicalMedicine 2023;58:101914.
[43] Bale JF Jr. Fetal infections and brain development. Clin Perinatol 2009;36:639–53.
[44] Barkovich AJ, Raybaud C. Pediatric neuroimaging. 6th edition. Philadelphia, Pa: Lippincott Williams & Wilkins; 2019.
[45] Ziai WC, Lewin JJ 3rd. Update in the diagnosis and management of central nervous system infections. Neurol Clin 2008;26:427–68.viii.
[46] Hamada S, Vearncombe M, McGeer A, et al. Neonatal group B streptococcal disease: incidence, presentation, and mortality. J Matern Fetal Neonatal Med 2008;21:53–7.
[47] Bartha AI, Yap KR, Miller SP, et al. The normal neonatal brain: MR imaging, diffusion tensor imaging, and 3D MR spectroscopy in healthy term neonates. AJNR Am J Neuroradiol 2007;28:1015–21.
[48] Shroff MM, Soares-Fernandes JP, Whyte H, et al. MR imaging for diagnostic evaluation of encephalopathy in the newborn. Radiographics 2010;30:763–80.
[49] Tkach JA, Merhar SL, Kline-Fath BM, et al. MRI in the neonatal ICU: initial experience using a small-footprint 1.5-T system. AJR Am J Roentgenol 2014;202:W95–105.
[50] Thiim KR, Singh E, Mukundan S, et al. Clinical experience with an in-NICU magnetic resonance imaging system. J Perinatol 2022;42:873–9.
[51] Ulmer S, Backens M, Ahlhelm FJ. Basic principles and clinical applications of magnetic resonance spectroscopy in neuroradiology. J Comput Assist Tomogr 2016;40:1–13.
[52] Xu D, Vigneron D. Magnetic resonance spectroscopy imaging of the newborn brain–a technical review. Semin Perinatol 2010;34:20–7.
[53] Oz G, Alger JR, Barker PB, et al. Clinical proton MR spectroscopy in central nervous system disorders. Radiology 2014;270:658–79.

[54] Lally PJ, Montaldo P, Oliveira V, et al. Magnetic resonance spectroscopy assessment of brain injury after moderate hypothermia in neonatal encephalopathy: a prospective multicentre cohort study. Lancet Neurol 2019;18:35–45.
[55] Wu YW, Monsell SE, Glass HC, et al. How well does neonatal neuroimaging correlate with neurodevelopmental outcomes in infants with hypoxic-ischemic encephalopathy? Pediatr Res 2023;94:1018–25.
[56] Proisy M, Mitra S, Uria-Avellana C, et al. Brain perfusion imaging in neonates: an overview. AJNR Am J Neuroradiol 2016;37:1766–73.
[57] Pai V, Krishnan P, Shroff M. Special considerations for cross-sectional imaging in the Child with neurovascular disease. Neuroimaging Clin N Am 2024;34:491–515.
[58] Proisy M, Bruneau B, Rozel C, et al. Arterial spin labeling in clinical pediatric imaging. Diagn Interv Imaging 2016;97:151–8.
[59] Wintermark P, Hansen A, Gregas MC, et al. Brain perfusion in asphyxiated newborns treated with therapeutic hypothermia. AJNR Am J Neuroradiol 2011;32:2023–9.
[60] De Vis JB, Hendrikse J, Petersen ET, et al. Arterial spin-labelling perfusion MRI and outcome in neonates with hypoxic-ischemic encephalopathy. Eur Radiol 2015; 25:113–21.
[61] Wu TW, McLean C, Friedlich P, et al. Brain temperature in neonates with hypoxic-ischemic encephalopathy during therapeutic hypothermia. J Pediatr 2014;165: 1129–34.
[62] Wu TW, J LW, Geisler RF, et al. An in vivo assessment of regional brain temperature during whole-body cooling for neonatal encephalopathy. J Pediatr 2020;220: 73–9.e3.
[63] Weis J, Covaciu L, Rubertsson S, et al. Noninvasive monitoring of brain temperature during mild hypothermia. Magn Reson Imaging 2009;27:923–32.
[64] Zenobi C, Wisnowski JL, Tamrazi B, et al. Effects of tissue temperature and injury on ADC during therapeutic hypothermia in newborn hypoxic-ischemic encephalopathy. AJNR Am J Neuroradiol 2022;43:462–7.
[65] Tusor N, Wusthoff C, Smee N, et al. Prediction of neurodevelopmental outcome after hypoxic-ischemic encephalopathy treated with hypothermia by diffusion tensor imaging analyzed using tract-based spatial statistics. Pediatr Res 2012;72:63–9.
[66] Ly MT, Nanavati TU, Frum CA, et al. Comparing tract-based spatial statistics and manual region-of-Interest labeling as diffusion analysis methods to detect white matter abnormalities in infants with hypoxic-Ischemic encephalopathy. J Magn Reson Imaging 2015;42:1689–97.
[67] Annink KV, de Vries LS, Groenendaal F, et al. Mammillary body atrophy and other MRI correlates of school-age outcome following neonatal hypoxic-ischemic encephalopathy. Sci Rep 2021;11:5017.
[68] Cao Z, Lin H, Gao F, et al. Microstructural alterations in projection and association fibers in neonatal hypoxia-ischemia. J Magn Reson Imaging 2023;57:1131–42.
[69] Sato J, Vandewouw MM, Bando N, et al. White matter alterations and cognitive outcomes in children born very low birth weight. Neuroimage Clin 2021;32:102843.
[70] Paydar A, Fieremans E, Nwankwo JI, et al. Diffusional kurtosis imaging of the developing brain. AJNR Am J Neuroradiol 2014;35:808–14.
[71] Jensen JH, Helpern JA, Ramani A, et al. Diffusional kurtosis imaging: the quantification of non-Gaussian water diffusion by means of magnetic resonance imaging. Magn Reson Med 2005;53:1432–40.
[72] Jensen JH, Helpern JA. MRI quantification of non-Gaussian water diffusion by kurtosis analysis. NMR Biomed 2010;23:698–710.
[73] Kimpton JA, Batalle D, Barnett ML, et al. Diffusion magnetic resonance imaging assessment of regional white matter maturation in preterm neonates. Neuroradiology 2021;63:573–83.
[74] Kidokoro H, Neil JJ, Inder TE. New MR imaging assessment tool to define brain abnormalities in very preterm infants at term. AJNR Am J Neuroradiol 2013; 34:2208–14.
[75] Kelly CE, Thompson DK, Chen J, et al. Axon density and axon orientation dispersion in children born preterm. Hum Brain Mapp 2016;37:3080–102.
[76] Shi J, Chang L, Wang J, et al. Initial application of diffusional kurtosis imaging in evaluating brain development of healthy preterm infants. PLoS One 2016;11: e0154146.
[77] Zhang C, Zhu Z, Wang K, et al. Assessment of brain structure and volume reveals neurodevelopmental abnormalities in preterm infants with low-grade intraventricular hemorrhage. Sci Rep 2024;14:5709.
[78] Ohki A, Saito S, Hata J, et al. Neurite orientation dispersion and density imaging for evaluating the severity of neonatal hypoxic-ischemic encephalopathy in rats. Magn Reson Imaging 2019;62:214–9.
[79] Xiao J, He X, Tian J, et al. Diffusion kurtosis imaging and pathological comparison of early hypoxic-ischemic brain damage in newborn piglets. Sci Rep 2020;10: 17242.
[80] Edwards AD, Rueckert D, Smith SM, et al. The developing human connectome project neonatal data release. Front Neurosci 2022;16:886772.
[81] Smyser CD, Wheelock MD, Limbrick DD Jr, et al. Neonatal brain injury and aberrant connectivity. Neuroimage 2019;185:609–23.
[82] Tymofiyeva O, Hess CP, Ziv E, et al. Towards the "baby connectome": mapping the structural connectivity of the newborn brain. PLoS One 2012;7:e31029.
[83] Spencer APC, Brooks JCW, Masuda N, et al. Disrupted brain connectivity in children treated with therapeutic hypothermia for neonatal encephalopathy. Neuroimage Clin 2021;30:102582.
[84] Spencer APC, Brooks JCW, Masuda N, et al. Motor function and white matter connectivity in children cooled for neonatal encephalopathy. Neuroimage Clin 2021;32:102872.

[85] Biswal B, Yetkin FZ, Haughton VM, et al. Functional connectivity in the motor cortex of resting human brain using echo-planar MRI. Magn Reson Med 1995; 34:537–41.
[86] Greicius MD, Krasnow B, Reiss AL, et al. Functional connectivity in the resting brain: a network analysis of the default mode hypothesis. Proc Natl Acad Sci U S A 2003;100:253–8.
[87] Beckmann CF, Smith SM. Tensorial extensions of independent component analysis for multisubject FMRI analysis. Neuroimage 2005;25:294–311.
[88] Power JD, Cohen AL, Nelson SM, et al. Functional network organization of the human brain. Neuron 2011;72:665–78.
[89] Bullmore E, Sporns O. Complex brain networks: graph theoretical analysis of structural and functional systems. Nat Rev Neurosci 2009;10:186–98.
[90] Zang Y, Jiang T, Lu Y, et al. Regional homogeneity approach to fMRI data analysis. Neuroimage 2004; 22:394–400.
[91] Jiang L, El-Metwally D, Sours Rhodes C, et al. Alterations in motor functional connectivity in neonatal hypoxic ischemic encephalopathy. Brain Inj 2022;36:287–94.
[92] Li HX, Yu M, Zheng AB, et al. Resting-state network complexity and magnitude changes in neonates with severe hypoxic ischemic encephalopathy. Neural Regen Res 2019;14:642–8.
[93] Wang Y, Wang Y, Hua G, et al. Changes of functional brain network in neonates with different degrees of hypoxic-ischemic encephalopathy. Brain Connect 2023; 13:427–35.
[94] Boerwinkle VL, Sussman BL, Manjon I, et al. Association of network connectivity via resting state functional MRI with consciousness, mortality, and outcomes in neonatal acute brain injury. Neuroimage Clin 2022; 34:102962.
[95] Hakansson G, Robertsson Grossmann K, Aden U, et al. Functional brain connectivity in early adolescence after hypothermia-treated neonatal hypoxic-ischemic encephalopathy. Pediatr Res 2025.
[96] Spencer APC, Goodfellow M, Chakkarapani E, et al. Resting-state functional connectivity in children cooled for neonatal encephalopathy. Brain Commun 2024;6: fcae154.
[97] Lee MH, Smyser CD, Shimony JS. Resting-state fMRI: a review of methods and clinical applications. AJNR Am J Neuroradiol 2013;34:1866–72.
[98] Ferrari M, Quaresima V. A brief review on the history of human functional near-infrared spectroscopy (fNIRS) development and fields of application. Neuroimage 2012;63:921–35.
[99] Zhang S, Peng C, Yang Y, et al. Resting-state brain networks in neonatal hypoxic-ischemic brain damage: a functional near-infrared spectroscopy study. Neurophotonics 2021;8:025007.
[100] Tang L, Kebaya LMN, Altamimi T, et al. Altered resting-state functional connectivity in newborns with hypoxic ischemic encephalopathy assessed using high-density functional near-infrared spectroscopy. Sci Rep 2024; 14:3176.
[101] Baranger J, Demene C, Frerot A, et al. Bedside functional monitoring of the dynamic brain connectivity in human neonates. Nat Commun 2021;12: 1080.
[102] Fortin JP, Parker D, Tunc B, et al. Harmonization of multi-site diffusion tensor imaging data. Neuroimage 2017;161:149–70.
[103] Bonthrone AF, Blesa Cabez M, Edwards AD, et al. Harmonizing multisite neonatal diffusion-weighted brain MRI data for developmental neuroscience. Dev Cogn Neurosci 2025;71:101488.
[104] Yu M, Linn KA, Cook PA, et al. Statistical harmonization corrects site effects in functional connectivity measurements from multi-site fMRI data. Hum Brain Mapp 2018;39:4213–27.
[105] Meyers B, Lee VK, Dennis L, et al. Harmonization of multi-center diffusion tensor tractography in neonates with congenital heart disease: optimizing post-processing and application of ComBat. Neuroimage Rep 2022;2.
[106] Vesoulis ZA, Trivedi SB, Morris HF, et al. Deep learning to optimize magnetic resonance imaging prediction of motor outcomes after hypoxic-ischemic encephalopathy. Pediatr Neurol 2023;149:26–31.
[107] Ouyang M, Whitehead MT, Mohapatra S, et al. Machine-learning based prediction of future outcome using multimodal MRI during early childhood. Semin Fetal Neonatal Med 2024;29:101561.
[108] Rosenberg MD, Casey BJ, Holmes AJ. Prediction complements explanation in understanding the developing brain. Nat Commun 2018;9:589.
[109] Howell BR, Styner MA, Gao W, et al. The UNC/UMN Baby Connectome Project (BCP): an overview of the study design and protocol development. Neuroimage 2019;185:891–905.
[110] Chen L, Wu Z, Hu D, et al. A 4D infant brain volumetric atlas based on the UNC/UMN baby connectome project (BCP) cohort. Neuroimage 2022;253: 119097.
[111] Huang H, Zhang J, Wakana S, et al. White and gray matter development in human fetal, newborn and pediatric brains. Neuroimage 2006;33:27–38.
[112] Feng L, Li H, Oishi K, et al. Age-specific gray and white matter DTI atlas for human brain at 33, 36 and 39 postmenstrual weeks. Neuroimage 2019; 185:685–98.
[113] HEALthy brain and Child development (HBCD) study. Available at: https://heal.nih.gov/research/infants-and-children/healthy-brain.
[114] Azzopardi DV, Strohm B, Edwards AD, et al. Moderate hypothermia to treat perinatal asphyxial encephalopathy. N Engl J Med 2009;361:1349–58.
[115] Azzopardi D, Brocklehurst P, Edwards D, et al. The TOBY Study. Whole body hypothermia for the

treatment of perinatal asphyxial encephalopathy: a randomised controlled trial. BMC Pediatr 2008;8:17.

[116] Gluckman PD, Wyatt JS, Azzopardi D, et al. Selective head cooling with mild systemic hypothermia after neonatal encephalopathy: multicentre randomised trial. Lancet 2005;365:663–70.

[117] Shankaran S, Laptook AR, Ehrenkranz RA, et al, National Institute of Child Health and Human Development Neonatal Research Network. Whole-body hypothermia for neonates with hypoxic-ischemic encephalopathy. N Engl J Med 2005;353:1574–84.

[118] Shankaran S, Laptook AR, Pappas A, et al, Eunice Kennedy Shriver National Institute of Child H, Human Development Neonatal Research N. Effect of Depth and duration of cooling on death or disability at age 18 Months among neonates with hypoxic-ischemic encephalopathy: a randomized clinical trial. JAMA 2017;318:57–67.

Advances in Clinical Radiology 7 (2025) 129–140
ADVANCES IN CLINICAL RADIOLOGY

Advances in Imaging the Glymphatic System

Jeremy Ford, MD, MBA[a,*], Neel Madan, MD[b], Christopher G. Filippi, MD[c], Karen Buch, MD[a]
[a]Department of Radiology, Massachusetts General Hospital, Boston, MA, USA; [b]Department of Radiology, Tufts Medical Center, Boston, MA, USA; [c]Department of Radiology, Hospital for Sick Children, Toronto, Ontario

KEY WORDS
• Glymphatic system • Cerebrospinal fluid clearance • Neuroimaging • Gadolinium-based contrast agents
• Diffusion MRI • Perivascular spaces • Brain waste clearance • Neurodegenerative diseases

KEY POINTS

- *The glymphatic system is essential for brain waste clearance*, utilizing cerebrospinal fluid to remove metabolic byproducts.
- *Innovative MRI techniques enable noninvasive assessment of glymphatic function*, including diffusion-weighted imaging, T1 mapping, dynamic contrast-enhanced MRI, and arterial spin labeling, each providing unique insights into brain fluid dynamics.
- *Intrathecal gadolinium-based contrast agent imaging directly visualizes glymphatic pathways*, revealing impaired clearance in conditions such as idiopathic normal pressure hydrocephalus, neurodegenerative diseases, and chronic poor sleep.
- *Perivascular space imaging and diffusion tensor image analysis along the perivascular space may serve as an indirect biomarker of glymphatic function.*

INTRODUCTION

Despite accounting for only 2% of the body's mass, the human brain consumes approximately 25% of the body's energy, making it the most metabolically active organ by weight. Like any energy-intensive system, the brain generates a substantial amount of metabolic waste—equivalent to its own weight of approximately 1.4 kg each year [1].

The proposed glymphatic system, a brain-wide fluid transport mechanism, has emerged as the leading hypothesis to address this waste clearance problem. Although the concept of interstitial fluid (ISF) drainage had been postulated for decades [2,3], it was not until 2012 that Nedergaard and Iliff [4] first characterized the glymphatic system as a structured pathway for cerebrospinal fluid (CSF) influx and ISF clearance.

The glymphatic system operates in a perivascular manner and relies on astroglial aquaporin-4 (AQP4) water channels for CSF-ISF exchange (Fig. 1). Nedergaard and other's research underscored the importance of sleep in glymphatic function, demonstrating that clearance is enhanced during slow-wave sleep, when interstitial spaces expand, facilitating greater fluid movement [5]. Iliff and colleagues [6] further extended these findings, linking glymphatic dysfunction to traumatic brain injury (TBI), stroke [7], and aging [8].

This article will explore the evolution of glymphatic system imaging, detailing the various techniques used

*Corresponding author. Massachusetts General Hospital, 55 Fruit Street, Boston, MA 02114. *E-mail address:* jnford@mgh.harvard.edu

https://doi.org/10.1016/j.yacr.2025.05.010 www.advancesinclinicalradiology.com
2589-8701/25/

ABBREVIATIONS

2D	2 dimensional
3D	3 dimensional
4D	4 dimensional
AP	anterior-posterior
AQP4	aquaporin-4
BBB	blood–brain barrier
CA	cerebral aqueduct
CSF	cerebrospinal fluid
DCE	dynamic contrast enhanced
DP-ASL	diffusion-prepared arterial spin labeling
DTI-ALPS	diffusion tensor image analysis along the perivascular space
DTI-ALPS	diffusion tensor imaging along the perivascular space
FMo	foramen of Monro
GBCAs	gadolinium-based contrast agents
IIH	idiopathic intracranial hypertension
iNPH	idiopathic normal pressure hydrocephalus
iNPH	idiopathic normal pressure hydrocephalus
ISF	interstitial fluid
IV	intravenous
LV	lateral ventricles
PC-MRI	phase-contrast MRI
PSD	parasagittal dural
PVS	perivascular spaces
SC	spinal canal
SI	superior-inferior
TBI	traumatic brain injury
TOF	time-of-flight

to assess CSF–ISF exchange, waste clearance, and their clinical relevance in central nervous system disorders. By integrating current physiologic knowledge with the latest imaging advancements, we aim to provide a comprehensive understanding of how the glymphatic system can be effectively studied and applied in clinical practice. Each imaging technique discussed here may assess either global glymphatic clearance or a specific component of the circuit (Table 1). Additionally, distinguishing whether a method primarily captures solvent dynamics (eg, water movement) or solute transport (eg, contrast agents) is crucial for interpreting results. While this list does not cover all available techniques—excluding, for example, radiotracer-based methods and intravoxel incoherent motion MRI—it highlights those with the greatest potential for clinical translation and application.

STRUCTURAL IMAGING

Perivascular spaces

Perivascular spaces (PVS), also known as Virchow–Robin spaces, are fluid-filled tunnels that accompany penetrating arteries and veins throughout the brain. These structures serve as key conduits for CSF–ISF exchange, forming a critical component of the glymphatic system. Abnormal PVS enlargement has been associated with small vessel disease, neuroinflammation, and neurodegenerative disorders [9].

In the study by Bouvy and colleagues [10], perivascular spaces (PVS) and their spatial relationship with penetrating blood vessels (Fig. 2) were examined, revealing that PVS visible on T2-weighted imaging are predominantly associated with perforating arteries rather than veins. This finding reinforces the periarterial nature of glymphatic influx pathways. In the basal ganglia, PVS were connected to the basal cisterns and followed the course of the lenticulostriate arteries, often exhibiting focal dilations. In the centrum semiovale, PVS tended to converge toward the ventricles but did not extend into the cortex.

PVS enlargement and glymphatic dysfunction can arise from several physiologic mechanisms. One major contributing factor is vascular stiffness and reduced arterial pulsatility, which diminishes the driving force for CSF influx into the brain, leading to stagnation of interstitial waste and PVS dilation [11]. Additionally, AQP-4 depolarization at the astrocyte endfeet [12] could diminish glymphatic influx from the periarterial side, leading to an enlarging fluid reservoir proximal to the glia limitans.

Given their role in brain fluid dynamics, PVS have become an important emerging biomarker. PVS are best visualized using 3D T2-weighted MRI, which provides high contrast between CSF and surrounding brain tissue, allowing for clear delineation of these spaces [9]. However, manual identification of PVS is labor-intensive and prone to interobserver variability. Consequently, automatic segmentation techniques have been developed to improve accuracy and reproducibility [13–15]. An important step forward in PVS segmentation is the use of 3D T1-weighted images [16], which is more commonly acquired in clinical settings than 3D T2-weighted imaging.

One key advantage of studying PVS is that large research and clinical imaging datasets are available, particularly since 3D T1-weighted imaging—which is commonly acquired in clinical MRI protocols—can be leveraged for segmentation and analysis. This allows for wide-scale population studies without the need for specialized imaging sequences.

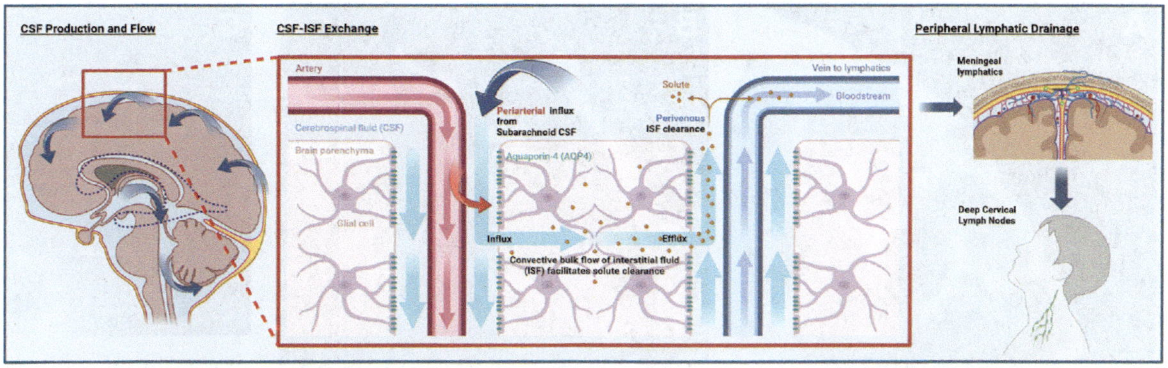

FIG. 1 Representation of the glymphatic system, illustrating cerebrospinal fluid (CSF) production, interstitial fluid (ISF) exchange, and peripheral lymphatic drainage. CSF is produced within the choroid plexus of the ventricular system and flows into the subarachnoid space before entering the brain parenchyma via periarterial spaces. Aquaporin-4 (AQP4) channels facilitate the convective mixing of CSF and ISF, promoting waste clearance along perivenous pathways. The waste-laden fluid is then drained into the meningeal lymphatics and ultimately reaches the deep cervical lymph nodes, where it enters systemic circulation. According to the glymphatic hypothesis, this system plays a crucial role in clearing metabolic byproducts, including amyloid-beta and tau, and is most active during sleep. (*Created in* BioRender. Ford, J. (2025) https://BioRender.com/vheq738.)

TABLE 1
Summary of common imaging modalities used to assess glymphatic function

Category	Imaging Modality	Measures Solute or Solvent?	Targeted Glymphatic Pathway Component
Structural imaging techniques	3 dimensional (3D) T1 or T2-weighted MRI	Solvent (CSF spaces)	Enlarged perivascular spaces (predominately periarterial), suggests diminished glymphatic influx and enlarged reservoir
	Parasagittal dural space MRI	Solvent (CSF volume)	Parasagittal dural space and transarachnoid CSF clearance in the distal glymphatic circuit
Diffusion/Perfusion/ Flow-based techniques	Phase-contrast MRI (PC-MRI), including 4 dimensional (4D)	Solvent (CSF flow)	Bulk CSF movement and velocity throughout the ventricular system
	Diffusion-prepared arterial spin labeling (DP-ASL)	Solvent (CSF perfusion interaction)	Convective flow/glymphatic influx at the blood–brain barrier
	Diffusion tensor image analysis along the perivascular space (DTI-ALPS)	Solvent (water diffusivity)	Perivenous ISF clearance
Gadolinium-based contrast agent techniques	Intrathecal gadolinium-enhanced MRI	Solute (tracer-based clearance)	CSF and glymphatic clearance pathways
	Intravenous gadolinium-enhanced MRI	Solute (tracer leakage)	Blood–brain barrier permeability and glymphatic solute transport

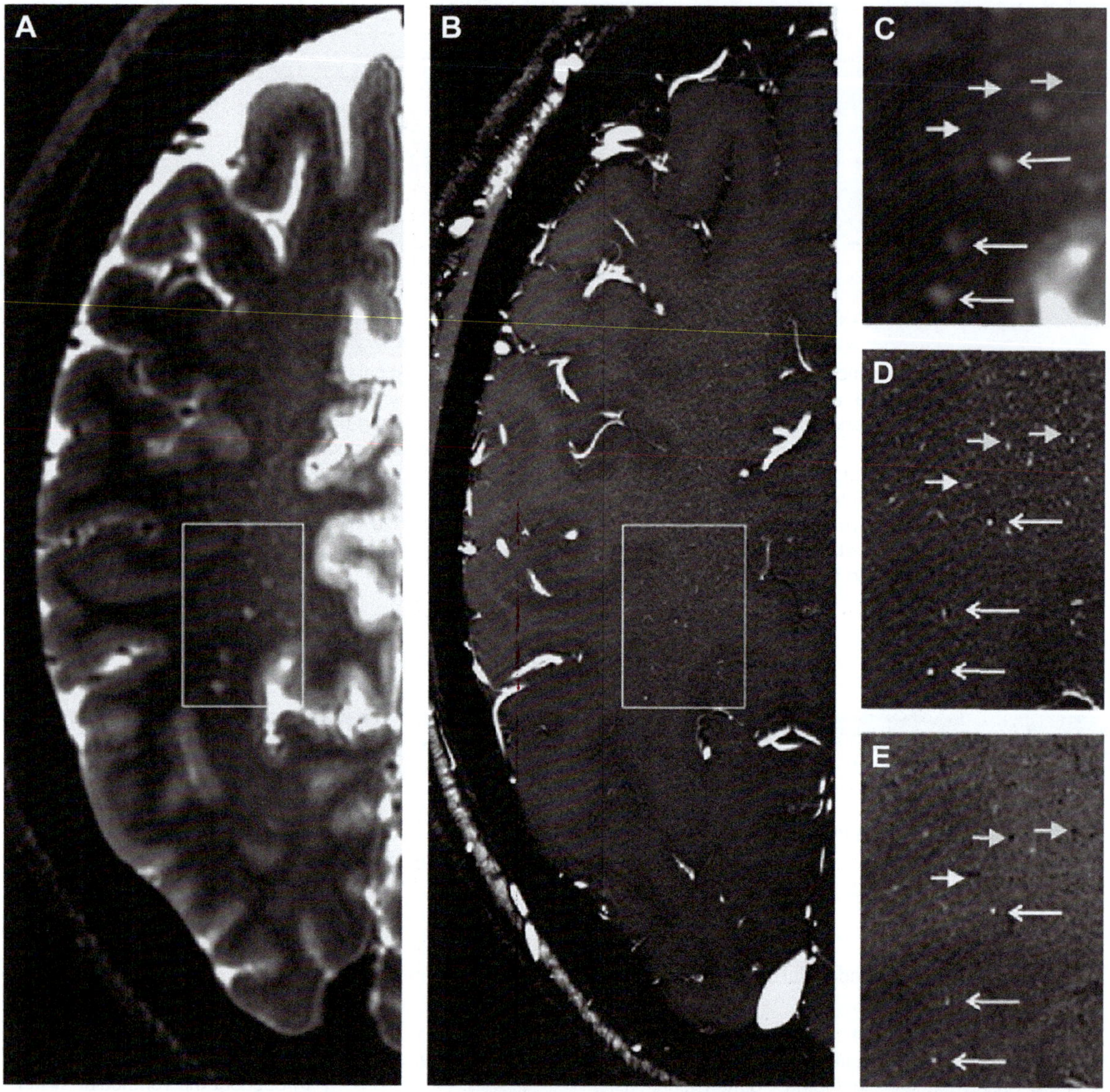

FIG. 2 Visualization of the relationship between perivascular spaces (PVS) and perforating arteries and veins using the 2 dimensional (2D) time-of-flight (TOF) sequence. Panels A and C display T2-weighted turbo spin echo (TSE) slices, 2 mm thick, highlighting PVS within the centrum semiovale. Panels B and D show the first echo of the 2D TOF sequence, where both perforating arteries and veins appear as bright structures (denoted by open and solid *arrows*, respectively). Panel E presents the third echo of the TOF sequence, where veins become dark (*solid arrows*), while arteries remain bright. Close examination reveals that PVS align with perforating arteries (*open arrows*) but not with veins (*solid arrows*). (Reprinted with permission.)

However, a major disadvantage is that PVS may not exhibit significant measurable changes over short time horizons, limiting their utility in longitudinal studies or intervention trials. This slow progression may reduce their sensitivity as early biomarkers for glymphatic dysfunction. Furthermore, while PVS are an important structural component of the glymphatic system, they only represent one aspect of the broader glymphatic pathway—primarily the periarterial CSF influx mechanism. Other glymphatic processes, such as ISF exchange and perivenous clearance, are not directly assessed by PVS imaging alone, necessitating complementary imaging techniques.

Parasagittal dural space

The parasagittal dural (PSD) space has recently emerged as an important anatomic region that is possibly relevant to glymphatic clearance. Located adjacent to the superior sagittal sinus, the PSD space can be visualized noninvasively using 3D T2-weighted MRI, which provides high contrast between CSF and surrounding dura. PSD volume can be quantified using deep-learning-based segmentation techniques applied to high-resolution MRI. These methods allow for automated, reproducible volumetric measurements, overcoming the limitations of manual segmentation. In a recent study, PSD volume was found to increase with age (Fig. 3) and correlated significantly with cerebral aqueductal CSF flow, reinforcing the hypothesis that PSD serves as a distal outlet for CSF clearance [17].

One of the main advantages of studying PSD in glymphatic research is that it can be readily measured using widely available 3D T1-weighted and T2-weighted MRI, making it accessible across large-scale research and clinical datasets. Another key advantage of PSD imaging is that it may reflect a later stage of glymphatic clearance, particularly the transarachnoid movement of CSF and metabolic waste products. Because the glymphatic system facilitates CSF influx along periarterial spaces and subsequent solute clearance along perivenous pathways, the final step in this clearance process involves the movement of CSF

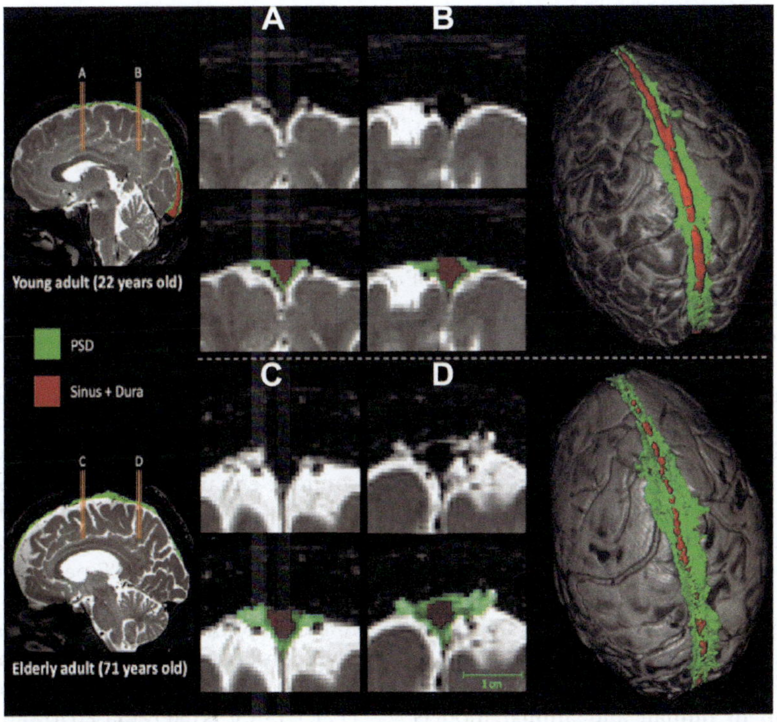

FIG. 3 Comparison of parasagittal dural (PSD) space volume between a young adult (top row) and an older adult (bottom row), as identified using an automatic segmentation method. Red regions represent voxels classified as the superior sagittal sinus and contributing veins, while green regions correspond to PSD space. The middle panels show selected cross-sectional slices taken from 2 different brain regions: (*A*, *C*) the posterior frontal lobe and (*B*, *D*) the anterior parietal lobe, where PSD volume expansion is most pronounced in the older adult. The right panels display 3D surface reconstructions of the brain, highlighting PSD structures in green. The images illustrate age-related enlargement of PSD space, which may reflect changes in cerebrospinal fluid (CSF) drainage or glymphatic function over time. (Reprinted under Creative Commons license.)

and waste from the parenchyma toward extracranial lymphatic drainage sites.

Despite its potential, PSD volume as a marker for glymphatic function has several limitations. One concern is that changes in PSD size likely occur over extended periods, making it a relatively static biomarker that may not capture acute fluctuations in glymphatic activity. This presents challenges for using PSD volume to evaluate short-term interventions aimed at modulating glymphatic flow, such as sleep modifications or pharmacologic treatments. Furthermore, while PSD enlargement may suggest alterations in glymphatic clearance, it remains unclear whether this reflects a failure of waste elimination or an adaptive response to altered CSF dynamics. Increased PSD volume could be compensatory, representing an alternative route for CSF egress rather than a strict indicator of glymphatic dysfunction.

DIFFUSION, PERFUSION, AND FLOW IMAGING

Phase contrast

Phase-contrast MRI (PC-MRI) is a well-established method for quantifying CSF flow dynamics in both clinical and research settings. By leveraging velocity-sensitive encoding gradients, PC-MRI provides direct measurements of CSF velocity, pulsatility, and directional flow patterns throughout the ventricular system [18]. The ability to visualize and measure bulk CSF movement makes PC-MRI a valuable tool for assessing neurofluid clearance mechanisms upstream of CSF–ISF exchange.

While not typically depicted as part of the canonical glymphatic pathway, the production and flow of CSF are critical to providing clean material for CSF–ISF exchange. The glymphatic system depends on a continuous supply of fresh CSF to drive perivascular fluid transport and facilitate the removal of metabolic waste. PC-MRI enables researchers to quantify CSF stroke volume, velocity, and pulsatility, providing insights into the overall efficiency of fluid circulation that underpins glymphatic clearance.

PC-MRI has been used to assess CSF transport and glymphatic function in human and animal models, demonstrating how factors like aging and neurodegenerative disease can reduce CSF velocity and impair waste clearance [19]. This suggests that PC-MRI could serve as a biomarker for upstream glymphatic dysfunction in conditions like Alzheimer's disease and idiopathic normal pressure hydrocephalus (iNPH).

Recent advancements in 4D PC-MRI have extended its applications beyond traditional 2D slice-based CSF flow measurements, enabling volumetric assessment of CSF circulation across multiple compartments with improved spatial and temporal resolution [20] (Fig. 4). However, challenges remain, particularly regarding low CSF velocities and long T1 relaxation times, which necessitate optimization of velocity-encoding parameters (Venc) and imaging protocols to maximize signal-to-noise ratio.

In clinical practice, PC-MRI is a tool for CSF flow characterization in hydrocephalus, aqueductal stenosis, and Chiari malformations, where abnormal pulsatility or restricted flow can indicate pathology [21]. As research progresses, PC-MRI may play a crucial role in noninvasive assessment of CSF and glymphatic function, with potential applications in distinguishing neurodegenerative diseases and iNPH. Continued refinements in spatial and temporal resolution, velocity sensitivity, and automated segmentation will further enhance PC-MRI's utility.

Diffusion-prepared arterial spin labeling

DP-ASL is an emerging noninvasive MRI technique to assess water exchange across the blood–brain barrier (k_W). Specifically, the diffusion preparation probes the movement of labeled water molecules between relatively high-diffusion compartments (such as intravascular and perivascular spaces) and low-diffusion compartments (such as the brain parenchyma). This technique, initially developed by Danny JJ Wang, Keith St Lawrence, and later also Xingfeng Shao [22], has undergone improvements in image quality and resolution [23].

While DP-ASL has been explored as a tool for measuring blood–brain barrier (BBB) permeability, the lack of clear association with K_{TRANS} from dynamic contrast enhanced (DCE) perfusion [24] suggested the technique was probing a different aspect of BBB function. Notably, gadolinium-based contrast agents (GBCAs) used with DCE perfusion do not have access to AQP-4 channels and may also be insensitive to small BBB disruptions. Given AQP-4's essential role in glymphatic influx at the glia limitans and its demonstrated depolarization in aging and Alzheimer's disease (AD) [12], DP-ASL is likely biased toward measuring water exchange at the glia limitans rather than purely transendothelial transport. Since DP-ASL primarily detects the transition of labeled water molecules from high-diffusion environments (such as intravascular and perivascular spaces) to lower diffusion environments (such as the brain parenchyma), it is inherently more sensitive to exchange at the perivascular–glial interface rather than at the endothelial barrier itself. This distinction is

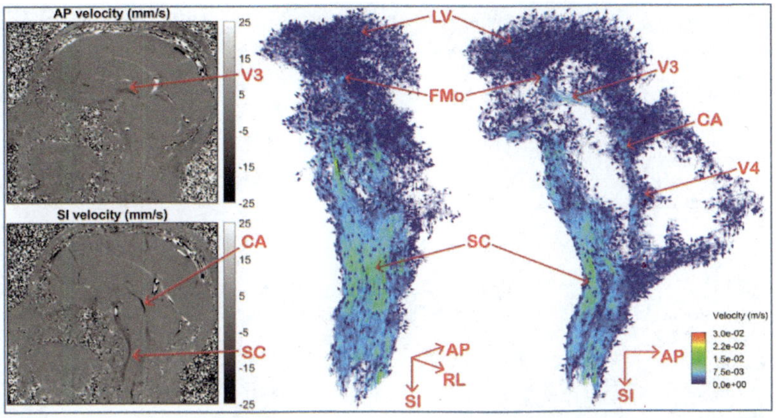

FIG. 4 This image shows velocity maps from a 4D flow MRI scan of cerebrospinal fluid (CSF), displayed in the sagittal view (left). The colors indicate CSF movement in the anterior-posterior (AP) and superior-inferior (SI) directions during the late diastolic phase of the cardiac cycle, highlighting CSF inflow into the third ventricle (V3), the cerebral aqueduct (CA), and the spinal canal (SC). On the right, velocity streamlines were created from the same 4D flow data, providing a visual representation of CSF motion at the same point in the cardiac cycle. The middle streamline image is rotated 45° to give an alternative perspective. Labels indicate key anatomic structures, including the fourth ventricle (V4), the foramen of Monro (FMo), and the lateral ventricles (LV). (Reprinted with permission.)

particularly important, as it positions DP-ASL as a technique that is better suited to capturing glymphatic inflow dynamics, in contrast to GBCA studies, which focus more directly on BBB permeability.

Recent studies have applied DP-ASL to evaluate BBB water exchange in the context of glymphatic function and sleep physiology. An effort at using concurrent MRI and electroencephalography (EEG) demonstrated that k_W tended to increase during slow wave sleep [25]. Also, multiple groups have shown that k_W measured with DP-ASL is lower among older individuals, suggesting diminished glymphatic influx with aging [26,27]. Furthermore, there is mounting evidence k_W tends to decrease with the presence of AD-type pathology [28,29], at least among healthy controls and in the mild cognitive impairment stage (Fig. 5).

Although DP-ASL holds promise as a noninvasive marker of BBB water exchange and glymphatic influx, its ability to comprehensively assess the entire glymphatic circuit is limited, necessitating the use of complementary imaging techniques for a more holistic evaluation. Additionally, in conditions where BBB disruption and leakage are more pronounced than AQP-4 depolarization, such as in TBI or neuroinflammatory disorders, DP-ASL's ability to measure glymphatic influx may be confounded by large-scale vascular permeability changes. Despite these limitations, DP-ASL remains a valuable tool in the imaging armamentarium, offering unique insights into perivascular water transport and its role in neurodegenerative and cerebrovascular diseases.

Diffusion tensor imaging along the perivascular space

The most widely used and controversial tool to probe glymphatic function is diffusion tensor imaging along the perivascular space (DTI-ALPS). Since its first description by Toshiaki Taoka [30], the use of the ALPS-index as a marker for glymphatic activity has been steadily growing, and since the 2020s, it may now account for nearly a quarter of published articles on the glymphatic system (Fig. 6) [31]. Reduced ALPS-indices have been found in a wide array of conditions, including neurodegeneration [32], after whole-brain radiation [33], demyelinating disorders [34], and idiopathic intracranial hypertension (IIH) [35]. This surge in adoption is largely driven by its ease of implementation, as it requires only standard DTI data, making it significantly more accessible than other techniques. However, even Taoka himself has cautioned against overinterpreting the ALPS index as a comprehensive measure of glymphatic function. In his 2024 review, he emphasized, "a higher ALPS-index indicates predominant Brownian motion of water molecules in the radial direction at the lateral ventricular body level, no more and no less" [36].

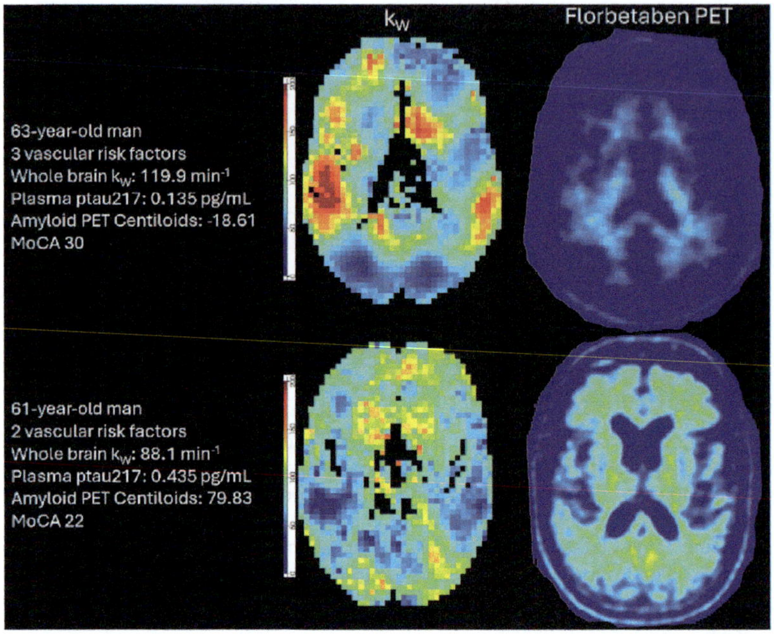

FIG. 5 The left column shows k_W maps, representing brain-wide water exchange rates (min^{-1}), while the right column shows corresponding florbetaben PET scans, a marker of amyloid deposition. The top row corresponds to a 63 year old cognitively normal (MoCA 30) man with 3 vascular risk factors, higher whole-brain k_W (119.9 min^{-1}), low plasma ptau217 (0.135 pg/mL), and negative amyloid PET (Centiloids: −18.61), indicating an absence of significant amyloid pathology. The bottom row represents a 61 year old man with MCI (MoCA 22) 2 vascular risk factors, lower whole-brain k_W (88.1 min^{-1}), elevated plasma ptau217 (0.435 pg/mL), and positive amyloid PET (Centiloids: 79.83), consistent with significant amyloid burden. This illuminates a potential relationship between glymphatic influx and amyloid deposition, whereby reduced water exchange may be associated with impaired clearance and increased amyloid accumulation.

DTI-ALPS quantifies water diffusion in specific white matter regions, particularly near the lateral ventricles, where medullary veins and perivascular spaces run orthogonally to major white matter tracts [30]. By leveraging this unique geometric orientation, the ALPS-index is calculated as the ratio of water diffusivity in the perivascular direction relative to diffusion perpendicular to white matter tracts. Importantly, DTI-ALPS is positioned along the veins, meaning it is biased toward assessing perivenous fluid efflux rather than periarterial influx.

Despite its potential, the interpretation and specificity of the ALPS-index face several challenges and limitations. Because the ALPS-index is based on white matter diffusion, it can be influenced by axonal degeneration and microstructural changes rather than reflecting perivascular fluid movement alone. For example, one group demonstrated that changes in radial asymmetry may account for at least some variation in the ALPS-index [37]. Another group found that crossing fibers significantly inflate ALP-indices, introducing a systematic bias that could explain some of the variability in previous glymphatic studies [38]. Collectively, these studies raise concerns about whether ALPS-index truly isolates perivascular water transport or if it also captures broader changes in white matter integrity.

Due to its ease-of-use, DTI-ALPS is expected to play an increasing role in probing glymphatic function and its role in brain health and disease, though its interpretation should remain circumspect and contextualized within broader glymphatic imaging approaches.

GADOLINIUM-BASED CONTRAST AGENT TECHNIQUES

Intrathecal gadolinium-based contrast agents

Intrathecal GBCAs have emerged as one of the most direct methods to assess glymphatic function in humans.

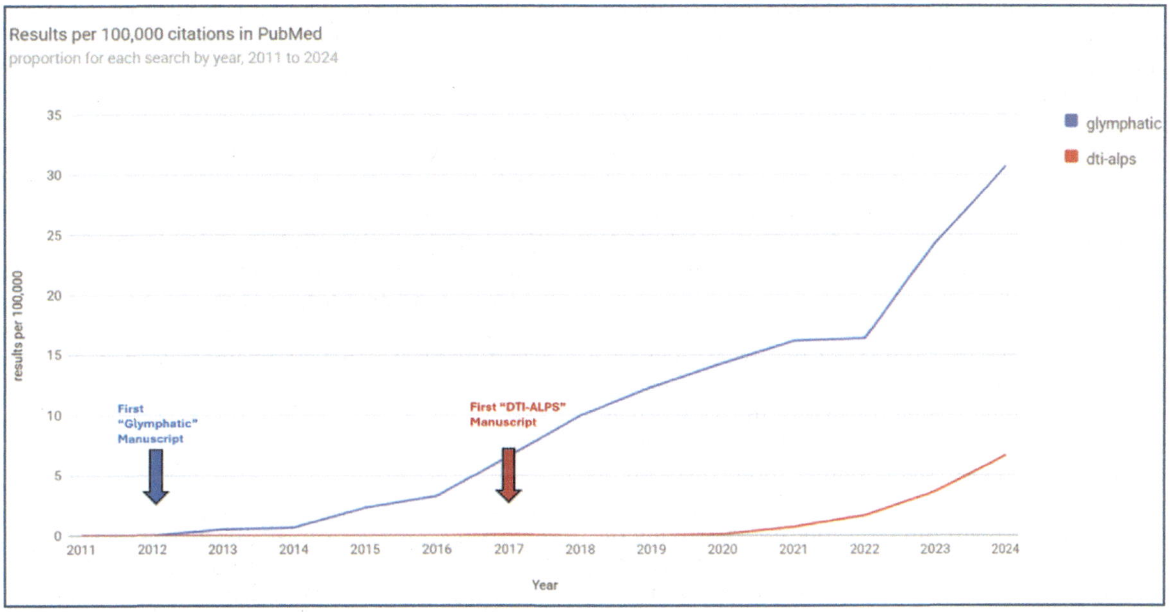

FIG. 6 This graph illustrates the increasing number of PubMed citations per 100,000 publications for the terms "glymphatic" (blue) and "DTI-ALPS" (red) from 2011 to 2024. The first glymphatic article was published in 2012 (*blue arrow*), marking the introduction of the glymphatic system concept. The first DTI-ALPS article appeared in 2017 (*red arrow*). Notably, all DTI-ALPS publications include the term "glymphatic," suggesting that the rise of DTI-ALPS research has been a significant driver of glymphatic-related publications, particularly in the 2020s. The continued expansion of DTI-ALPS studies may indicate increasing interest in noninvasive imaging of glymphatic function and its role in neurologic disorders. Generated from PubMed by Year [31].

Unlike other neuroimaging techniques that infer glymphatic activity from surrogate measures such as diffusion or structural changes, intrathecal GBCA-enhanced MRI directly tracks the movement of a tracer through CSF compartments and perivascular pathways. This method has been instrumental in elucidating glymphatic clearance pathways, particularly in pathologic conditions such as iNPH, IIH, and neurodegenerative diseases.

Several studies have validated the use of intrathecal GBCA to visualize glymphatic function. Ringstad and others [39] demonstrated that following intrathecal administration of gadobutrol, the contrast agent distributes throughout the brain in a centripetal manner, moving along perivascular pathways and reaching deep brain structures. Their findings provided evidence that the glymphatic system is active in humans and plays a crucial role in CSF–ISF exchange and waste clearance. This technique was applied to patients with iNPH, showing that these individuals exhibit delayed glymphatic clearance, particularly in the entorhinal cortex, suggesting an impaired waste elimination mechanism in this form of dementia [40]. Another study found that in individuals with chronic poor sleep, glymphatic enhancement following GBCA administration was significantly reduced, reinforcing the link between sleep glymphatic clearance [40]. Another group demonstrated the value of quantitative MRI with this technique, utilizing serial T1 mapping [41].

Despite its advantages, intrathecal GBCA imaging carries certain risks and limitations. The technique is invasive, requiring a lumbar puncture for contrast administration. Moreover, concerns have been raised about potential neurotoxicity associated with intrathecal GBCAs, although studies indicate that macrocyclic agents such as gadobutrol are relatively stable and safe when used at appropriate doses.

Intravenous gadolinium-based contrast agents

The use of intravenous (IV) GBCAs for glymphatic imaging has generated increasing interest due to its noninvasive administration and potential to reveal

CSF–ISF dynamics over extended time frames. Unlike intrathecal GBCA, which directly enters the CSF, IV GBCA must traverse the BBB before reaching the brain's fluid compartments. This passage is thought to occur via the choroid plexus and, potentially, through subtle BBB permeability variations in the aging and diseased brain. Several studies have demonstrated delayed GBCA enhancement in perivascular spaces and brain parenchyma hours after administration, suggesting that IV contrast can serve as an indirect marker of glymphatic function.

A study by Deike-Hofmann and colleagues [42] explored the delayed clearance of IV GBCA using T2-weighted fluid-attenuated inversion recovery (FLAIR) imaging, revealing signal increases in perivascular spaces, the choroid plexus, and cranial nerve perineural sheaths several hours after administration. These findings suggest that IV GBCA follows a pathway similar to ISF and CSF, contributing to our understanding of solute transport in the brain. However, compared to intrathecal GBCA, which provides a direct window into glymphatic exchange, IV GBCA imaging is more dependent on factors such as BBB integrity, systemic circulation, and renal clearance.

While IV GBCA techniques offer the advantage of avoiding invasive lumbar punctures, they also face key limitations. The signal detected in glymphatic regions is often weaker and more diffuse compared to intrathecal administration, necessitating optimized MRI sequences for adequate visualization. Studies have highlighted that long echo-time 3D-FLAIR sequences are among the most sensitive for detecting low GBCA concentrations in the glymphatic system [43]. Additionally, IV administration does not selectively target the glymphatic system, making it challenging to differentiate glymphatic transport from passive diffusion or BBB leakage.

In summary, both intrathecal and IV GBCA techniques provide unique insights into glymphatic function, with intrathecal administration offering more direct and detailed visualization, while IV methods provide a noninvasive alternative with broader systemic implications. As research continues to evolve, these techniques may further elucidate glymphatic dynamics and their impact on brain health, potentially guiding new therapeutic interventions for neurologic disorders.

SUMMARY

Imaging of the glymphatic system has become feasible, with various imaging modalities providing valuable insights into brain fluid dynamics and waste clearance. Structural MRI techniques, such as T1-weighted imaging and PSD space imaging, have advanced our comprehension of glymphatic-associated anatomic changes. Diffusion-based methods, including DTI-ALPS and DP-ASL, offer indirect assessments of perivascular water transport. Among the most direct techniques, GBCA imaging—both intrathecal and IV—has facilitated detailed visualization of solute transport through glymphatic pathways. Future research should aim to refine imaging protocols, integrate multimodal approaches, and translate glymphatic imaging into clinical practice to improve the diagnosis and treatment of neurologic disorders associated with impaired waste clearance.

CLINICS CARE POINTS

- *Glymphatic imaging techniques should be interpreted within their specific methodological limitations*—While techniques like DTI-ALPS, IV GBCA, and phase-contrast MRI provide insights into fluid transport, each measures different aspects of glymphatic function and should not be used interchangeably.
- *Intrathecal GBCA remains the most direct method for assessing glymphatic clearance*—Despite its invasiveness, lumbar intrathecal contrast-enhanced MRI provides the clearest visualization of CSF–ISF exchange, though safety concerns about neurotoxicity must be carefully considered.
- *IV GBCA methods reflect BBB permeability more than glymphatic transport*—Enhancement patterns in perivascular spaces following IV contrast should be interpreted with caution, as they may indicate vascular leakage rather than glymphatic activity.
- *Diffusion-based imaging (DTI-ALPS) offers an accessible but indirect measure of glymphatic function*—This method is widely used but may be confounded by white matter microstructural changes and fiber orientation effects, necessitating careful interpretation in clinical settings.

DISCLOSURE

Jeremy Ford has received research funding from the Radiological Society of North America and the Alzheimer's Drug Discovery Foundation, United States. Otherwise, Jeremy Ford has nothing to disclose. Nel Madan has nothing to disclose. Christopher Filippi received a grant from the American Society of Neuroradiology on Glympathic Flow. Karen Buch: Nothing to Disclose.

REFERENCES

[1] Ray LA, Heys JJ. Fluid flow and mass transport in brain tissue. Fluids 2019;4(4):196.

[2] Zhang E, Richards HK, Kida S, et al. Directional and compartmentalised drainage of interstitial fluid and cerebrospinal fluid from the rat brain. Acta Neuropathol 1992;83:233–9.

[3] Weller RO. Pathology of cerebrospinal fluid and interstitial fluid of the CNS: significance for Alzheimer disease, prion disorders and multiple sclerosis. J Neuropathol Exp Neurol 1998;57(10):885–94.

[4] Iliff JJ, Wang M, Liao Y, et al. A paravascular pathway facilitates CSF flow through the brain parenchyma and the clearance of interstitial solutes, including amyloid β. Sci Transl Med 2012;4(147):147ra111.

[5] Hablitz LM, Plʼ V, Giannetto M, et al. Circadian control of brain glymphatic and lymphatic fluid flow. Nat Commun 2020;11(1):4411.

[6] Iliff JJ, Chen MJ, Plog BA, et al. Impairment of glymphatic pathway function promotes tau pathology after traumatic brain injury. J Neurosci 2014;34(49):16180–93.

[7] Wang M, Iliff JJ, Liao Y, et al. Cognitive deficits and delayed neuronal loss in a mouse model of multiple microinfarcts. J Neurosci 2012;32(50):17948–60.

[8] Kress BT, Iliff JJ, Xia M, et al. Impairment of paravascular clearance pathways in the aging brain. Ann Neurol 2014;76(6):845–61.

[9] Yu L, Hu X, Li H, et al. Perivascular spaces, glymphatic system and MR. Front Neurol 2022;13:844938.

[10] Bouvy WH, Biessels GJ, Kuijf HJ, et al. Visualization of perivascular spaces and perforating arteries with 7 T magnetic resonance imaging. Investig Radiol 2014;49(5):307–13.

[11] Mestre H, Kostrikov S, Mehta RI, et al. Perivascular spaces, glymphatic dysfunction, and small vessel disease. Clin Sci 2017;131(17):2257–74.

[12] Zeppenfeld DM, Simon M, Haswell JD, et al. Association of perivascular localization of aquaporin-4 with cognition and Alzheimer disease in aging brains. JAMA Neurol 2017;74(1):91–9.

[13] Pham W, Lynch M, Spitz G, et al. A critical guide to the automated quantification of perivascular spaces in magnetic resonance imaging. Front Neurosci 2022;16:1021311.

[14] Sinclair B, Vivash L, Moses J, et al. Perivascular space identification nnunet for generalised usage (PINGU). arXiv preprint 2024 arXiv:2405.08337.

[15] Ballerini L, Lovreglio R, Valdś Hernńdez MDC, et al. Perivascular spaces segmentation in brain MRI using optimal 3D filtering. Sci Rep 2018;8(1):2132.

[16] Barisano G, Iv M, Choupan J, et al. Robust, fully-automated assessment of cerebral perivascular spaces and white matter lesions: a multicentre MRI longitudinal study of their evolution and association with risk of dementia and accelerated brain atrophy. EBioMedicine 2025;111.

[17] Hett K, McKnight CD, Eisma JJ, et al. Parasagittal dural space and cerebrospinal fluid (CSF) flow across the lifespan in healthy adults. Fluids Barriers CNS 2022;19(1):24.

[18] Rivera-Rivera LA, Vikner T, Eisenmenger L, et al. Four-dimensional flow MRI for quantitative assessment of cerebrospinal fluid dynamics: status and opportunities. NMR Biomed 2023;37(7):e5082.

[19] Ding G, Li L, Chopp M, et al. Velocity of cerebrospinal fluid in the aqueduct measured by phase-contrast MRI in rat. NMR Biomed 2024;37(12):e5233.

[20] Vikner T, Johnson KM, Cadman RV, et al. CSF dynamics throughout the ventricular system using 4D flow MRI: associations to arterial pulsatility, ventricular volumes, and age. Fluids Barriers CNS 2024;21(1):68.

[21] Elsafty HG, ELAggan A, Yousef M, et al. Cerebrospinal fluid flowmetry using phase-contrast MRI technique and its clinical applications. Tanta Medical Journal 2018;46(2):121–32.

[22] Wang J, Fernńdez-Seara MA, Wang S, et al. When perfusion meets diffusion: in vivo measurement of water permeability in human brain. J Cerebr Blood Flow Metabol 2007;27(4):839–49.

[23] Shao X, Zhao C, Shou Q, et al. Quantification of blood–brain barrier water exchange and permeability with multidelay diffusion-weighted pseudo-continuous arterial spin labeling. Magn Reson Med 2023;89(5):1990–2004.

[24] Shao X, Jann K, Ma SJ, et al. Comparison between blood-brain barrier water exchange rate and permeability to Gadolinium-based contrast agent in an elderly cohort. Front Neurosci 2020;14:1236.

[25] Yook S, Shao X, Chai Y, et al. Human brain MRI reveals more active glymphatic flow in deeper delta sleep. J Neurol Sci 2023;455.

[26] Shao X, Shou Q, Felix K, et al. Age-related decline in blood-brain barrier function is more pronounced in males than females in parietal and temporal regions. Elife 2024;13:RP96155.

[27] Ford JN, Zhang Q, Sweeney EM, et al. Quantitative water permeability mapping of blood-brain-barrier dysfunction in aging. Front Aging Neurosci 2022;14:867452.

[28] Uchida Y, Kan H, Sakurai K, et al. APOE ε4 dose associates with increased brain iron and β-amyloid via blood–brain barrier dysfunction. J Neurol Neurosurg Psychiatr 2022;93(7):772–8.

[29] Gold BT, Shao X, Sudduth TL, et al. Water exchange rate across the blood-brain barrier is associated with CSF amyloid-β42 in healthy older adults. Alzheimers Dement 2021;17(12):2020–9.

[30] Taoka T, Masutani Y, Kawai H, et al. Evaluation of glymphatic system activity with the diffusion MR technique: diffusion tensor image analysis along the perivascular space (DTI-ALPS) in Alzheimer's disease cases. Jpn J Radiol 2017;35:172–8.

[31] Sperr E. PubMed by Year. 2016. Available at: http://esperr.github.io/pubmed-by-year/. Accessed February 15, 2025.

[32] Steward CE, Venkatraman VK, Lui E, et al. Assessment of the DTI-ALPS parameter along the perivascular space in older adults at risk of dementia. J Neuroimaging 2021; 31(3):569–78.

[33] Saraf A, Ford J, Parsons M, et al. Association of ALPS-index and glymphatic flow with neurocognitive changes in patients receiving brain irradiation: secondary analysis of a prospective study. Int J Radiat Oncol Biol Phys 2024;120(2):e269–70.

[34] Bayoumi A, Hasan KM, Thomas JA, et al. Glymphatic dysfunction in multiple sclerosis and its association with disease pathology and disability. Multiple Sclerosis Journal 2024;30(13):1609–19.

[35] Bouffard MA, Avanaki MA, Ford JN, et al. MRI indices of glymphatic function correlate with disease duration in idiopathic intracranial hypertension. J Neuro Ophthalmol 2024. https://doi.org/10.1097/WNO.0000000000002259.

[36] Taoka T, Ito R, Nakamichi R, et al. Diffusion tensor image analysis ALong the perivascular space (DTI-ALPS): revisiting the meaning and significance of the method. Magn Reson Med Sci 2024;23:268–90.

[37] Wright AM, Wu YC, Chen NK, et al. Exploring radial asymmetry in MR diffusion tensor imaging and its impact on the interpretation of glymphatic mechanisms. J Magn Reson Imag 2024;60(4):1432–41.

[38] Georgiopoulos C, Werlin A, Lasic S, et al. Diffusion tensor imaging along the perivascular space: the bias from crossing fibres. Brain Communications 2024;6(6): fcae421.

[39] Ringstad G, Valnes LM, Dale AM, et al. Brain-wide glymphatic enhancement and clearance in humans assessed with MRI. JCI insight 2018;3(13).

[40] Eide PK, Ringstad G. Delayed clearance of cerebrospinal fluid tracer from entorhinal cortex in idiopathic normal pressure hydrocephalus: a glymphatic magnetic resonance imaging study. J Cerebr Blood Flow Metabol 2019;39(7):1355–68.

[41] Watts R, Steinklein JM, Waldman L, et al. Measuring glymphatic flow in man using quantitative contrast-enhanced MRI. Am J Neuroradiol 2019;40(4):648–51.

[42] Deike-Hofmann K, Reuter J, Haase R, et al. Glymphatic pathway of gadolinium-based contrast agents through the brain: overlooked and misinterpreted. Investig Radiol 2019;54(4):229–37.

[43] Mijnders LS, Steup FW, Lindhout M, et al. Optimal sequences and sequence parameters for GBCA-enhanced MRI of the glymphatic system: a systematic literature review. Acta Radiologica 2021;62(10):1324–32.

Advances in Clinical Radiology 7 (2025) 141–155
ADVANCES IN CLINICAL RADIOLOGY

Up to Date Imaging Evaluation of Pediatric Syndromes Associated with Neoplasms

What Radiologists Need to Know

Jessica Kurian, MD[a,*], Rita Maria Lahoud, MD[b], Nathan C. Hull, MD[c], Edward Y. Lee, MD[d]
[a]Department of Radiology, Westchester Medical Center, 100 Woods Road, Valhalla, NY 10595, USA; [b]Department of Radiology, Tufts Medical Center, 800 Washington St, #299, Boston, MA 02111, USA; [c]Department of Radiology, Mayo Clinic, 200 First Street Southwest, Rochester, MN 55905, USA; [d]Department of Radiology, Boston Children's Hospital and Harvard Medical School, 300 Longwood Avenue, Boston, MA 02115, USA

KEYWORDS
• Cancer predisposition syndrome • Neoplasm • Malignancy • Children • Whole body MRI

KEY POINTS
- Children with cancer predisposition syndromes develop organ-specific neoplasms at an earlier age than seen in the general population.
- In selected cancer predisposition syndromes, the recommended annual screening requires whole-body MRI.
- A combination of ultrasound, computed tomography, and MRI is used in surveillance protocols for early detection of cancer, as well as staging and monitoring of disease.

INTRODUCTION

Cancer predisposition syndromes (CPS) are hereditary disorders characterized by genetic mutations that increase the risk of developing cancer. In CPS, tumors arise in specific organs, anatomic locations, or tissue types, and some CPS also predispose patients to a broader spectrum of malignancies [1] (Table 1). CPS is suspected when a child presents with any of the following: cancer at an unusually young age, multifocal cancers, unique types of cancer, family history of related cancers, or physical stigmata of a CPS. Most CPS result from loss-of-function mutations of tumor suppressor genes, which inhibit cell growth, although some CPS result from gain-of-function mutations of oncogenes, which promote cell growth.

Imaging is used in CPS for the workup of primary cancers, as well as for cancer surveillance, which usually begins in childhood and sometimes lasts throughout the lifespan. Surveillance is focused on cancers that present in children, and also cancers known to be particularly aggressive [2]. Patient outcomes may be improved by early detection, since tumors are identified at a smaller size and before they metastasize [2]. Survival benefits have been demonstrated in patients with Beckwith-Wiedemann syndrome and Li-Fraumeni syndrome [3,4].

Radiological evaluation is indispensable in the workup of CPS patients. This article reviews the relevant imaging modalities used in CPS management, as well as the specific clinical and radiologic features of

*Corresponding author. *E-mail address:* jessy.kurian@gmail.com

https://doi.org/10.1016/j.yacr.2025.06.001 www.advancesinclinicalradiology.com
2589-8701/25/

ABBREVIATIONS	
ACC	adrenal cortical carcinoma
AFP	serum alpha-fetoprotein
AML	angiomyolipomas
BWS	Beckwith-Wiedemann syndrome
CNS	central nervous system
CPS	cancer predisposition syndromes
CT	computed tomography
DWI	diffusion weighted imaging
ELST	endolymphatic sac tumor
FLAIR	fluid-attenuated inversion recovery
GIST	gastrointestinal stromal tumor
HB	hemangioblastoma
LAM	lymphangioleiomyomatosis
LFS	Li-Fraumeni syndrome
MEN	multiple endocrine neoplasia
MPNST	malignant peripheral nerve sheath tumor
MTC	medullary thyroid carcinoma
NET	neuroendocrine tumor
NF1	neurofibromatosis type 1
NF2	neurofibromatosis type 2
PPB	pleuropulmonary blastoma
RML	radial migration line
SEGA	subependymal giant cell astrocytoma
SEN	subependymal nodule
TSC	tuberous sclerosis complex
US	ultrasound
VHL	von Hippel-Lindau
WBMRI	Whole-body MRI

various CPS that are reliant on imaging in the pediatric population.

IMAGING TECHNIQUES

The currently used imaging modalities in CPS include ultrasound (US), computed tomography (CT), magnetic resonance imaging (MRI), and PET/CT. In children with a palpable lesion or possible abdominal mass, US is the initial test and can be targeted to the area of concern. US is also a workhorse in surveillance of CPS, as it is often used to screen for solid organ tumors. CT is used for characterization and staging of new malignancies, as well as screening for thoracic malignancies. However, due to potentially harmful ionizing radiation exposure associated with CT, it must be used carefully by following the As Low As Reasonably Achievable (ALARA) principle, particularly in some CPS that are radiosensitive.

Whole-body MRI (WBMRI) provides global assessment of the entire body in a single examination, made possible by a large field of view. Other benefits of WBMRI include high tissue contrast and lack of ionizing radiation. However, the limiting factors of WBMRI include cost, longer examination time, need for anesthesia or sedation (particularly in young children), motion-sensitivity, and reduced spatial resolution when compared to site-specific MRI due to the large field of view. WBMRI is also suboptimal for imaging of small lung nodules ($\leq$4 mm), small lymph nodes, skin lesions, thyroid lesions, and some skeletal lesions [5–7]. Despite these drawbacks, WBMRI currently remains a robust technique for screening of neoplasms and characterization of multifocal disease that is seen in CPS [5,8]. The American Association for Cancer Research recommends WBMRI in the surveillance of selected CPS, including Li-Fraumeni syndrome (LFS), neurofibromatosis types 1 and 2 (NF1 and NF2), schwannomatosis, hereditary retinoblastoma, constitutional mismatch repair deficiency syndrome, and hereditary paraganglioma pheochromocytoma syndrome [5,9].

WBMRI can be successfully performed with free breathing and without gadolinium. 1.5-Tesla (T) field strength allows better fat suppression, less susceptibility artifact, and less distortion. However, 3.0-T is also acceptable, and offers higher signal-to-noise ratio and faster acquisition [5,10]. Although WBMRI protocols vary among practices, typical sequences include coronal short tau inversion recovery, coronal T1, and axial diffusion weighted imaging (DWI) or DWI with background suppression [5–7,10,11]. The large coverage area is obtained by scanning multiple contiguous stations from vertex to toes, with a small overlap between stations, and with the patient's hands by their sides. Whole-body images can be displayed by stitching together the coronal stations. The targeted table time is 30 to 40 minutes, which can be accomplished using multichannel and in-table coils, sliding table platforms, fast motion-resistant sequences, and parallel imaging [5,10,12,13].

FEATURES OF CANCER PREDISPOSITION SYNDROMES

Neurofibromatosis type I

Neurofibromatosis is comprised of a group of syndromes with benign and malignant nervous system tumors, and includes NF1, NF2, and schwannomatosis. The most common of these is NF1, also known as von Recklinghausen's disease. NF1 is autosomal dominant,

TABLE 1
Neoplastic and nonneoplastic features of cancer predisposition syndromes

Syndrome	Most Frequent Neoplasms	Additional Neoplasms	Nonneoplastic Features
NF 1	Neurofibroma Plexiform neurofibroma Malignant peripheral nerve sheath tumor Optic pathway glioma	Sarcomas Endocrine, skin, breast, genitourinary, abdominopelvic, and hematopoietic neoplasms	Iris hamartomas (Lisch nodules) Café-au-lait macules Inguinal & axillary freckling Osseous lesions (sphenoid dysplasia and tibial pseudoarthrosis) Interstitial lung disease, vascular dysplasia
BWS	Hepatoblastoma Wilms tumor	Neuroblastoma Adrenal cortical carcinoma Pheochromocytoma Rhabdomyosarcoma	Macrosomia Hemihypertrophy Organomegaly Macroglossia Dysmorphic facies Abdominal wall defects Cardiac anomalies Hyperinsulinism Renal findings (hydronephrosis, calyceal diverticula, medullary cysts, and nephrolithiasis)
LFS	Osteosarcoma Rhabdomyosarcoma Adrenocortical carcinoma CNS tumors Breast cancer Leukemia	Gastric, colon, thyroid, lung, ovarian, and skin cancers	
MEN 1	Parathyroid adenoma/hyperplasia Pituitary neoplasms (esp. prolactinoma) Pancreatic and duodenal neuroendocrine tumors (esp. gastrinoma)	CNS neoplasms Leiomyoma	Cutaneous lesions (e.g. angiofibroma)
MEN 2	MEN2A: Medullary thyroid carcinoma, parathyroid adenoma/hyperplasia, and pheochromocytoma MEN2B: Medullary thyroid carcinoma and pheochromocytoma	MEN2B: Mucosal neuromas and intestinal ganglioneuromas	MEN2B: Marfanoid habitus
DICER1 Syndrome	PPB Gynecologic tumors (Sertoli-Leydig cell tumor of ovary) Renal cystic nephroma	Cervical embryonal rhabdomyosarcoma	Lung cysts Thyroid nodules
TSC	Subependymal giant cell astrocytoma Cardiac rhabdomyoma Renal angiomyolipoma	Pancreatic neuroendocrine tumors Hepatic angiomyolipoma Perivascular epithelioid tumors	Skin lesions (hypomelanotic macules, Shagreen patch, and others) RMLs Cortical/subcortical tubers Subependymal nodules Retinal hamartomas LAM Splenic hamartoma Vascular aneurysms Myocardial fat foci Sclerotic bone lesions Renal cysts

(*continued on next page*)

TABLE 1
(continued)

Syndrome	Most Frequent Neoplasms	Additional Neoplasms	Nonneoplastic Features
VHL Disease	HB (CNS and retina) Endolymphatic sac tumor Pheochromocytoma Extra-adrenal paraganglioma Pancreatic neuroendocrine tumor Clear cell RCC Epididymal or adnexal papillary cystadenoma		Renal and pancreatic cysts

Abbreviation: CNS, central nervous system.

but half of cases are sporadic mutations. Mutation of the NF1 gene, a tumor suppressor gene encoding neurofibromin, triggers the Ras pathway, which leads to cellular proliferation [14].

NF1 is distinguished by mesodermal and neuroectodermal dysplasia [14]. According to the revised National Institutes of Health criteria, diagnosis of NF1 is made in patients meeting 2 or more of the following criteria: 6 or more café-au-lait macules, axillary or inguinal freckling, 2 or more Lisch nodules, 2 or more neurofibromas or 1 plexiform neurofibroma, optic glioma, and a distinctive osseous lesion, as well as a parent with NF1 or demonstration of a pathogenic NF1 variant (Fig. 1) [15]. Other findings seen in NF1 include focal areas of signal intensity (FASI) in the brain, brainstem gliomas, abdominopelvic neoplasms (pheochromocytoma/paraganglioma and gastrointestinal stromal tumor [GIST]), rhabdomyosarcoma, interstitial lung disease, vascular dysplasia (arterial stenoses, moya moya, and aneurysms), and skeletal lesions (anterolateral tibial bowing/pseudoarthrosis, sphenoid wing dysplasia, scoliosis, nonossifying fibromas) [14].

Neurofibromas are the most common neoplasm in NF1, consisting of benign nerve sheath tumors that can involve spinal nerve roots, as well as superficial or deep soft tissues [16]. The 3 types of neurofibroma include localized neurofibroma (most common), plexiform neurofibroma, and diffuse neurofibroma. MRI is the preferred imaging modality, as neurofibromas typically appear as nonspecific masses on US and CT. On MRI, lesions are typically fusiform in shape, intermediate to low signal intensity on T1, hyperintense on T2, and have variable enhancement qualities. T2 images may demonstrate a classic *target sign* with central low signal and peripheral high signal. Plexiform neurofibromas consist of lobular tortuous multispacial nerve lesions, with a *bag of worms* appearance and multiple target signs (Fig. 2) [14,17]. Diffuse neurofibromas are usually seen in children and young adults, and on

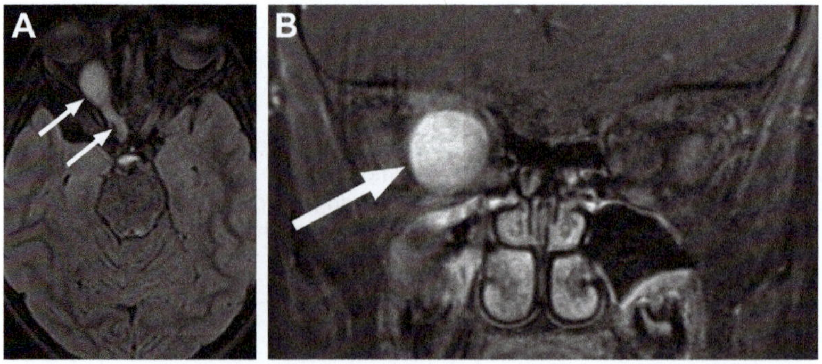

FIG. 1 10-year-old male with NF1 and optic pathway glioma. (**A**) Axial FLAIR image and (**B**) coronal postcontrast T1-weighted fat suppressed MR image show a fusiform expansile enhancing mass (*arrows*) of the intraorbital segment of the right optic nerve.

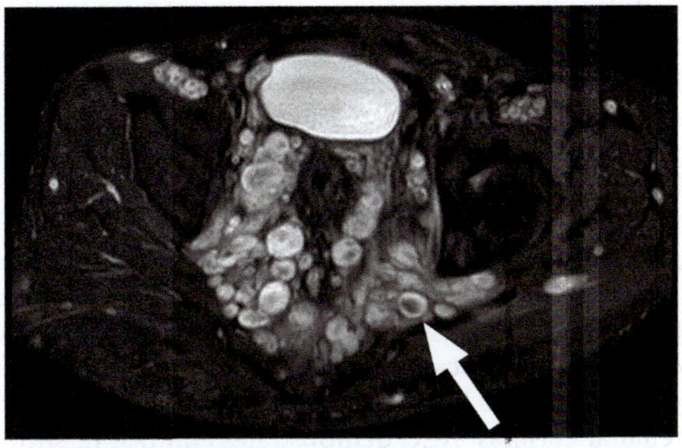

FIG. 2 18-year-old male with NF1 and plexiform neurofibromas. Axial T2-weighted fat suppressed MR image demonstrates numerous tortuous lobular lesions associated with the lumbosacral plexus, with a *bag of worms* appearance. Innumerable target signs (*arrow* on example) are present. Individual neurofibromas are also noted in the soft tissues.

imaging they appear as ill-defined reticulated lesions of skin and subcutaneous fat [18].

Malignant peripheral nerve sheath tumor (MPNST) is seen in 8% to 13% of NF1 patients, making it the most common malignancy of NF1 [19]. Patients with a large plexiform neurofibroma burden are at greater risk for MPNST, and children have a worse prognosis than adults [20,21]. It is thought that plexiform neurofibromas give rise to MPNST, which presents as a painful rapidly growing lesion, sometimes with focal neurologic signs, although some MPNST are asymptomatic [22]. MRI features that favor MPNST over benign neurofibroma include heterogeneous T1 signal, cystic degeneration or necrosis, infiltrative margins, and perilesional edema (Fig. 3) [23,24]. On 18-fluorodeoxygluocose (FDG) PET/CT, MPNST demonstrates greater uptake and heterogeneity compared to neurofibroma, although standardized uptake values significantly overlap [18].

Screening practices for MPNST in NF1 lack an established consensus. Some institutions obtain WBMRI to detect MPNST, monitor progression, and assess global neurofibroma burden [18,22,25]. Site-specific MRI is obtained for suspected MPNST, GIST, and brain tumors. Clinical surveillance includes physical examination (particularly neurologic and dermatologic checkups), blood pressure checks (vascular complications), and annual ophthalmologic examination (optic glioma and orbital lesions, among others.) [19,22].

Beckwith-Wiedemann syndrome

Beckwith-Wiedemann syndrome (BWS) is characterized by the early onset of embryonal tumors. BWS is also the most common overgrowth syndrome, with a spectrum ranging from classic BWS to isolated hemihypertrophy [26]. Typical features of BWS include macroglossia, hemihypertrophy, macrosomia, and abdominal wall defects (umbilical hernia, omphalocele, and diastasis recti) [27–29]. Other findings can include dysmorphic facies, organomegaly, cardiac anomalies, and hyperinsulinism [27].

BWS is typically recognized at birth, with 85% resulting from sporadic mutations, and 15% inherited in an autosomal dominant pattern [28,30]. The majority (up to 90%) of BWS involve mutations that affect the imprinting control regions on chromosome 11p15.5, altering the expression of various genes involved in cell cycle progression and somatic growth regulation [27,28]. Additionally, it is worth noting that there is a 10-fold increased risk with assisted reproductive techniques [28].

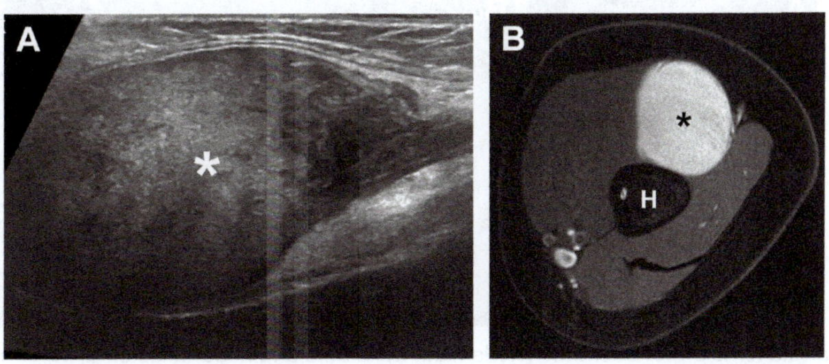

FIG. 3 15-year-old female with NF 1 and malignant peripheral nerve sheath tumor. (**A**) Sagittal US demonstrates a large heterogeneous mass (*asterisk*) in the left arm. (**B**) Axial post-contrast T1-weighted fat suppressed MR image shows an avidly enhancing mass (*asterisk*) anterior to the humerus (*H*).

The most common neoplasms in BWS are Wilms tumor (which can be bilateral) and hepatoblastoma (Figs. 4 and 5). Other neoplasms seen in BWS include neuroblastoma, adrenal cortical carcinoma (ACC), and rhabdomyosarcoma [27,29]. The highest risk for cancer in BWS patients is in the first 2 years of life, and most cancers develop before the age of 7 years [27,28]. The lifetime probability of cancer is 10%, and even higher in some subtypes of BWS [27,28]. Imaging features of neoplasms in BWS will parallel those of sporadic neoplasms in nonsyndromic patients. In approximately 25% of BWS patients, nonneoplastic findings are seen in the kidneys, including hydronephrosis, calyceal diverticula, medullary cysts, and nephrolithiasis [30,31].

Standard surveillance in BWS consists of serum alpha-fetoprotein (AFP) levels along with abdominal US, performed every 3 months up to the age of 3 years, followed by renal US until the age of 7 years [26–28]. AFP levels are inherently high in infants and should be interpreted carefully in this age group [26].

Li-Fraumeni syndrome

LFS is a multifaceted CPS, signified by early-onset of neoplasms in various tissue types. LFS patients are also predisposed to radiation-induced cancers [6]. The inheritance pattern is autosomal dominant, and 75% of LFS result from mutations in the tumor suppressor gene p53, which is involved in DNA repair [32]. The overall risk of cancer is greater than 90% in females and greater than 70% in males, and 50% of LFS patients develop an invasive cancer by the age of 30 [6,33]. Neoplasms commonly seen in children and young adults with LFS include soft tissue sarcomas (especially rhabdomyosarcoma), osteosarcoma, ACC, and central nervous system (CNS) tumors (glioblastoma, medulloblastoma, choroid plexus carcinoma, and primitive neuroectodermal tumor) (Figs. 6 and 7) [6,17]. Older patients are also susceptible to gastrointestinal cancers, breast cancer, and melanoma [34].

ACC is a hallmark cancer of LFS, and on MRI appears as an enhancing mass, which may demonstrate heterogeneous signal, necrosis, and hemorrhage (Fig. 7) [6,8]. Invasion of the renal vein, inferior vena cava, and adjacent structures may be seen, as well as hepatic metastases [6,8]. On CT, in contrast to benign adrenal adenomas, ACC demonstrates contrast retention (less washout) on delayed phase images. Imaging features of other LFS neoplasms are also equivalent to their sporadic analogs.

LFS surveillance includes physical examination, imaging, and laboratory studies, which are based on the modified Toronto protocol [34]. Screening includes repeated abdomen-pelvis US (every 3–4 months), annual brain MRI, and annual WBMRI.

Multiple endocrine neoplasias

Multiple endocrine neoplasias (MEN1, MEN2) are autosomal dominant syndromes distinguished by multiple endocrine gland tumors. In MEN type 1, also known as Wermer syndrome, the affected gene is MEN1, encoding the tumor suppressor menin [29]. In MEN type 2 the affected gene is MEN2, encoding the *RET* proto-oncogene [29]. MEN4, also known as *CDKN1B*-related MEN, has also been identified as a third type of MEN; however, there is currently a scarcity of data regarding this entity [35].

The diagnosis of MEN1 is usually established by age 40 to 50 years, with the most common presentation

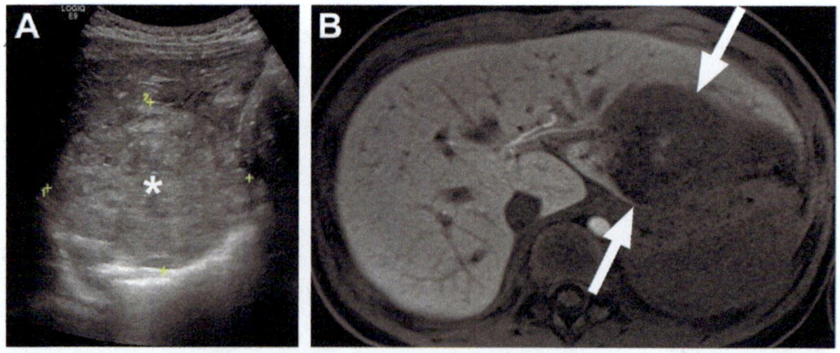

FIG. 4 2-year-old female with Beckwith-Wiedemann syndrome and hepatoblastoma. (**A**) Sagittal US image demonstrates a hyperechoic solid mass (*asterisk*) in the left hepatic lobe. (**B**) Axial hepatobiliary phase post-contrast T1-weighted fat suppressed MR image with gadoexetate disodium (Eovist) shows low signal intensity of the mass (*arrows*) relative to the background liver.

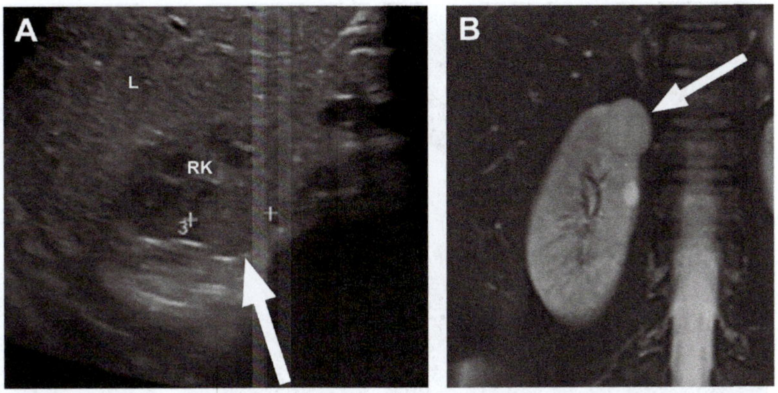

FIG. 5 3-year-old female with Beckwith-Wiedemann syndrome and Wilms tumor. (**A**) Transverse US image demonstrates a solid isoechoic lesion (*arrow*) in the upper pole of the right kidney RK L = liver. (**B**) Coronal T2-weighted fat suppressed MR image demonstrates a well-circumscribed hyperintense renal mass (*arrow*). A small cyst is incidentally noted in the medial right kidney.

being primary hyperparathyroidism; however, it can manifest as early as age 5 years [35–38]. The *3Ps* of MEN1 include parathyroid gland adenomas or hyperplasia, anterior pituitary gland adenomas (most commonly prolactinoma), and pancreatic neuroendocrine tumors (NET, most commonly gastrinoma). Evaluation of the parathyroid gland using US can show an adenoma situated posterior to the thyroid gland, consisting of an ovoid hypoechoic well-circumscribed nodule, often with visualization of a conspicuous feeding vessel (a branch of the inferior thyroidal artery.) [17,36,39] To detect small or ectopic parathyroid adenomas, nuclear scintigraphy with 99m-Technetium-sestamibi is more sensitive [17,39]. Parathyroid adenomas demonstrate characteristic early arterial enhancement and washout on multiphase CT, which is sometimes used preoperatively to precisely localize adenomas in the neck or superior mediastinum [36,39].

Pancreatic NET in MEN1 can be identified with CT, MRI, endoscopic US, or nuclear scintigraphy (Fig. 8). On multiphasic CT or MRI, pancreatic NET classically appears hypervascular in the arterial phase, although some will show atypical enhancement patterns [39,40]. MRI is more sensitive than CT, as some lesions are seen only on DWI [36,39]. Both imaging and tissue sampling can be obtained using endoscopic US. [39]. PET/CT with ^{68}Ga-DOTA peptide radiotracers is also used for imaging of pancreatic NET in MEN1, and is thought to be more sensitive than ^{111}In-pentetreotide scan [39,41].

MEN2 includes MEN2A, MEN2B, and familial medullary thyroid carcinoma. The characteristic tumors of

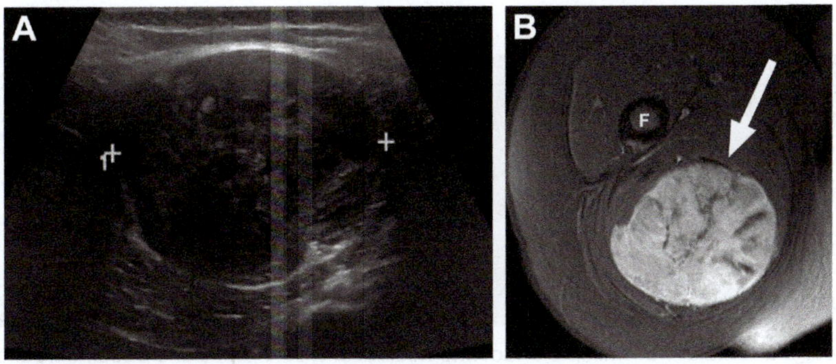

FIG. 6 3-year-old male with Li-Fraumeni syndrome and rhabdomyosarcoma. (**A**) Transverse ultrasound image of the right thigh demonstrates a hypoechoic, heterogeneous solid mass (calipers). (**B**) Axial post-contrast T1-weighted fat suppressed MR image demonstrates an avidly enhancing mass (*arrow*). F, Femur.

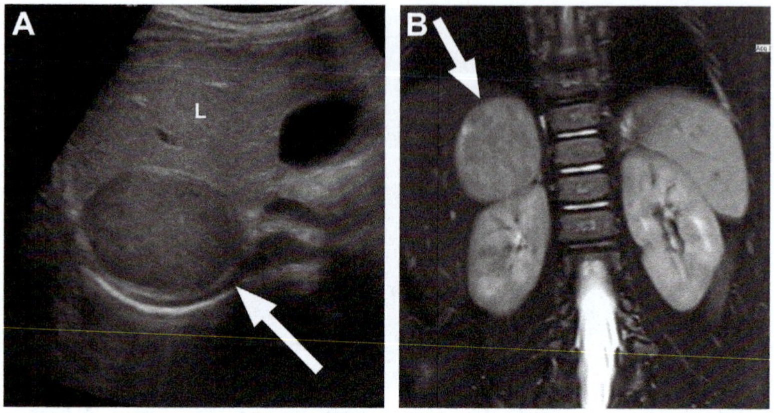

FIG. 7 2-year-old female with Li-Fraumeni syndrome and adrenocortical carcinoma. (**A**) Transverse ultrasound image demonstrates a solid mass (*arrow*) in the right upper quadrant. L, liver. (**B**) Coronal T2-weighted fat suppressed MR image shows a heterogeneously hyperintense right adrenal gland mass (*arrow*).

MEN2A are medullary thyroid carcinoma (MTC), adrenal pheochromocytoma, and parathyroid adenoma/hyperplasia. MTC and pheochromocytoma are also seen in MEN2B, in addition to mucosal neuromas, intestinal ganglioneuromas, and marfanoid habitus [39]. MTC on US appears similar to other malignant thyroid neoplasms, with a hypoechoic solid mass, spiculated margins, taller-than-wide orientation, and microcalcification or macrocalcification (Fig. 9) [39]. 80% of pheochromocytomas in MEN2 are bilateral [39]. On CT or MRI these lesions show avid enhancement, with larger lesions having necrosis or cystic change, as well as *light bulb* hyperintensity on T2-weighted MRI and delayed washout on adrenal protocol CT [36,39]. Nuclear medicine studies including ^{123}I-metaiodobenzylguanidine (MIBG) and ^{18}F-fluoro-L-3,4-dihydroxyphenylalanine (FDOPA) PET/CT are helpful for pheochromocytoma staging [36,39].

A variety of screening regimens for MEN1 and MEN2 can be found in the literature [39]. In MEN1, these usually include biochemical testing, abdominal MRI and/or endoscopic US, and brain/pituitary MRI, while MEN2 includes biochemical testing, abdominal CT or MRI, and thyroid US. Thyroidectomy is performed prophylactically in children with MEN2 [35,36].

DICER1 syndrome (pleuropulmonary blastoma syndrome)

DICER1 is an autosomal dominant syndrome characterized by pleuropulmonary blastoma (PPB), in addition to other neoplastic, hamartomatous and hyperplastic lesions. After PPB, the most common neoplasms in *DICER1* syndrome are renal cystic nephroma and gynecologic tumors (Sertoli-Leydig cell

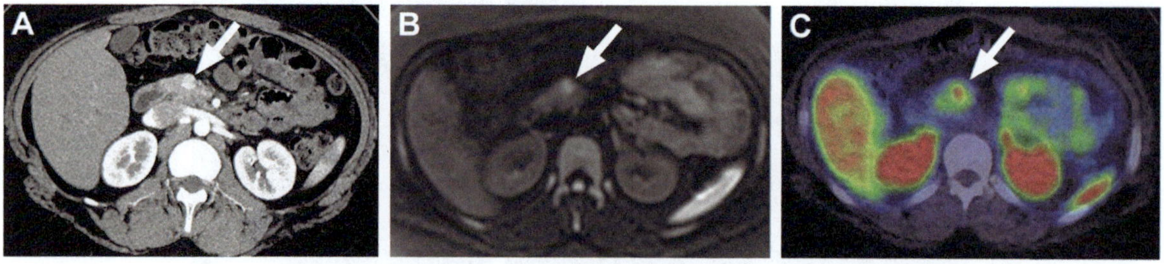

FIG. 8 13-year-old female with multiple endocrine neoplasia type 1 and pancreatic neuroendocrine tumor. (**A**) Axial post-contrast CT image shows an enhancing mass (*arrow*) in the head of the pancreas. (**B**) Axial diffusion weighted MR image shows that the mass restricts diffusion. (**C**) Axial image from ^{68}Ga-DOTATATE PET/CT scan shows avidity of the mass.

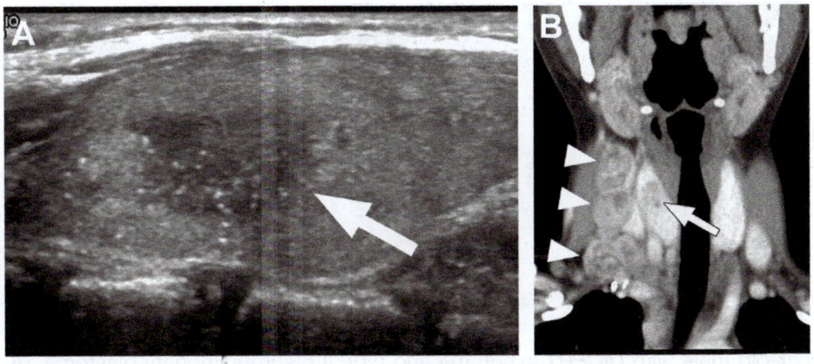

FIG. 9 15-year-old female with multiple endocrine neoplasia type 2B and medullary thyroid carcinoma. (**A**) Sagittal ultrasound image of the right thyroid lobe demonstrates a solid hypoechoic nodule (*arrow*) with irregular margins and microcalcifications. (**B**) Coronal post-contrast CT of the neck demonstrates a hypodense mass (*arrow*) in the right thyroid lobe, as well as multiple metastatic cervical lymph nodes (*arrowheads*).

tumor and cervical rhabdomyosarcoma) [42] Mutations in the DICER1 gene affect an enzyme that modulates various protein-encoding genes [43]. Lung cysts and thyroid nodules can occur in unaffected carriers [42,44]. The cancer risk in *DICER1* syndrome is 5% before the age of 10 years and 19% by the age of 50 years [42].

PPB is a rare embryonal malignancy arising from pleural surfaces and lung parenchyma, usually presenting before the age of 6 years, and may even be seen on prenatal imaging [45,46]. There are 3 forms of PPB: Type I (purely cystic), type II (mixed solid and cystic), and type III (purely solid). Type Ir (regressed version of type I) is also recognized as a cystic tumor without malignant cells. On chest radiograph performed for a patient with fever and cough, the solid tissue-containing types II and III can unknowingly be interpreted as pneumonia [44]. PPB is usually imaged with CT, although MRI can also depict necrosis, hemorrhage, restricted diffusion, and local invasion [45]. Type I PPB appears as a unilocular or multilocular cyst with thin septations, and may be difficult to distinguish from a cystic congenital pulmonary airway malformation on imaging [44,45]. Type II appears as a cyst containing nodular or botryoid solid tissue, which can invade the mediastinum, diaphragm, and chest wall, sometimes accompanied by a pleural effusion (Fig. 10). Type III appears as a fully solid lesion, and large tumors may demonstrate necrosis, mediastinal shift, and local invasion along with a pleural effusion [44,45].

DICER1 syndrome surveillance regimens vary, but most begin in infancy and require serial chest radiographs and a baseline chest CT [42,44,47,48]. Additional imaging includes serial US (abdominal, pelvic, and thyroid) beginning in childhood [42,48].

Tuberous sclerosis complex

Tuberous sclerosis complex (TSC), also known as Bourneville disease, is characterized by tumors and hamartomatous lesions of the brain, chest, and abdomen. The inheritance pattern is autosomal dominant, with mutations occurring on the TSC1 gene for hamartin or the TSC2 gene for tuberin, which trigger the mammalian target of rapamycin (mTOR) pathway and lead to unregulated cell growth [49,50]. Major diagnostic findings in TSC include cutaneous lesions, retinal hamartomas, subependymal nodules (SEN), subependymal giant cell astrocytoma (SEGA), cortical and subcortical tubers, radial migration lines (RML), angiomyolipomas (AML, most commonly renal), lymphangioleiomyomatosis (LAM), and cardiac rhabdomyoma [51]. TSC is usually diagnosed within the first year of life but can present at any age [52].

CNS lesions of TSC are well-demonstrated on MRI [49]. RMLs extend between the periventricular white matter and the brain cortex, often forming a comet tail extending from a tuber [17,49]. Cortical/subcortical tubers are seen in over 90% of patients, consisting of wedge-shaped lesions expanding a gyrus with overlying cortical thickening (Fig. 11). More than 90% of tubers are nonenhancing, and some can be cystic [17,49,50]. Folial retraction and *zebra* enhancement pattern can be seen in tubers of the cerebellum [17,49]. In children lesser than 6 months of age, tubers are hyperintense on T1-weighted images due to incomplete myelination, but in older children and adults, tubers are hyperintense on fluid-attenuated inversion recovery

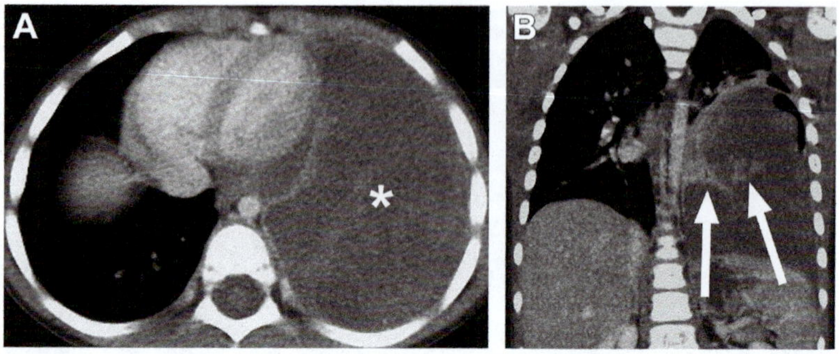

FIG. 10 3-year-old male with *DICER1* syndrome and type II pleuropulmonary blastoma. (**A**) Axial and (**B**) coronal post-contrast chest CT images demonstrate a large hypoattenuating mass (*asterisk*) occupying the left hemithorax, resulting in rightward mediastinal shift. Enhancing nodular components (*arrows*) are present internally.

(FLAIR) [49]. SENs are seen as nodules lining the lateral ventricles, most commonly at the caudothalamic groove or foramen of Monro [49]. Calcification of SENs is depicted well on CT (Fig. 12) [49]. SEGA is thought to arise from SEN and can lead to obstructive hydrocephalus, often presenting in early childhood (see Fig. 11). In distinction to SEN, SEGA are larger (>10–13 mm), and may demonstrate intense enhancement and rapid growth [17,49].

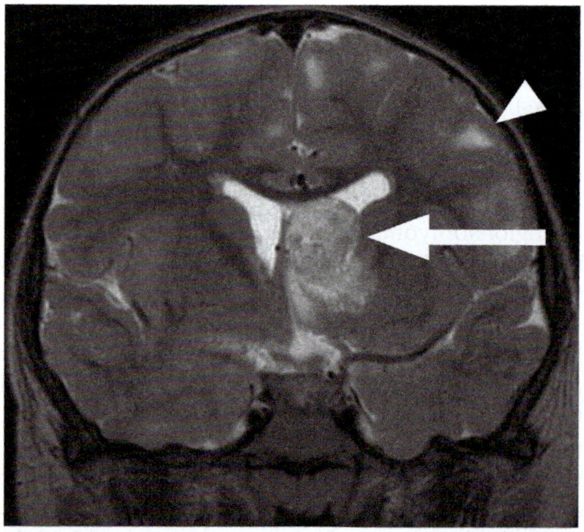

FIG. 11 3-year-old male with tuberous sclerosis complex, multiple tubers, and subependymal giant cell astrocytoma (SEGA). Coronal T2-weighted MR image shows a SEGA as a solid mass (*arrow*) in the left lateral ventricle at the foramen of Monro, deviating the septum pellucidum. Multiple wedge-shaped subcortical tubers (*arrowhead* on example) are also present.

As a result of the proximity of the TSC2 gene to the polycystic kidney disease-1 gene on the same chromosome, renal cysts are frequent in TSC [49,50]. Renal AMLs are also common, seen in about 80% of TSC, with risk of hemorrhage in lesions bigger than 4 cm,

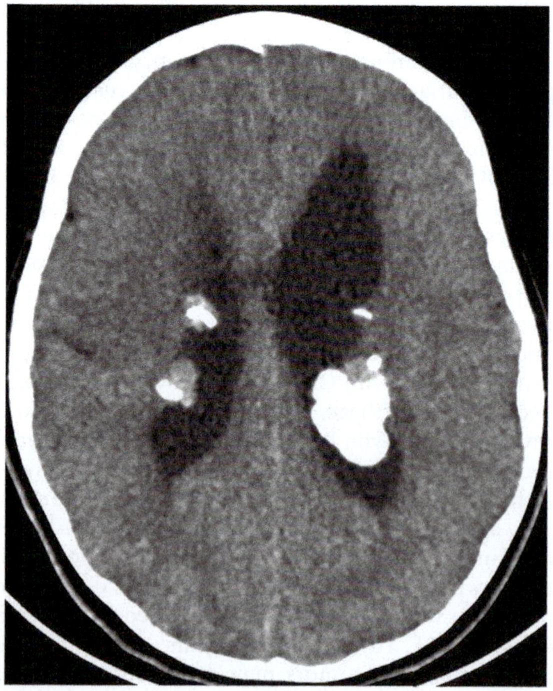

FIG. 12 9-year-old male with tuberous sclerosis complex and subependymal nodules. Axial noncontrast CT image of the head shows calcified nodules of varying sizes along the ependymal surfaces. The lateral ventricles are noted to be dilated.

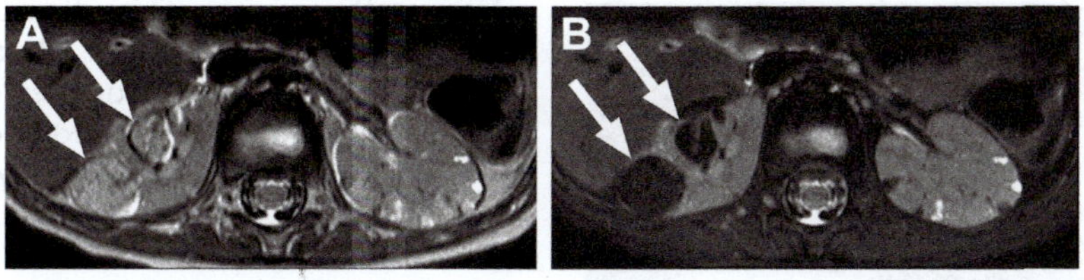

FIG. 13 3-year-old male with tuberous sclerosis complex and renal angiomyolipomas. (**A**) Axial T2-weighted MR image and (**B**) axial T2-weighted fat suppressed MR image demonstrate two right renal masses (*arrows*) with signal dropout on fat suppressed images, indicating the presence of fat. Additional smaller angiomyolipomas and cysts are noted in the left kidney.

or if aneurysms greater than 5 mm are seen [49,50]. Renal AMLs are usually hyperechoic on US and may show posterior acoustic shadowing, along with macroscopic fat (<-10–20 Hounsfield units) on unenhanced CT [49,50]. On MRI, fatty tissue can be identified by hypointensity on fat-suppressed sequences, and *india ink* artifact on opposed-phase T1-weighted images (Fig. 13). The *lipid poor* type of AML can present a diagnostic challenge in TSC, as they are indistinguishable from renal cell carcinoma (RCC) due to lack of visible macroscopic fat [49,50,53]. Imaging features that support a diagnosis of lipid poor AML over RCC include hyperdensity on unenhanced CT, hypointensity on T2-weighted nonfat-suppressed MRI, and prolonged enhancement on postcontrast imaging [50,54]. Although the risk of RCC in TSC patients is equivalent to the general population, it often presents at younger ages (mean 28 years) and may show less aggressive growth [49,54].

LAM, usually seen in female patients with TSC, consists of multiple thin-walled pulmonary cysts, which are at risk for rupture leading to chylothorax or pneumothorax [49,50]. Multifocal micronodular pneumocyte hyperplasia is another pulmonary feature of TSC and consists of multiple subcentimeter ground-glass or solid pulmonary nodules [49,54]. Other findings seen on imaging of TSC include hepatic AML, pancreatic NET, splenic hamartoma, perivascular epithelioid tumors (PEComas), intrabdominal LAM, vascular aneurysms, myocardial fat foci, and sclerotic bone lesions [49–51,54].

Screening strategies for TSC include blood pressure checks, neuropsychiatric screening, physical examination (dermatologic, dental, and ophthalmologic), renal function tests, pulmonary function tests, and electroencephalography [51]. Imaging includes echocardiogram, brain MRI, and abdominal MRI, as well as baseline chest CT for females and symptomatic males [51].

von Hippel–Lindau disease

von Hippel-Lindau (VHL) disease is an autosomal dominant syndrome with the propensity for multiple CNS and non-CNS tumors. Typical findings include

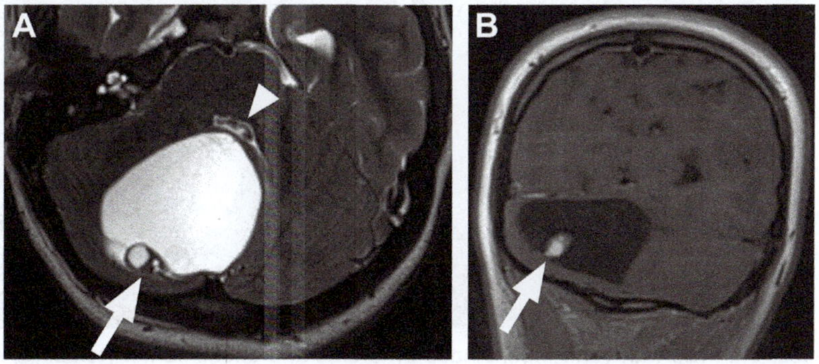

FIG. 14 12-year-old male with von Hippel-Lindau syndrome and hemangioblastoma. (**A**) Axial T2-weighted MR image and (**B**) coronal post-contrast T1-weighted MR image show a right cerebellar cystic mass with an internal enhancing nodule (*arrows*). There is mass effect on the fourth ventricle (*arrowhead*).

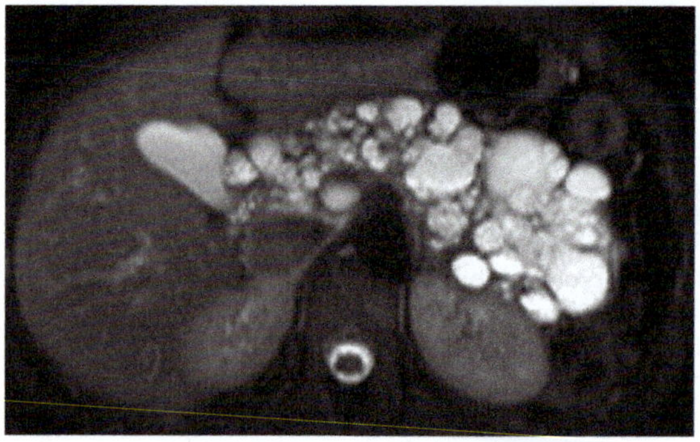

FIG. 15 17-year-old female with von Hippel-Lindau syndrome and pancreatic cysts. Axial T2-weighted fat suppressed MR image shows innumerable pancreatic cysts.

hemangioblastoma (HB) (retina, brain, brainstem, and spinal cord), endolymphatic sac tumor (ELST) of the temporal bone, pheochromocytoma or extra-adrenal paraganglioma, pancreatic NET, clear cell RCC, epididymal or adnexal papillary cystadenoma, and renal and pancreatic cysts [55]. VHL tumor suppressor gene mutations lead to endothelial proliferation and angiogenesis, which correlates with the hypervascular nature of VHL tumors [56,57]. The average age at diagnosis is 24 to 26 years; however, VHL can present at any age [56].

The most common feature of VHL is multiple HBs, with 75% developing in the cerebellum and 25% in the spinal cord [29]. HB of the retina is seen in 50% of patients and is commonly bilateral [29]. On MRI, HB usually consists of a well-circumscribed cyst with an enhancing mural nodule, abutting the pial surface (Fig. 14), although one-quarter of HBs may consist of just an enhancing solid nodule [17,56,57]. Peritumoral edema and prominent flow voids may be seen [17,56]. Syrinx is a common finding with spinal HB [57].

Bilateral ELST is pathognomonic of VHL and consists of a locally aggressive neoplasm arising from the endolymphatic sac within the petrous bone [17]. On CT, these lesions cause a moth-eaten pattern of bone destruction, and contain a spiculated tumor matrix [17]. High signal on T1-weighted MRI can be seen due to hemorrhage, and enhancement is usually intense, sometimes with a *paint brush* or stippled pattern [17,56,57]. Epididymal papillary cystadenoma in VHL resembles ESLT pathologically, and presents on US as a mixed solid-cystic lesion with Doppler flow [56,57].

A variety of pancreatic lesions are seen in VHL, including simple cysts (Fig. 15), serous cystadenomas, and NETs (see earlier section on MEN for imaging findings of NET). VHL is also associated with renal cysts and clear cell RCC, which tends to be bilateral and multicentric [56]. Pheochromocytomas linked to VHL also tend to be bilateral and multicentric (imaging also described in MEN section) (Fig. 16).

Surveillance in VHL includes blood pressure checks, ophthalmologic examinations, audiologic examinations, urinary or plasma-free metanephrine levels, and MRI of the brain, spine, and abdomen [55,56].

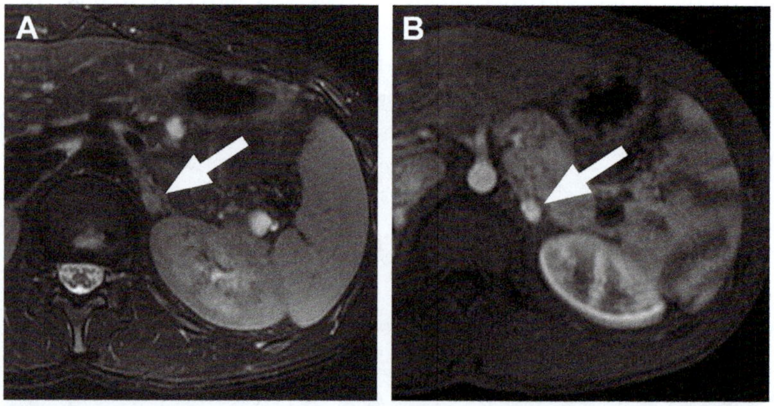

FIG. 16 17-year-old male with von Hippel-Lindau syndrome and pheochromocytoma. (**A**) Axial T2-weighted fat suppressed MR image shows a mass (*arrow*) with high signal intensity in the left adrenal gland. (**B**) Axial post-contrast T1-weighted fat suppressed MR image shows early avid enhancement of the mass (*arrow*).

SUMMARY

Imaging evaluation is requisite for the screening and diagnosis of benign and malignant tumors seen in children with CPS. Surveillance imaging is particularly important for the detection of early-onset and aggressive malignancies in CPS, and includes US, WBMRI and/or single-site MRI, and sometimes CT, which are performed at repeated time intervals throughout the lifespan. Annual WBMRI is recommended in certain childhood CPS, as it provides an all-inclusive total body assessment. The radiologist plays an important role in the optimal management of children with CPS, and familiarity with the imaging characteristics of typical neoplasms and other stigmata of CPS is necessary for early cancer detection and accuracy of diagnosis.

CLINICS CARE POINTS

- Cancer predisposition syndromes involve genetic mutations that increase the risk of developing cancer in specific organs, tissue types, or anatomic locations, often at an unusually young age
- Each cancer predisposition syndrome is uniquely characterized by distinctive neoplasms, and sometimes by non-neoplastic physical stigmata
- Ultrasound, computed tomography, and magnetic resonance imaging are the most common imaging modalities used in surveillance protocols for CPS
- Whole-body MRI provides a global assessment in a single examination, and is used to screen for neoplasms in selected cancer predisposition syndromes, such as Li-Fraumeni syndrome, neurofibromatosis, and several others.

DISCLOSURE

The authors have nothing to disclose.

REFERENCES

[1] Imyanitov EN, Kuligina ES, Sokolenko AP, et al. Hereditary cancer syndromes. World J Clin Oncol 2023;14:40–68.

[2] Brodeur GM, Nichols KE, Plon SE, et al. Pediatric cancer predisposition and surveillance: an overview, and a tribute to alfred G. Knudson Jr. Clin Cancer Res 2017;23:e1–5.

[3] Villani A, Shore A, Wasserman JD, et al. Biochemical and imaging surveillance in germline TP53 mutation carriers with Li-Fraumeni syndrome: 11 year follow-up of a prospective observational study. Lancet Oncol 2016;17:1295–305.

[4] McNeil DE, Brown M, Ching A, et al. Screening for Wilms tumor and hepatoblastoma in children with Beckwith-Wiedemann syndromes: a cost-effective model. Med Pediatr Oncol 2001;37:349–56.

[5] Greer MC, Voss SD, States LJ. Pediatric cancer predisposition imaging: focus on whole-body MRI. Clin Cancer Res 2017;23:e6–13.

[6] Gosangi B, Dixe de Oliveira Santo I, Keraliya A, et al. Li-fraumeni syndrome: imaging features and guidelines. Radiographics 2024;44:e230202.

[7] Tewattanarat N, Junhasavasdikul T, Panwar S, et al. Diagnostic accuracy of imaging approaches for early tumor detection in children with Li-Fraumeni syndrome. Pediatr Radiol 2022;52:1283–95.

[8] Consul N, Amini B, Ibarra-Rovira JJ, et al. Li-fraumeni syndrome and whole-body MRI screening: screening guidelines, imaging features, and impact on patient management. AJR Am J Roentgenol 2021;216:252–63.

[9] Greer MC, States LJ, Malkin D, et al. Update on whole-body MRI surveillance for pediatric cancer predisposition syndromes. Clin Cancer Res 2024;30:5021–33.

[10] Kraus MS, Yousef AA, Cote SL, et al. Improving protocols for whole-body magnetic resonance imaging: oncological and inflammatory applications. Pediatr Radiol 2023;53:1420–42.

[11] Schooler GR, Davis JT, Daldrup-Link HE, et al. Current utilization and procedural practices in pediatric whole-body MRI. Pediatr Radiol 2018;48:1101–7.

[12] Goo HW. Whole-body MRI in children: current imaging techniques and clinical applications. Korean J Radiol 2015;16:973–85.

[13] Eutsler EP, Khanna G. Whole-body magnetic resonance imaging in children: technique and clinical applications. Pediatr Radiol 2016;46:858–72.

[14] Wang MX, Dillman JR, Guccione J, et al. Neurofibromatosis from head to toe: what the radiologist needs to Know. Radiographics 2022;42:1123–44.

[15] Legius E, Messiaen L, Wolkenstein P, et al. Revised diagnostic criteria for neurofibromatosis type 1 and Legius syndrome: an international consensus recommendation. Genet Med 2021;23:1506–13.

[16] Wilson MP, Katlariwala P, Low G, et al. Diagnostic accuracy of MRI for the detection of malignant peripheral nerve sheath tumors: a systematic review and meta-analysis. AJR Am J Roentgenol 2021;217:31–9.

[17] Batchala PP, Eluvathingal Muttikkal TJ, Mukherjee S. Imaging of tumor syndromes. Radiol Clin North Am 2021;59:471–500.

[18] Liu J, Huang JN, Wang MH, et al. Image-based differentiation of benign and malignant peripheral nerve sheath tumors in neurofibromatosis type 1. Front Oncol 2022;12:898971.

[19] Friedman JM. Neurofibromatosis 1. In: Adam MP, Feldman J, Mirzaa GM, et al, editors. GeneReviews. Seattle: University of Washington; 2022. Available at: https://www.ncbi.nlm.nih.gov/books/NBK1109/. Accessed January 29, 2025.

[20] Nguyen R, Jett K, Harris GJ, et al. Benign whole body tumor volume is a risk factor for malignant peripheral nerve sheath tumors in neurofibromatosis type 1. J Neuro Oncol 2014;116:307–13.
[21] Martin E, Coert JH, Flucke UE, et al. Neurofibromatosis-associated malignant peripheral nerve sheath tumors in children have a worse prognosis: a nationwide cohort study. Pediatr Blood Cancer 2020;67:e28138.
[22] Evans DGR, Salvador H, Chang VY, et al. Cancer and central nervous system tumor surveillance in pediatric neurofibromatosis 2 and related disorders. Clin Cancer Res 2017;23:e54–61.
[23] Broski SM, Johnson GB, Howe BM, et al. Evaluation of (18)F-FDG PET and MRI in differentiating benign and malignant peripheral nerve sheath tumors. Skelet Radiol 2016;45:1097–105.
[24] Wasa J, Nishida Y, Tsukushi S, et al. MRI features in the differentiation of malignant peripheral nerve sheath tumors and neurofibromas. AJR Am J Roentgenol 2010;194:1568–74.
[25] Kang E, Kim YM, Choi Y, et al. Whole-body MRI evaluation in neurofibromatosis type 1 patients younger than 3 years old and the genetic contribution to disease progression. Orphanet J Rare Dis 2022;17:24.
[26] Kalish JM, Becktell KD, Bougeard G, et al. Update on surveillance for Wilms tumor and hepatoblastoma in Beckwith-Wiedemann Syndrome and other predisposition syndromes. Clin Cancer Res 2024;30(23):5260–9.
[27] Wang KH, Kupa J, Duffy KA, et al. Diagnosis and management of beckwith-wiedemann syndrome. Front Pediatr 2019;7:562.
[28] Borjas Mendoza PA, Daley SF, Mendez MD. Beckwith-wiedemann syndrome. In: StatPearls. 2024. Available at: https://www.ncbi.nlm.nih.gov/books/NBK558993/. Accessed January 29, 2025.
[29] Monsalve J, Kapur J, Malkin D, et al. Imaging of cancer predisposition syndromes in children. Radiographics 2011;31:263–80.
[30] Wong CA, Cuda S, Kirsch A. A review of the urologic manifestations of Beckwith-Wiedemann syndrome. J Pediatr Urol 2011;7:140–4.
[31] Choyke PL, Siegel MJ, Oz O, et al. Nonmalignant renal disease in pediatric patients with Beckwith-Wiedemann syndrome. AJR Am J Roentgenol 1998;171:733–7.
[32] Malkin D, Li FP, Strong LC, et al. Germ line p53 mutations in a familial syndrome of breast cancer, sarcomas, and other neoplasms. Science 1990;250:1233–8.
[33] Guha T, Malkin D. Inherited TP53 mutations and the Li-Fraumeni syndrome. Cold Spring Harb Perspect Med 2017;7.
[34] Kratz CP, Achatz MI, Brugieres L, et al. Cancer screening recommendations for individuals with Li-Fraumeni syndrome. Clin Cancer Res 2017;23:e38–45.
[35] Wasserman JD, Tomlinson GE, Druker H, et al. Multiple endocrine neoplasia and hyperparathyroid-jaw tumor syndromes: clinical features, genetics, and surveillance recommendations in childhood. Clin Cancer Res 2017;23:e123–32.
[36] Grajo JR, Paspulati RM, Sahani DV, et al. Multiple endocrine neoplasia syndromes: a comprehensive imaging review. Radiol Clin North Am 2016;54:441–51.
[37] Pieterman CRC, van Leeuwaarde RS, van den Broek MFM, et al. Multiple endocrine neoplasia type 1. In: Feingold KR, Anawalt B, Blackman MR, et al, editors. Endotext. South dartmouth. MDText.com, Inc.; 2021. Available at: https://www.ncbi.nlm.nih.gov/books/NBK481897/. Accessed January 29, 2025.
[38] McDonnell JE, Gild ML, Clifton-Bligh RJ, et al. Multiple endocrine neoplasia: an update. Intern Med J 2019;49:954–61.
[39] Ali A, Revels J, Wang DT, et al. Multimodality imaging review of multiple endocrine neoplasia. AJR Am J Roentgenol 2021;217:245–56.
[40] Khanna L, Prasad SR, Sunnapwar A, et al. Pancreatic neuroendocrine neoplasms: 2020 update on pathologic and imaging findings and classification. Radiographics 2020;40:1240–62.
[41] Sadowski SM, Millo C, Cottle-Delisle C, et al. Results of (68)Gallium-DOTATATE PET/CT scanning in patients with multiple endocrine neoplasia type 1. J Am Coll Surg 2015;221:509–17.
[42] Stewart DR, Best AF, Williams GM, et al. Neoplasm risk among individuals with a pathogenic germline variant in DICER1. J Clin Oncol 2019;37:668–76.
[43] Bueno MT, Martinez-Rios C, la Puente Gregorio A, et al. Pediatric imaging in DICER1 syndrome. Pediatr Radiol 2017;47:1292–301.
[44] Guillerman RP, Foulkes WD, Priest JR. Imaging of DICER1 syndrome. Pediatr Radiol 2019;49:1488–505.
[45] Leung SS, Donuru A, Kandula V, et al. Multimodality imaging of pleuropulmonary blastoma: pearls, pitfalls, and differential diagnosis. Semin Ultrasound CT MR 2022;43:61–72.
[46] Dehner LP, Schultz KA, Hill DA. Pleuropulmonary blastoma: more than a lung neoplasm of childhood. Mo Med 2019;116:206–10.
[47] Caroleo AM, De Ioris MA, Boccuto L, et al. DICER1 syndrome and cancer predisposition: from a rare pediatric tumor to lifetime risk. Front Oncol 2020;10:614541.
[48] Schultz KAP, Williams GM, Kamihara J, et al. DICER1 and associated conditions: identification of at-risk individuals and recommended surveillance strategies. Clin Cancer Res 2018;24:2251–61.
[49] Krishnan A, Kaza RK, Vummidi DR. Cross-sectional imaging review of tuberous sclerosis. Radiol Clin North Am 2016;54:423–40.
[50] Manoukian SB, Kowal DJ. Comprehensive imaging manifestations of tuberous sclerosis. AJR Am J Roentgenol 2015;204:933–43.
[51] Northrup H, Aronow ME, Bebin EM, et al. Updated international tuberous sclerosis complex diagnostic criteria and surveillance and management recommendations. Pediatr Neurol 2021;123:50–66.

[52] Ebrahimi-Fakhari D, Mann LL, Poryo M, et al. Incidence of tuberous sclerosis and age at first diagnosis: new data and emerging trends from a national, prospective surveillance study. Orphanet J Rare Dis 2018;13:117.

[53] Jinzaki M, Silverman SG, Akita H, et al. Renal angiomyolipoma: a radiological classification and update on recent developments in diagnosis and management. Abdom Imaging 2014;39:588–604.

[54] Morin CE, Morin NP, Franz DN, et al. Thoracoabdominal imaging of tuberous sclerosis. Pediatr Radiol 2018;48:1307–23.

[55] Rednam SP, Erez A, Druker H, et al. Von hippel-lindau and hereditary pheochromocytoma/paraganglioma syndromes: clinical features, genetics, and surveillance recommendations in childhood. Clin Cancer Res 2017;23:e68–75.

[56] Shanbhogue KP, Hoch M, Fatterpaker G, et al. von Hippel-Lindau Disease: Review of Genetics and Imaging. Radiol Clin North Am 2016;54:409–22.

[57] Ganeshan D, Menias CO, Pickhardt PJ, et al. Tumors in von Hippel-Lindau Syndrome: From Head to Toe-Comprehensive State-of-the-Art Review. Radiographics 2018;38:849–66.

Advances in Clinical Radiology 7 (2025) 157–173

ADVANCES IN CLINICAL RADIOLOGY

Technical Advances in Pediatric Musculoskeletal Imaging

Theory to Daily Clinical Practice

Emilio J. Inarejos Clemente, MD[a,*], Maria Navallas, MD[a], Angel M. Lancharro-Zapata, MD[b], Jordi Català March, MD[c], Abbey J. Winant, MD[d], Edward Y. Lee, MPH, MD[d]

[a]Department of Radiology, Sant Joan de Deu Barcelona Hospital, Av. Sant Joan de Deu, 2, Esplugues de Llobregat, Barcelona 08950 Spain; [b]Department of Radiology, Hospital Materno-Infantil Gregorio Marañon, O'Donnell 48, Madrid 28009 Spain; [c]Department of Radiology, Instituts Guirado. Muntaner 531, Barcelona 08022 Spain; [d]Department of Radiology, Boston Children's Hospital and Harvard Medical School, 300 Longwood Avenue, Boston, MA 02115, USA

KEYWORDS

- Advanced imaging techniques • Dynamic contrast-enhanced MRI • Diffusion-weighted imaging
- Whole body MRI • Pediatric MSK

KEY POINTS

- Advanced imaging techniques, including dynamic contrast-enhanced MRI, diffusion-weighted imaging, and whole-body MRI, have improved the accuracy of pediatric musculoskeletal imaging, enabling earlier diagnosis and treatment monitoring.
- Ultrasound advancements, such as contrast-enhanced ultrasound and microvascular imaging, enhance soft tissue and vascular assessment, reducing the need for ionizing radiation.
- Dixon-based MRI techniques improve fat and water separation, allowing better assessment of bone marrow infiltration and soft tissue composition.
- Artificial intelligence-driven imaging solutions facilitate automated detection, lesion characterization, and workflow optimization in pediatric musculoskeletal radiology.

INTRODUCTION

Pediatric musculoskeletal imaging plays a crucial role in diagnosing and managing a wide range of pediatric musculoskeletal conditions, from congenital abnormalities to acquired diseases, such as infections, trauma, tumors, and inflammatory disorders. The optimal imaging modality depends on the specific clinical scenario, balancing diagnostic accuracy, safety, and patient comfort. Historically, conventional radiography and ultrasound have been the primary tools in pediatric musculoskeletal disorder assessment [1]. However, new imaging technologies, such as computed tomography (CT), MRI, and artificial intelligence (AI)-assisted diagnostic tools, have transformed the field, making it easier to detect and characterize musculoskeletal conditions at an early stage, as well as providing key information for pediatric patient management [2].

Musculoskeletal imaging is essential in many clinical areas. In oncology, it enables early detection, staging, and monitoring of treatment response in soft tissue sarcomas and bone sarcomas. MRI, particularly diffusion-weighted imaging (DWI) and dynamic contrast-enhanced (DCE) techniques, provides valuable information about tumor cellularity, vascularity,

*Corresponding author. *E-mail address:* emilioinarejos@gmail.com

https://doi.org/10.1016/j.yacr.2025.06.002 www.advancesinclinicalradiology.com
2589-8701/25/

ABBREVIATIONS

ADC	apparent diffusion coefficient
AI	artificial intelligence
CEUS	contrast-enhanced ultrasound
CT	computed tomography
DCE-MRI	dynamic contrast-enhanced MRI
DWI	diffusion-weighted imaging
FLAIR FS	fluid-attenuated inversion recovery with fat suppression
JIA	juvenile idiopathic arthritis
MRS	magnetic resonance spectroscopy
PCCT	photon-counting computed tomography
REACT	Relaxation-enhanced Angiography without Contrast and Triggering
SMI	superb microvascular imaging
SWE	shear wave elastography
TIC	time-intensity curve
WB-MRI	whole-body MRI

and response to therapy. CT, especially photon-counting and spectral CT, enhances bone lesion detection, and allows for the use of algorithms to detect bone marrow edema in cases where MRI is not available or is contraindicated.

Infections of the musculoskeletal system, including osteomyelitis, septic arthritis, and soft tissue abscesses, require prompt and accurate imaging for diagnosis and management. MRI with DWI and DCE sequences is highly sensitive for detecting early bone marrow changes and differentiating between infectious and inflammatory conditions [3]. CEUS and microvascular imaging techniques also have utility in assessing soft tissue infections, in particular for guiding percutaneous interventions such as drainage or biopsy [1].

This article discusses advancements in pediatric musculoskeletal imaging, highlighting novel imaging techniques with an emphasis on clinical applications in oncology, infection, trauma, and inflammatory conditions in the pediatric population.

ADVANCES IN ULTRASOUND

Contrast-enhanced ultrasound

Contrast-enhanced ultrasound (CEUS) uses intravenous microbubble contrast agents that remain intravascular, allowing for real-time assessment of blood flow dynamics without the nephrotoxic effects associated with iodinated intravenous CT contrast agents or gadolinium-based MRI contrast media. The microbubbles oscillate at a frequency detectable by ultrasound probes in response to ultrasound waves, demonstrating vascularity and providing detailed insights into tissue perfusion and microvascularity. CEUS is particularly beneficial for pediatric patients with renal insufficiency or contrast allergies, as it provides an alternative to the iodinated or gadolinium-based contrast agents typically used in CT and MRI. Moreover, CEUS can be an invaluable tool in critically ill children who cannot undergo transport to CT or MRI due to their clinical condition [4].

In the evaluation of infections, CEUS allows for the differentiation between fluid collections, such as abscesses, and solid masses, providing detailed information about vascularity [5]. For example, in osteomyelitis, CEUS can identify hypervascular areas around the bone, which are suggestive of early infection, and can guide drainage procedures. Similarly, in soft tissue infections, CEUS can identify areas of increased blood flow (hyperemia), detect irregular peripheral enhancement suggesting abscess formation, differentiate phlegmon from abscess, and monitor response to antibiotic treatment. Sonographically, infected tissue typically demonstrates increased vascularity with heterogeneous enhancement, while abscesses appear as nonenhancing central areas with rim enhancement.

In the assessment of vascular anomalies, CEUS provides valuable information on lesion vascularity and hemodynamics, aiding in differentiation between low-flow and high-flow vascular anomalies. Low-flow venous malformations typically demonstrate slow, progressive contrast enhancement with persistent late-phase retention (Fig. 1). In contrast, high-flow arteriovenous malformations exhibit rapid contrast uptake with early arterial phase enhancement and quick washout, consistent with arteriovenous shunting. CEUS also helps evaluate treatment response after sclerotherapy or embolization by assessing residual perfusion within the lesion [6].

In addition, CEUS has shown promise in the assessment of soft tissue tumors, due to its ability to characterize tumor vascularity, which can help differentiate benign versus malignant lesions [7]. For example, soft tissue sarcomas often exhibit increased vascularization, which can be detected and delineated with CEUS. CEUS can complement other imaging techniques by providing functional information about blood flow patterns that can be helpful in tumor staging, treatment planning, and monitoring treatment response. The ability to assess real-time perfusion with CEUS makes it a valuable complement to MRI and CT, especially for pediatric patients, where reducing ionizing radiation exposure and need for sedation is of paramount importance.

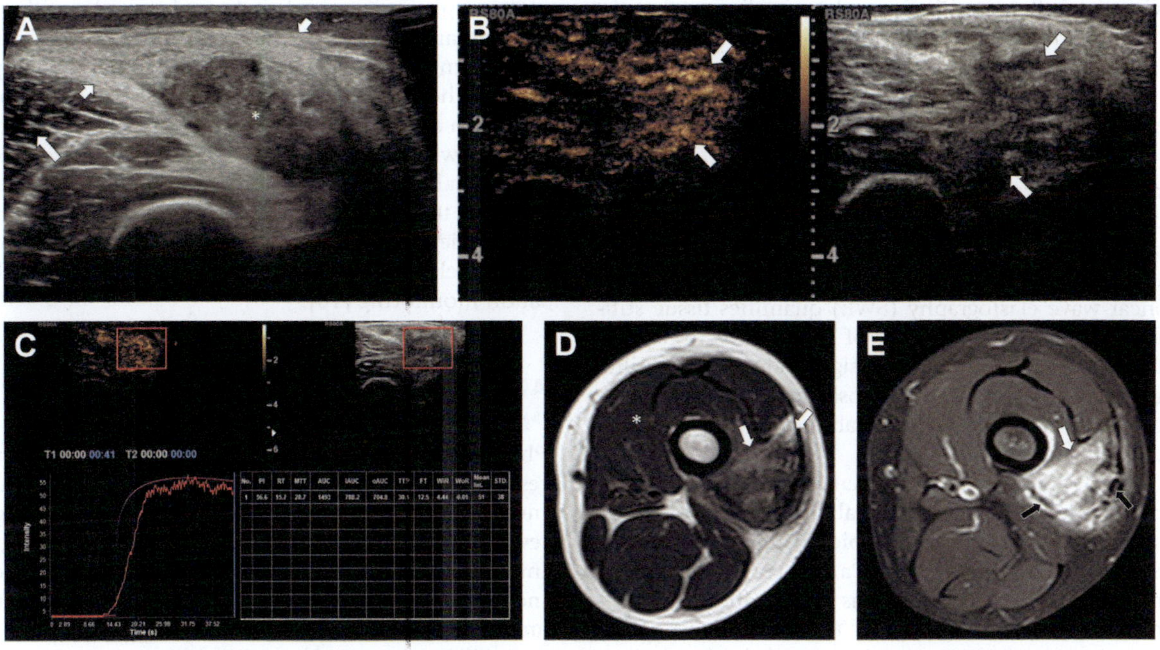

FIG. 1 Fibroadipose vascular anomaly in a 9-year-old male who presented with a slow growing mass on the thigh associated with discoloration of the skin. (**A**) Transverse gray-scale ultrasound image of the left thigh shows a heterogeneous, hypoechoic, and ill-defined mass (*asterisk*) involving the vastus lateralis. There is surrounding hyperechogenicity (*short arrows*) suggestive of fatty infiltration. Note normal echogenicity of the vastus medialis (*long arrow*). (**B**) Transverse CEUS dual image of the lesion acquired 24 seconds after intravenous microbubble agent (2.5 mL) administration shows a prominent nodular enhancement of the hypoechoic component of the mass (*arrows*). (**C**) Analysis of the enhancement shows early, rapid enhancement followed by a plateau phase (*red curve*). This plateau enhancement curve indicates that the lesion demonstrates sustained enhancement over time, a characteristic pattern often seen in benign lesions. The red square box shows the area where the enhancement is calculated. (**D**) Axial T1-weighted MR image shows fatty infiltration (*arrow*) of the lesion. Note normal intensity of the remainder musculature (*asterisk*). (**E**) Axial enhanced T1-weighted, fat-suppressed MR image shows marked heterogenous enhancement (*white arrow*) of the lesion. Note internal vessels (*black arrows*). Combining different imaging techniques, such as ultrasound, CEUS, and MRI, improves the characterization of vascular anomalies in pediatric patients.

Microvascular imaging

Microvascular imaging techniques, such as superb microvascular imaging (SMI), use advanced Doppler filtering to detect slow-flowing blood vessels that are typically missed by conventional Doppler techniques [8]. By eliminating motion artifacts and improving spatial resolution, SMI can be used in pediatric musculoskeletal imaging for the assessment of synovial inflammation, neovascularization, and early-stage osteomyelitis.

In pediatric patients with juvenile idiopathic arthritis (JIA), early detection of synovitis is crucial for timely intervention and improved long-term joint outcomes. SMI not only enhances visualization of synovial blood flow but also enables quantification of vascularity, allowing for comparison of inflammation levels over time (Fig. 2). In fact, a large study comparing SMI with power Doppler ultrasound in assessing synovitis of the knee in JIA patients found that SMI demonstrated superior sensitivity for detecting synovial inflammation [8].

In addition, microvascular imaging has been proved useful in detecting inflammatory activity in children with juvenile localized scleroderma [9]. Furthermore, SMI has been found to be as sensitive as CEUS for detecting synovial vascularity in rheumatoid arthritis, without the need for contrast agents. Consequently, SMI is a valuable tool for monitoring disease activity and treatment response in pediatric patients, because it allows for noninvasive, reproducible assessments of synovial inflammation in a chronic disease that requires frequent monitoring for treatment response [10–12].

Ultrasound elastography

Ultrasound elastography is a noninvasive imaging technique that evaluates tissue stiffness by measuring mechanical or shear wave propagation. In ultrasound strain elastography, external compression is applied to assess tissue displacement. In contrast, ultrasound shear wave elastography (SWE) quantifies tissue stiffness based on the velocity of shear waves traversing the tissue. This method has significant clinical utility in assessing various musculoskeletal conditions due to its noninvasive nature and ability to provide quantitative data.

Elastography helps characterize soft tissue masses by differentiating benign from malignant lesions based on stiffness. Benign lipomas typically appear soft, with SWE values around 5 to 10 kPa, whereas malignant tumors like soft tissue sarcomas exhibit increased stiffness, often exceeding 50 kPa. These differences reflect variations in tissue composition, with benign lesions showing lower elasticity and malignant tumors demonstrating increased rigidity due to high cellularity and desmoplastic reaction (Fig. 3). This differentiation assists clinicians in determining the need for biopsy or further intervention [13].

In cases of muscle injuries, elastography may be helpful for detecting fibrosis and scar formation during the healing process. Increased tissue stiffness can indicate the presence of fibrotic changes or scar tissue, which may impact muscle function and inform rehabilitation strategies.

Ultrasound elastography is particularly useful for assessing myopathies, detecting early fibrosis in muscular disorders, and evaluating the mechanical properties of tendons and ligaments. In neuromuscular diseases such as Duchenne muscular dystrophy, elastography can reveal increased muscle stiffness due to early fibrosis before changes become evident on conventional imaging [14]. In inflammatory myopathies, it helps differentiate edematous, inflamed muscle which appears softer from fibrotic or fatty-replaced muscle, which demonstrates increased stiffness [15]. Additionally, elastography provides valuable information on tendon and ligament integrity, identifying areas of decreased elasticity in tendinopathy or chronic injury, helping with treatment planning and rehabilitation monitoring [16].

ADVANCES IN COMPUTED TOMOGRAPHY

Photon-counting computed tomography

Photon-counting computed tomography (PCCT) represents a paradigm shift in CT imaging by directly measuring individual X ray photons and their energy levels. Unlike conventional CT, which uses energy-integrating detectors that sum the total energy of incoming photons, photon-counting detectors count and sort photons based on their energy levels. PCCT technique reduces image noise, enhances soft tissue contrast, and provides spectral information, allowing differentiation between various tissue types [17].

In pediatric musculoskeletal imaging, PCCT improves the detection of subtle bone abnormalities while reducing radiation dose. This is particularly useful in conditions, such as osteogenesis imperfecta, congenital skeletal dysplasias, and post-traumatic fractures, where minimizing radiation exposure is important given the frequency of imaging [18]. In addition, PCCT allows for enhanced visualization of growth plate physiology and early detection of osteochondral lesions.

Furthermore, in fetal imaging, PCCT has the potential to detect bone dysplasias earlier in development, providing information for prenatal diagnosis and management. By delivering higher resolution images with

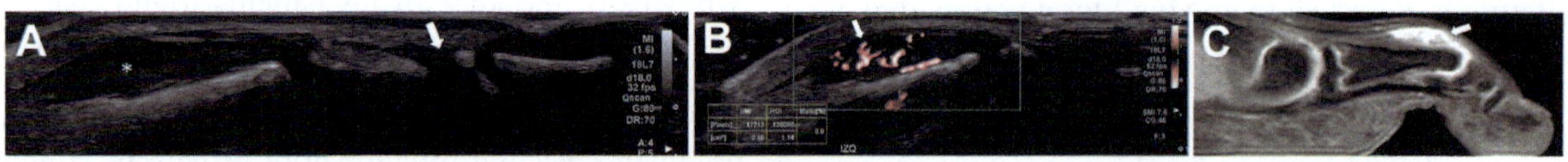

FIG. 2 JIA in a 12-year-old girl who presented with inflammation of the second digit. (**A**) Longitudinal gray-scale ultrasound image shows hypoechogenic material (*asterisk*) in the proximal interphalangeal joint suggestive of synovitis. The distal interphalangeal joint is normal (*arrow*). (**B**) Longitudinal microvascular ultrasound image shows moderate hypervascularity (*arrow*), with a ratio of 9%, indicating the degree of colored pixels within the green box. (**C**) Sagittal enhanced T1-weighted, fat suppressed MR image confirms moderate thickening and enhancement of the synovium (*arrow*), suggestive of active synovitis. Microvascular ultrasound allows quantification of synovitis by measuring the percentage of vascularity, providing an objective parameter to monitor inflammation over time and assess treatment response.

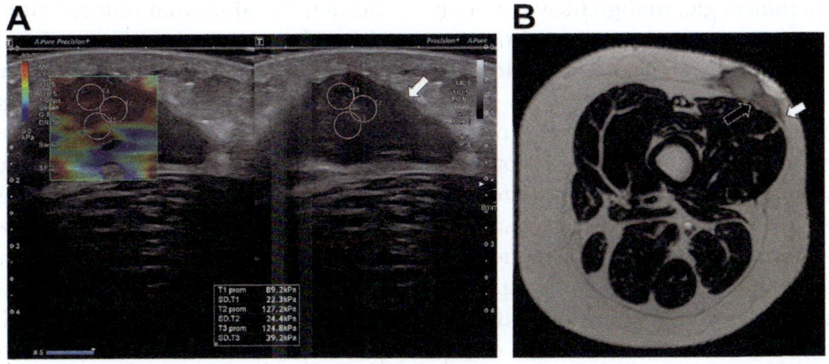

FIG. 3 Soft tissue sarcoma involving the subcutaneous tissue of the thigh in a 14-year-old boy who presented with a slow-growing mass. (**A**) Transverse SWE ultrasound image shows an ill-defined and hypoechogenic lesion (*arrow*) with values ranging from 89 to 127 kPa. This findings suggest the presence of a solid and stiff mass. (**B**) Axial T1-weighted MR image confirms the presence of a mass with spiculated margins (*white arrow*) in close relation to the muscular fascia (*black arrow*). SWE provides quantitative stiffness assessment, helping differentiate soft tissue sarcomas from benign lesions and serving as a potential tool for monitoring disease progression.

lower radiation exposure, this technology could play a crucial role in detecting fetal skeletal abnormalities with greater accuracy.

Spectral computed tomography

Spectral CT, also known as dual-energy CT, differentiates tissues based on their atomic composition by acquiring images at 2 different energy levels. This allows for material decomposition and characterization of musculoskeletal structures. The physics behind spectral CT relies on the differential attenuation of X rays at different energy levels, which improves tissue contrast and reduces beam-hardening artifacts.

Applications in pediatric musculoskeletal imaging include detecting bone marrow edema, differentiating urate from calcium deposits in metabolic bone diseases, and assessing cartilage integrity [19]. This technique is particularly valuable in JIA by enhancing visualization of bone marrow edema, subtle erosions, and synovial composition for early diagnosis and monitoring. This is especially useful in patients who cannot undergo MRI, as spectral CT provides a viable alternative for evaluating bone marrow abnormalities with improved sensitivity, reducing time and risk. In osteomyelitis, spectral CT improves detection of early marrow involvement, differentiates infected from reactive bone, and helps with the visualization of periosteal reaction and sequestra [20].

Furthermore, spectral CT can be beneficial in trauma cases, particularly for detecting bone marrow edema in the vertebral bodies [21]. Unlike traditional CT, which relies on density differences that may not be sufficient to identify marrow abnormalities, spectral CT enhances detection by using material decomposition and virtual noncalcium images to highlight edema.

ADVANCES IN MRI

Advances in MRI have substantially enhanced its diagnostic capabilities in pediatric musculoskeletal imaging, particularly through the development of T1 and T2 Dixon techniques. These methods separate water and fat signals, producing images with distinct contrasts that are invaluable for evaluating bone marrow composition and detecting fatty infiltration in muscles.

T1 and T2 Dixon techniques

The Dixon technique is an MRI method that exploits the differences in resonance frequencies between water and fat protons to generate separate images of each component. By acquiring images at multiple echo times, this technique effectively distinguishes between water and fat signals, producing clear and detailed depictions of musculoskeletal structures. This capability is particularly valuable in pediatric imaging, where minimizing scan time and maximizing image quality are essential [22,23].

In pediatric patients, quantitative Dixon imaging can assess bone marrow fat fraction, a key parameter in diagnosing conditions such as marrow infiltration in leukemia or evaluating marrow reconversion [24]. By measuring the proportion of fat and water in the bone marrow, clinicians can monitor disease progression and therapy response. This is particularly useful in the context of hematologic malignancies, where changes in marrow fat content can serve as a surrogate marker for tumor infiltration or recovery following treatment.

In pediatric oncology, particularly in cases of neuroblastoma, a common extracranial solid tumor that frequently metastasizes to the bone marrow, detecting bone marrow infiltration is crucial for accurate staging and treatment planning. Traditional MRI sequences, such as T1-weighted and T2-weighted imaging, may not reliably differentiate between red marrow and infiltrated marrow, particularly when subtle changes occur. However, the Dixon technique enhances sensitivity in identifying bone marrow infiltration by providing clear differentiation between normal and infiltrated marrow.

On T1-weighted Dixon images, normal bone marrow typically appears isointense to fat, while areas of marrow infiltration, such as those affected by metastatic disease, typically appear iso to hypointense due to decreased fat content. On T2-weighted Dixon images, normal marrow is usually hyperintense, while infiltrated marrow may appear hypointense or slightly hyperintense, depending on the type of infiltration [25]. This allows for more accurate detection and characterization of bone marrow involvement in pediatric cancers, including neuroblastoma and leukemia.

The ability of Dixon imaging to distinguish between red marrow and infiltrated marrow is particularly enhanced when in-phase and out-of-phase images are used. In-phase images display a more homogeneous signal between fat and water protons, whereas out-of-phase images cause a fat-water signal difference. In healthy red marrow, both in-phase and out-of-phase Dixon images show hypointensity, reflecting the high fat content of the marrow. However, in cases of marrow infiltration, such as with leukemia or metastasis, the infiltration typically leads to decreased fat content, causing an absence of signal (eg, signal dropout) change in the out-of-phase images, while a relative hypointensity may persist in the in-phase images (Fig. 4). This allows for a clearer differentiation between normal red marrow and areas of infiltration, which is often challenging using conventional T1-weighted or T2-weighted sequences alone.

Diffusion-weighted imaging

DWI and apparent diffusion coefficient (ADC) mapping are now considered essential techniques in pediatric musculoskeletal imaging, providing functional information beyond conventional MRI sequences. DWI evaluates the movement of water molecules within tissues, while ADC quantifies this diffusion, offering numerical values that reflect cellularity and tissue integrity. These techniques aid in diagnosis, treatment planning, and response assessment for oncologic, infectious, and inflammatory conditions.

In pediatric bone and soft tissue sarcomas, volumetric ADC mapping has proven superior to traditional region-of-interest analysis by capturing the heterogeneity of the entire tumor. Tumors with high cellularity, such as rhabdomyosarcoma and Ewing sarcoma, demonstrate restricted diffusion, with low ADC values typically ranging between 0.6 and 1.1×10^{-3} mm^2/s, while post-treatment necrotic areas show increased ADC values due to loss of viable tumor cells [26]. Studies have shown that ADC histograms of the tumor provide a more comprehensive evaluation of treatment response than conventional cross-sectional analysis (Fig. 5 and 6). Additionally, combining DWI with DCE-MRI enhances tumor characterization, improving differentiation between viable tumor tissue, necrosis, and post-treatment changes.

DWI and ADC mapping are also crucial in the evaluation of musculoskeletal infections, particularly in osteomyelitis and soft tissue abscesses [27]. Restricted diffusion, seen as high signal intensity on DWI and low ADC values ($<1.0 \times 10^{-3}$ mm^2/s), is a hallmark of abscess formation, whereas reactive or inflammatory changes in cellulitis display facilitated diffusion with higher ADC values ($>1.5 \times 10^{-3}$ mm^2/s) (Fig. 7). In osteomyelitis, affected bone marrow shows decreased ADC values due to increased cellular infiltration, helping differentiate it from reactive bone marrow edema, which exhibits higher ADC values [28,29]. Furthermore, ADC mapping aids in distinguishing chronic osteomyelitis, where fibrosis leads to increased ADC, from active infection, where restricted diffusion persists (Fig. 8).

In inflammatory conditions, such as JIA, DWI, and ADC provide additional information regarding synovial inflammation and disease activity. Synovitis typically exhibits intermediate ADC values ($1.2–1.5 \times 10^{-3}$ mm^2/s), which can help differentiate it from infectious arthritis or neoplastic processes. The integration of these techniques into pediatric musculoskeletal MRI protocols enhances the accuracy of disease detection, staging, and treatment monitoring, offering a noninvasive and radiation-free comprehensive musculoskeletal evaluation [30].

The combination of Dixon techniques with DWI further improves diagnostic accuracy for bone marrow infiltration, particularly in pediatric patients with hematologic malignancies. While conventional MRI sequences often lack the sensitivity required to differentiate red

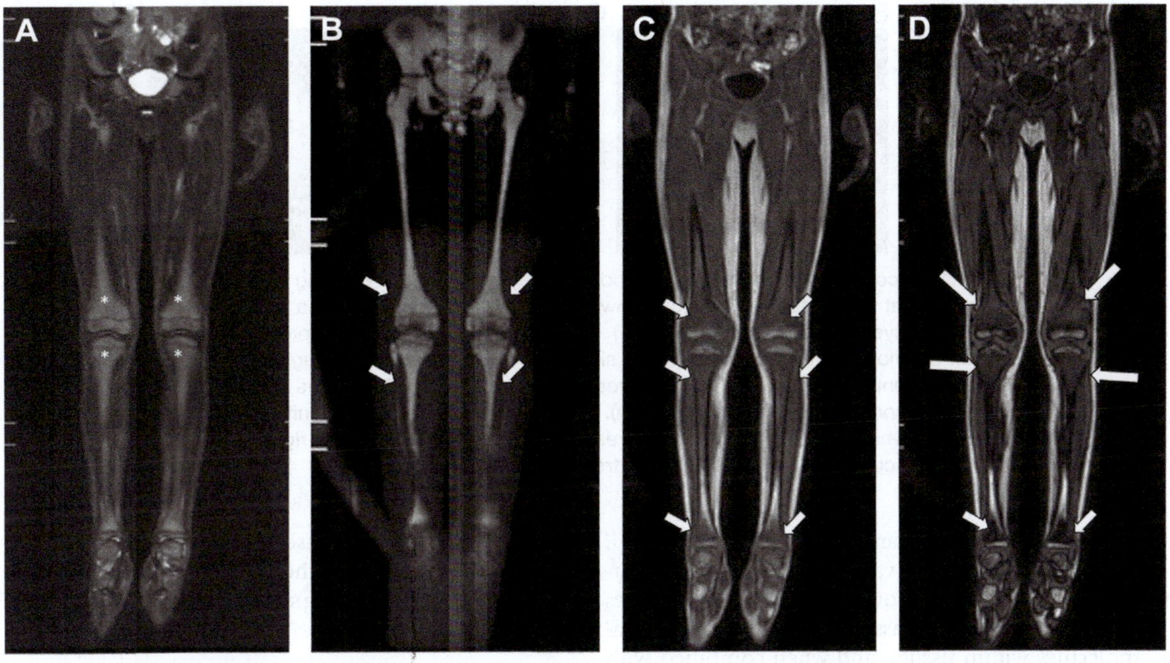

FIG. 4 Secondary myelodysplastic syndrome in a 13-year-old boy with previous rhabdomyosarcoma. (**A**) Coronal stir MR image shows diffuse hyperintensity (*asterisk*) of the bone marrow. (**B**) Coronal DWI MR image shows pathologic restriction (*arrows*) of the bone marrow in general. (**C**) Coronal T1 in phase MR image shows isointensity (*arrows*) to the muscle of the metaphyseal regions of the lower extremities. (**D**) Coronal T1 out of phase MR image shows hypointensity (*short arrows*) of the metaphysis the both distal tibia. However, there is isointensity (*long arrows*) on the metaphysis around the knee. Signal decay or drop-out in T1 Dixon out-of-phase imaging is characteristic of normal red bone marrow. The absence of this signal change, particularly in the metaphysis around the knee, suggests pathologic infiltration, as seen in secondary myelodysplastic syndrome.

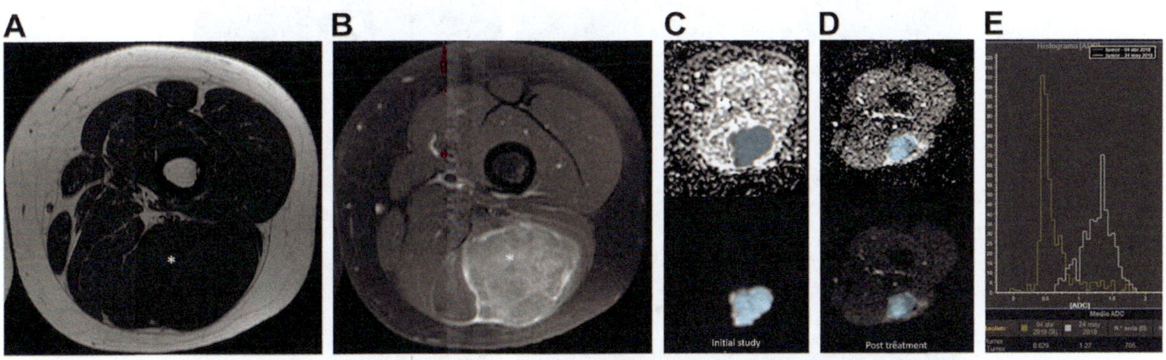

FIG. 5 Alveolar rhabdomyosarcoma involving the long head of the biceps femoris muscle in a 14-year-old boy. (**A**) Axial T1-weighted MR image shows a well-defined and isointense mass (*asterisk*). (**B**) Axial enhanced T1-weighted, fat-suppressed MR image shows heterogeneous enhancement of the mass (*asterisk*). (**C**, **D**) Volumetry of ADC applied on restricted areas of the tumor shows volume decrease after chemotherapy (blue colored area). (**E**) Histograms of ADC show initial mean values of 0.63 (yellow histogram), which increase to 1.27 after 2 months of treatment (white histogram). This right displacement of the histogram along the curve suggests response to treatment. ADC volumetry and histogram analysis can effectively assess tumor response to chemotherapy in pediatric musculoskeletal tumors.

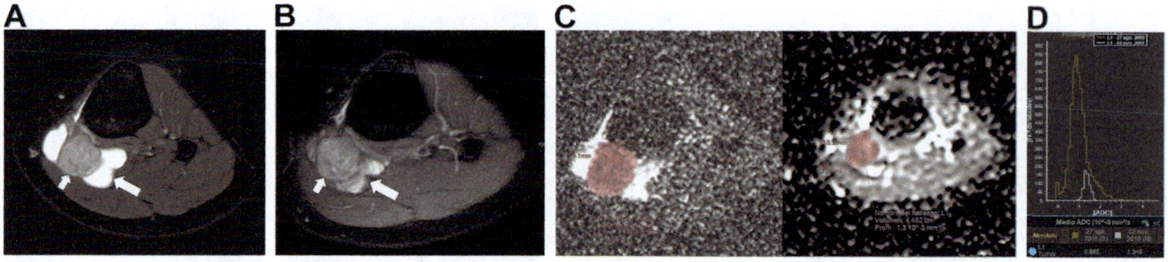

FIG. 6 Synovial sarcoma in a 15-year-old girl who presented with a slow growing mass on the knee. (**A**) Axial T2-weighted, fat suppressed MR image shows a bilobed lesion, containing a heterogeneous solid (*short arrow*) and a cystic component (*long arrow*). (**B**) Axial T2-weighted, fat suppressed MR image performed after chemotherapy shows decrease in size of the cystic component (*long arrow*) with persistence of the solid component (*short arrow*). (**C**, **D**) Volumetric determination of ADC shows reduction of 50% of the volume of the solid component (pink-colored area). (**D**) Histograms of ADC show initial mean values of 0.99 (yellow histogram), which increase to 1.35 after treatment (white histogram). This right displacement of the histogram along the curve suggests response to treatment.

marrow from infiltrated marrow, the addition of DWI, with the calculation of ADC values, allows for better characterization of bone marrow changes. DWI provides functional information by assessing the diffusion of water molecules within tissues, and when combined with Dixon imaging, it offers a more robust approach to detecting and differentiating infiltrative lesions from areas of red marrow reconversion. This is crucial in evaluating conditions like leukemia, lymphoma, and other marrow-infiltrative diseases, as the ADC values can correlate with cellularity and the degree of infiltration, making this multimodal imaging strategy a powerful tool in pediatric oncology.

Dynamic contrast-enhanced MRI and time-intensity curve analysis

DCE-MRI is a complementary tool in pediatric musculoskeletal imaging, particularly for evaluating bone

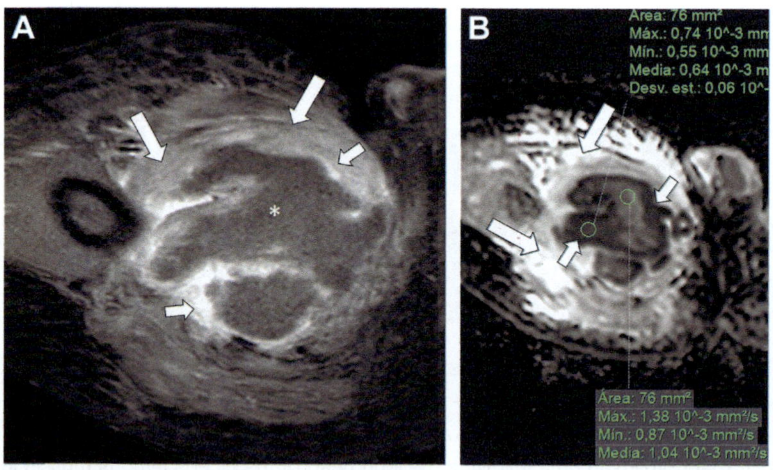

FIG. 7 Soft tissue abscess involving the proximal thigh in a 4-year-old girl who presented with fever and a reddish mass. (**A**) Axial enhanced T1-weighted, fat-suppressed MR image shows a heterogenous and ill-defined abscess, with peripheral enhancement (*short arrows*) and internal necrosis (*asterisk*). Note inflammation (*long arrows*) of the surrounding musculature. (**B**) Axial ADC map MR image shows restricted diffusion (*short arrows*). Reactive or inflammatory changes in the periphery of the abscess are represented by areas with facilitated diffusion (*long arrows*). ADC mapping can help differentiate the necrotic core of an abscess from the surrounding inflammatory tissue.

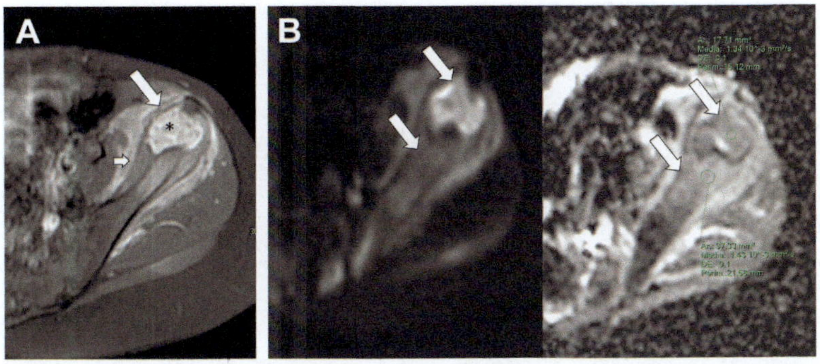

FIG. 8 Chronic osteomyelitis in a 10-year-old boy who presented with pain on the left iliac bone. (**A**) Axial enhanced T1-weighted, fat-suppressed MR image shows a heterogeneous bone lesion within the left iliac bone (*long arrow*), that present a thick periosteal reaction (*short arrow*). Note a heterogeneous enhancing tissue within the lesion (*asterisk*), suggestive of granulation tissue. (**B**) Axial DWI and ADC maps MR images show facilitated diffusion (*arrows*) both, in the iliac bone and within the lesion. ADC mapping aids in distinguishing chronic osteomyelitis, where fibrosis and granulation tissue lead to increased ADC, from active infection, where restricted diffusion persists. ADC mapping helps differentiate chronic osteomyelitis from active infection by identifying increased ADC in fibrosis and granulation tissue.

sarcomas, such as osteosarcoma and Ewing sarcoma, or soft tissue sarcomas, such as rhabdomyosarcoma. This technique assesses tissue perfusion by sequentially acquiring images after contrast administration, providing essential information regarding tissue vascularity, tumor characteristics, and the assessment of treatment response [31].

Time-intensity curves (TICs) classifies the enhancement patterns over time, which can help distinguish between different tissue types and help to characterize malignant or benign lesions infections [32]. The following are the main types of TICs:

1. *Type I: No Enhancement*—Typically observed in necrotic tissue, where there is little to no enhancement after contrast administration.
2. *Type II: Progressive Enhancement*—Seen in benign and inflammatory processes, where there is a steady increase in signal intensity, often indicating slow tumor growth or inflammation.
3. *Type III: Plateau*—Features a rapid initial enhancement followed by a plateau. This pattern is commonly associated with malignant tumors, reflecting their higher vascularity and more aggressive nature.
4. *Type IV: Plateau and Delayed Washout*—Typically seen in malignant tumors, where the initial enhancement is followed by a plateau, and then a delayed washout, reflecting more complex vascular structures in highly aggressive tumors.
5. *Type V: Variable Enhancement*—Represents heterogeneous enhancement patterns, often seen in granulation tissue, fibrosis, or complex lesions that may require biopsy for further characterization.

In the context of pediatric bone sarcomas or soft tissue sarcomas, DCE-MRI and TIC analysis are essential for distinguishing between benign and malignant lesions, evaluating tumor aggressiveness, and monitoring treatment response, when combined with conventional MRI sequences. Malignant tumors typically show a Type III or Type IV TIC, with rapid enhancement and either a plateau or delayed washout, which suggests high tumor vascularity and aggressive behavior (Fig. 9). Additionally, combining DCE-MRI with other imaging modalities, such as DWI improves the characterization of these tumors and helps track changes over time [33].

In the evaluation of musculoskeletal infections, DCE-MRI plays a critical role in differentiating between osteomyelitis, abscess formation, and post-treatment granulation tissue [34]. In acute osteomyelitis, infected bone and adjacent soft tissues exhibit rapid contrast uptake due to hyperemia and increased vascular permeability, often followed by a washout phase, resembling the TIC patterns seen in malignancies. However, granulation tissue, which forms during the healing process, typically demonstrates a more gradual and progressive enhancement (Type II TIC), reflecting lower vascular permeability compared with active infection (Fig. 10). Studies have shown that combining DCE-MRI with DWI further improves differentiation, as osteomyelitis frequently presents with restricted diffusion due to high cellularity, whereas granulation tissue exhibits

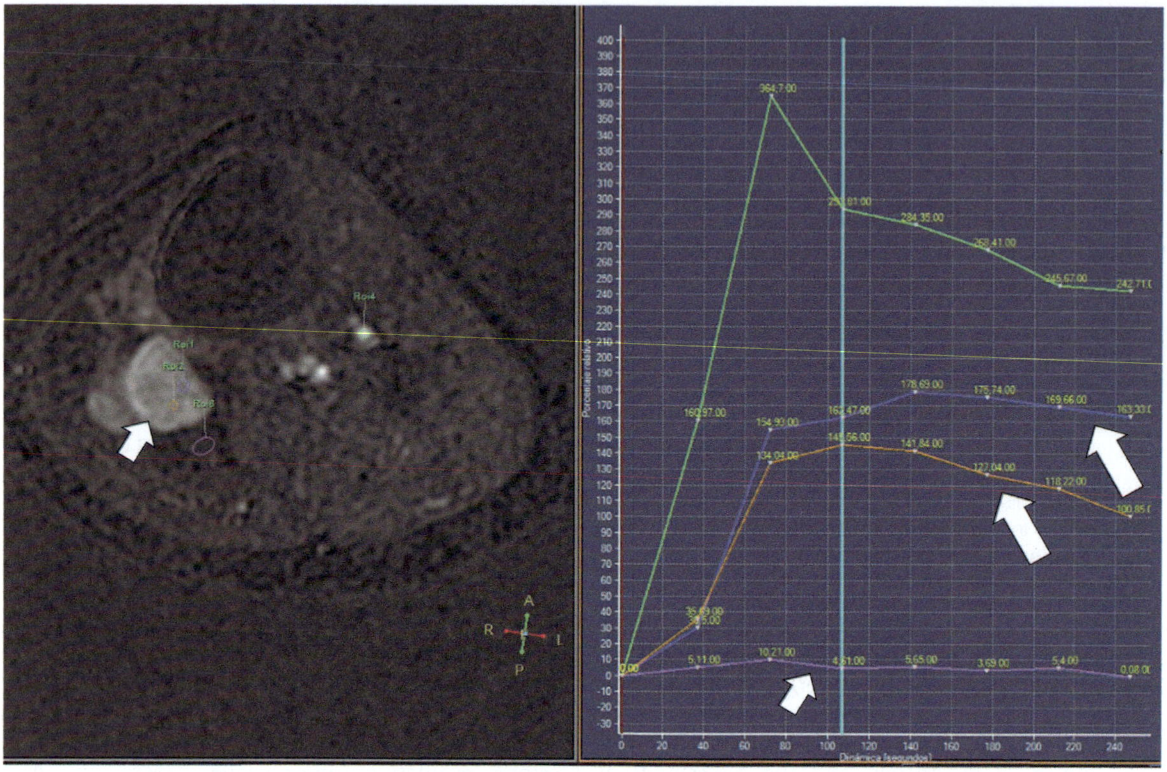

FIG. 9 Same patient as in Fig. 6. (**A**) Axial DCE-MR image shows arterial enhancement of the solid component (*short arrow*). TICs performed on the solid component show type III and type IV profiles (*long arrows*), while TICs performed on the cystic component show type I profile (*short arrow*). TICs classify the enhancement patterns over time, which can help distinguish between different tissue types. Green curve represent the normal arterial uptake.

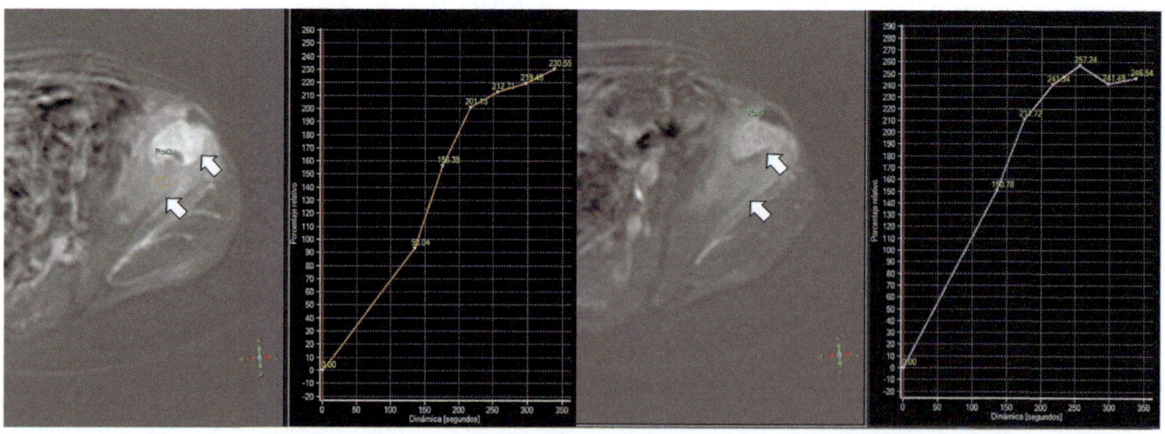

FIG. 10 Same patient as in Fig. 8. (**A**) Axial DCE-MR image shows diffuse enhancement of the iliac bone and of the heterogeneous lesion (*short arrows*). TIC performed in the bone and within the lesion show type II profile or progressive enhancement (*orange and purple curves*). Granulation tissue, which forms during the healing process, typically demonstrates a more gradual and progressive enhancement (Type II TIC), reflecting lower vascular permeability compared with active infection.

less restriction. This distinction is crucial in guiding treatment decisions, preventing unnecessary interventions, and ensuring accurate monitoring of therapeutic response in pediatric patients with suspected musculoskeletal infections.

Whole-body MRI

Whole-body MRI (WB-MRI) has emerged as an invaluable tool in pediatric musculoskeletal imaging, offering comprehensive, noninvasive assessments without the risks associated with ionizing radiation. This is particularly useful for evaluating multifocal oncologic or rheumatologic conditions, among other entities.

Recent technological advancements have substantially enhanced the utility of WB-MRI. The integration of DWI sequences provides functional information by assessing the movement of water molecules within tissues, which is crucial for detecting early inflammatory changes and monitoring disease progression. Studies have demonstrated that WB-MRI, when combined with DWI, offers comparable accuracy to traditional imaging modalities like PET/CT, with the added benefit of avoiding ionizing radiation (Fig. 11) [35].

In the context of chronic nonbacterial osteomyelitis, WB-MRI can identify multiple asymptomatic lesions, guiding biopsy, and treatment decisions. The ability to detect lesions in prestructural inflammatory stages allows for early intervention, potentially altering the disease course. Similarly, in juvenile spondyloarthritis, WB-MRI assesses the extent of joint and entheseal involvement, aiding in early diagnosis and monitoring therapeutic response. Functional MR sequences, such as WB-DWI and T2 Dixon [25,36], are also helpful in differentiating between active inflammation and chronic lesions, providing information useful in determining which patients need active treatment.

Volumetric MRI analysis is essential in NF1 for detecting and monitoring neurofibromas, particularly plexiform neurofibromas. This method provides precise measurements of tumor size and volume, enabling early detection of growth and facilitating timely intervention. A study comparing 2 volumetric analysis methods found that both yielded consistent results, underscoring the reliability of this approach in clinical settings [37].

In NF1, plexiform neurofibromas can cause substantial morbidity, and monitoring their progression is crucial. Volumetric MRI allows for the assessment of tumor growth over time, aiding in treatment planning and evaluation of therapeutic efficacy. Volumetric measurements are effective in tracking changes in tumor volume, which is vital for managing NF1-related complications. Additionally, incorporating DWI can help differentiate benign plexiform neurofibromas from malignant transformation, such as malignant peripheral nerve sheath tumors, by assessing tissue diffusivity and detecting early signs of malignancy.

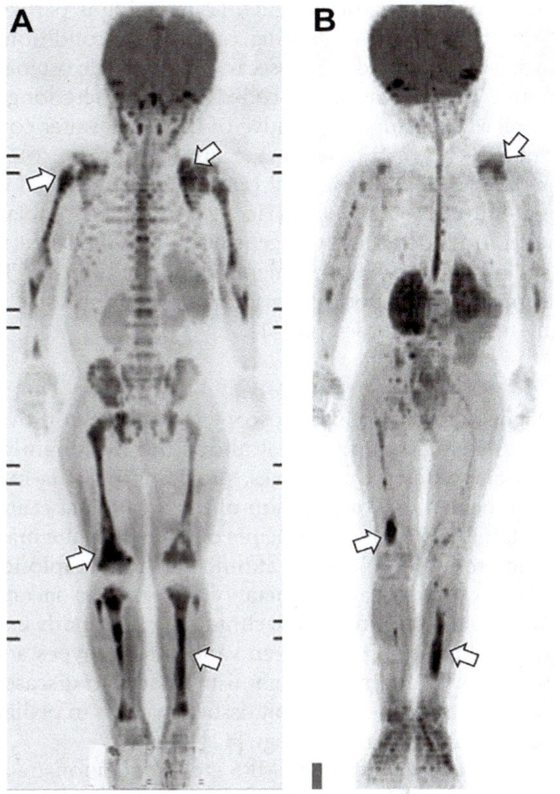

FIG. 11 Myeloblastic leukemia in a 3-year-old girl who presented with multiple bruises and malaise. (**A**) Whole-body DWI MR image reconstruction shows pathologic restriction (*arrows*) of the bone marrow involving the axial and the appendicular skeleton. (**B**) Whole-body DWI MR image reconstruction performed after 2 cycles of chemotherapy shows substantial reduction of the bone marrow involvement, with scattered areas of residual tumor (*arrows*). Whole-body DWI-MRI can provide comparable information to PET-CT in assessing bone marrow infiltration, though PET-CT remains the reference standard.

T2 mapping for cartilage assessment

T2 mapping in pediatric musculoskeletal imaging is a noninvasive method to assess cartilage health, detect early degenerative changes, and monitor the effectiveness of therapeutic interventions [38,39]. T2 mapping quantifies the T2 relaxation time of tissues, providing detailed information about cartilage composition and integrity. In pediatric patients, T2 mapping is particularly valuable for evaluating cartilage in conditions, such as osteochondritis dissecans and juvenile osteoarthritis. T2 maps are color-coded images where longer T2 relaxation times, indicative of increased water content and early cartilage damage, appear in warm colors (red/yellow), while normal cartilage is represented in cooler tones (blue/green) (Fig. 12). Increased T2 relaxation times detect early degeneration in articular cartilage in patients with JIA, highlighting the utility of T2 mapping in monitoring disease progression and assessing treatment efficacy [40,41].

Magnetic resonance spectroscopy

Magnetic resonance spectroscopy (MRS) is a noninvasive imaging technique that allows the measurement of metabolites within tissues, providing insights into the biochemical composition of the area being examined. It is based on the principle of MR, where the magnetic properties of certain atomic nuclei are exploited to detect and quantify metabolites, such as lactate, choline, and creatine. This technique is particularly useful in distinguishing between various tissue types and evaluating changes in metabolism related to diseases, including infections and soft tissue sarcomas in pediatric musculoskeletal radiology [42].

In soft tissue sarcomas, MRS typically demonstrates elevated levels of choline-containing compounds, which are associated with increased cell membrane turnover and indicative of malignancy [43]. For instance, a study published in *European Journal of Radiology* found that the presence of a choline peak in MRS spectra was a marker of malignancy in bone and soft tissue tumors, with a sensitivity of 72.2% and specificity of 83.3% [44].

MRS has also been used to detect metabolic changes in inflammatory processes [45]. In infections, MRS may show elevated levels of lactate and a decrease in choline, reflecting tissue hypoxia and an altered metabolic state due to infection-induced inflammation. For example, in osteomyelitis, MRS can help distinguish infection from other conditions by identifying these specific metabolic shifts. In contrast, in tumors like soft tissue sarcomas, MRS typically demonstrates increased choline levels, associated with high cellular turnover and malignancy. This difference allows MRS to potentially differentiate between infectious processes and malignant lesions, improving diagnostic accuracy and treatment monitoring.

Relaxation-enhanced angiography without contrast and triggering

Relaxation-enhanced angiography without contrast and triggering (REACT) is an advanced MRI technique designed to visualize blood vessels without the need for intravenous contrast agents or cardiac gating. REACT leverages differences in tissue relaxation times to produce high-contrast images of vascular structures, making it particularly useful for patients where contrast is contraindicated. REACT employs a magnetization-prepared 3-dimensional nonbalanced dual-echo Dixon method, enabling free-breathing, nongated imaging with robust fat suppression over large fields of view. This technique has shown promise in assessing conditions such as

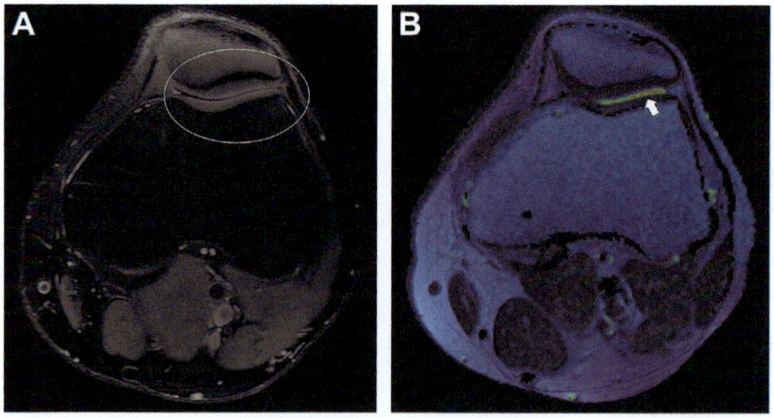

FIG. 12 Early onset of patellar chondromalacia in a 16-year-old girl who presented with anterior knee pain. (**A**) Axial T2-weighted, fat-suppressed MR image shows normal signal intensity of the patellar and trochlear cartilage (*white area*). (**B**) Axial T2 maps-weighted MR image shows red/yellow color in the surface of the patellar cartilage (*arrow*), indicative of increased water content and early cartilage damage.

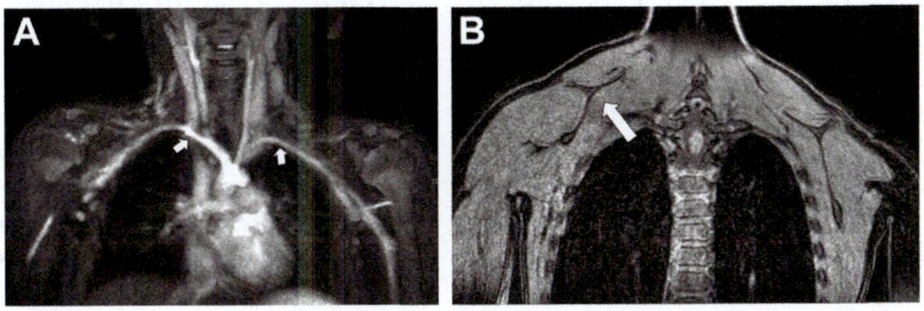

FIG. 13 Sprengel's deformity in a 13-year-old boy who presented with deformity of the scapula. (**A**) REACT shows normal original of the subclavian arteries (*short arrows*). (**B**) Coronal T1 DIXON, fat-suppressed MR image, shows elevation of the right scapular, suggestive of Sprengel's deformity (*long arrow*). The REACT MR technique is highly useful in preoperative cases, such as Sprengel's deformity, as it allows for the assessment of anatomic variants, thereby improving surgical accuracy and planning.

Sprengel's deformity (Fig. 13), thoracic outlet syndrome, central vein stenosis, renal artery stenosis, and vascular malformations [46].

In pediatric imaging, REACT offers substantial advantages by eliminating the need for intravenous contrast administration, thereby reducing procedure complexity and potential risks associated with gadolinium-based agents. Studies have demonstrated that REACT provides image quality comparable to traditional contrast-enhanced MR venography, making it a valuable tool for evaluating central venous structures in children and young adults [47].

Fluid-attenuated inversion recovery with fat suppression

Fluid-attenuated inversion recovery with fat suppression (FLAIR FS) is emerging as a valuable noncontrast MRI technique in pediatric musculoskeletal imaging, particularly for evaluating inflammatory joint conditions. This sequence was originally designed for neuroimaging, but

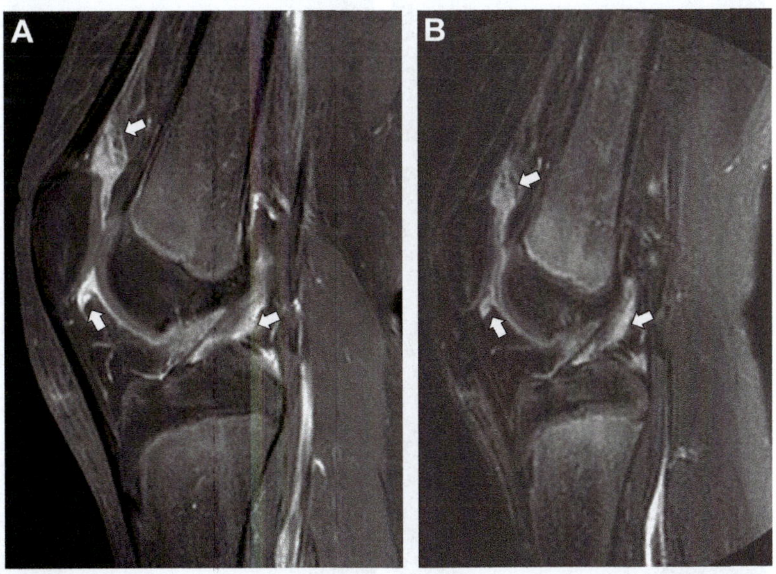

FIG. 14 JIA in a 7-year-old girl who presented with knee pain and inflammation. (**A**) Sagittal enhanced T1-weighted, fat-suppressed MR image shows thickening and enhancement of the synovium (*arrows*). (**B**) Sagittal FLAIR fat-suppressed MR image shows thickening of the synovium (*arrows*). The primary benefit of FLAIR FS is its ability to suppress both free fluid and fat signals, providing improved delineation of synovial thickening and inflammation.

now it has been adapted for musculoskeletal applications, offering enhanced visualization of synovial pathology without the need of intravenous contrast agents [48].

The primary benefit of FLAIR FS is its ability to suppress both free fluid and fat signals, providing improved delineation of synovial thickening and inflammation. This feature makes it particularly useful in conditions where conventional noncontrast sequences may fail to distinguish synovial pathology from joint effusions. In pediatric imaging, where minimizing intravenous contrast use is a priority, FLAIR FS presents a promising alternative for detecting and monitoring joint inflammation, especially in children with JIA. This sequence effectively highlights inflamed synovium without the confounding effects of joint fluid, producing results comparable to contrast-enhanced imaging (Fig. 14). Additionally, FLAIR FS has utility that extends to other inflammatory arthropathies, including spondyloarthritis and osteoarthritis, where it aids in detecting subtle inflammatory changes (fluid-attenuated inversion-recovery sequence with fat suppression as an alternative to contrast-enhanced MRI in pediatric synovitis).

ARTIFICIAL INTELLIGENCE AND DEEP LEARNING IN MUSCULOSKELETAL IMAGING

AI and deep learning have substantially transformed pediatric musculoskeletal imaging by enhancing diagnostic accuracy, streamlining workflows, and providing quantitative assessments [49]. These technologies utilize complex algorithms to analyze imaging data, facilitating the detection, and characterization of various musculoskeletal conditions. In addition, advanced MRI acceleration technology that builds on the established compressed SENSE technique, enhances image quality and boosts reconstruction speed by integrating AI algorithms early in the reconstruction process. This decrease in acquisition time is especially important in children to reduce the need for sedation.

Fracture detection and classification

AI algorithms have been developed to assist in the detection and classification of fractures in pediatric patients [50]. By analyzing radiographic images, AI systems can

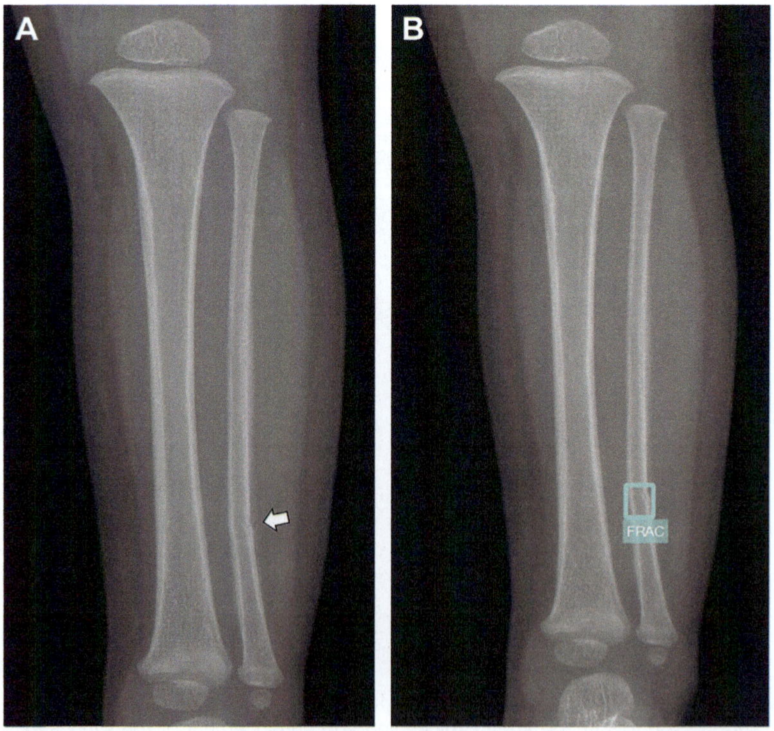

FIG. 15 Green stick fracture in a 17-month-old boy who presented with limping and difficulty to walk. (**A**) Frontal radiograph of the left leg shows a green stick fracture (*arrow*) involving the distal fibula. (**B**) The fracture (box) has been detected by the AI software.

identify subtle fractures that may be overlooked by the human eye. For instance, deep learning models have been trained to detect fractures in children, demonstrating high sensitivity and specificity (Fig. 15). These tools aid in prompt diagnosis and may reduce interobserver variability among radiologists.

Bone age assessment

Assessing bone age is crucial in evaluating growth disorders in children. Traditional methods involve manual analysis of hand and wrist radiographs, which can be time-consuming and subject to observer variability. AI-based systems have been developed to automate this process, providing rapid and consistent assessments. These systems utilize deep learning algorithms to compare patient images with reference standards, facilitating the diagnosis of endocrine diseases, such as growth hormone deficiencies or precocious puberty [51].

Detection of bone marrow infiltration

In pediatric oncology, early detection of bone marrow infiltration is vital for the diagnosis and management of hematologic malignancies. AI algorithms have been applied to MRI data to identify patterns suggestive of marrow infiltration [52]. By analyzing signal intensities and distribution patterns on sequences, such as T1-weighted and T2-weighted images, these systems can assist radiologists in distinguishing between normal and pathologic marrow, thereby facilitating early intervention.

Despite substantial progress in other imaging modalities, conventional radiography in pediatric musculoskeletal applications has seen limited advancements in recent years. Aside from the integration of AI for improved fracture detection, there have been no major breakthroughs in radiographic techniques specifically designed for musculoskeletal disorders or tumors.

While radiography remains a fundamental tool for evaluating fractures and bone abnormalities, innovations have primarily focused on MRI and CT, with radiography largely maintaining its traditional role. However, AI-driven applications are increasingly being explored to automate measurements and angle assessments, potentially saving time and improving diagnostic efficiency in clinical practice.

SUMMARY

Advancements in pediatric musculoskeletal imaging have substantially improved the detection, diagnosis, and management of a wide range of musculoskeletal pathologies in the pediatric population. The integration of cutting-edge techniques, such as photon-counting CT, spectral CT, and advanced MRI modalities, including DWI, and dynamic studies, has expanded diagnostic imaging capabilities in oncology, infections, trauma, and inflammatory conditions. These technologies provide insights into tumor characteristics, bone marrow changes, and soft tissue abnormalities, facilitating timely and accurate clinical decision-making. Furthermore, the use of AI-assisted tools and fast MRI sequences has decreased scan time, streamlined diagnostic workflows, and reduced patient discomfort. Continued improvements in imaging technologies continue to evolve, they promise to further improve the diagnosis and management of pediatric musculoskeletal disorders, resulting in improved outcomes for pediatric patients.

CLINICS CARE POINTS

- Selecting the appropriate imaging modality is critical for balancing diagnostic accuracy, safety, and patient comfort, particularly in pediatric musculoskeletal conditions.
- Whole-body MRI is a powerful tool for detecting multifocal bone involvement in rheumatologic and oncologic conditions, potentially serving as an alternative to PET-computed tomography in specific scenarios.
- Dynamic contrast-enhanced-MRI and volumetric determination of apparent diffusion coefficient are valuable for tumor characterization and assessing treatment response in pediatric patients.
- Contrast-enhanced ultrasound provides real-time vascular assessment without nephrotoxic contrast agents, making it useful for evaluating infections, vascular anomalies, and soft tissue tumors in children.
- Artificial intelligence-based imaging applications enhance fracture detection, automate bone age assessment, and support early diagnosis of bone marrow infiltration, improving clinical workflow.

DISCLOSURE

The authors declare no conflict of interest.

REFERENCES

[1] van Holsbeeck M, Soliman S, Van Kerkhove F, et al. Advanced musculoskeletal ultrasound techniques: what are the applications? AJR Am J Roentgenol 2021;216(2):436–45.

[2] Recht MP, White LM, Fritz J, et al. Advances in musculoskeletal imaging: recent developments and predictions for the future. Radiology 2023;308(2):e230615.
[3] Jardon M, Alaia EF. Approach to imaging modalities in the setting of suspected infection. Skelet Radiol 2024; 53(10):1957–68.
[4] Squires JH, McCarville MB. Contrast-enhanced ultrasound in children: implementation and key diagnostic applications. AJR Am J Roentgenol 2021;217(5):1217–31.
[5] Ntoulia A, Barnewolt CE, Doria AS, et al. Contrast-enhanced ultrasound for musculoskeletal indications in children. Pediatr Radiol 2021;51(12):2303–23.
[6] Wiesinger I, Jung W, Zausig N, et al. Evaluation of dynamic effects of therapy-induced changes in microcirculation after percutaneous treatment of vascular malformations using contrast-enhanced ultrasound (CEUS) and time intensity curve (TIC) analyses. Clin Hemorheol Microcirc 2018;69(1–2):45–57.
[7] Wang P, Wu M, Li A, et al. Diagnostic value of contrast-enhanced ultrasound for differential diagnosis of malignant and benign soft tissue masses: a meta-analysis. Ultrasound Med Biol 2020;46(12):3179–87.
[8] Alis D, Erol BC, Akbas S, et al. Superb microvascular imaging compared with power Doppler ultrasound in assessing synovitis of the knee in juvenile idiopathic arthritis: a preliminary study. J Ultrasound Med 2020; 39(1):99–106.
[9] Chen X, Zhou L, Xia Y, et al. Superb microvascular imaging for evaluating the activity of juvenile localised scleroderma: a preliminary study. Eur Radiol 2024;34-(10):6376–83.
[10] Gitto S, Messina C, Chianca V, et al. Superb microvascular imaging (SMI) in the evaluation of musculoskeletal disorders: a systematic review. La radiologia medica 2020;125(5):481–90.
[11] Santos JA, Tee CA, Galsim RJG, et al. Musculoskeletal ultrasound using superb microvascular imaging documents treatment response to biosimilar infliximab in rheumatoid arthritis. BMJ Case Rep 2021;14(2):e239112.
[12] Diao XH, Shen Y, Chen L, et al. Superb microvascular imaging is as sensitive as contrast-enhanced ultrasound for detecting synovial vascularity in rheumatoid arthritis. Quant Imaging Med Surg 2022;12(5):2866–76.
[13] Drakonaki EE, Allen GM, Wilson DJ. Ultrasound elastography for musculoskeletal applications. Br J Radiol 2012;85(1019):1435–45.
[14] Pichiecchio A, Alessandrino F, Bortolotto C, et al. Muscle ultrasound elastography and MRI in preschool children with Duchenne muscular dystrophy. Neuromuscul Disord 2018;28(6):476–83.
[15] Alfuraih AM, O'Connor P, Tan AL, et al. Muscle shear wave elastography in idiopathic inflammatory myopathies: a case-control study with MRI correlation. Skelet Radiol 2019;48(8):1209–19.
[16] Snoj Ž, Wu CH, Taljanovic MS, et al. Ultrasound elastography in musculoskeletal radiology: past, present, and future. Semin Musculoskelet Radiol 2020;24(2):156–66.
[17] Vosshenrich J, O'Donnell T, Fritz J. Photon-counting CT in musculoskeletal imaging-10 key questions answered. Semin Roentgenol 2024;59(4):378–86.
[18] Baffour FI, Glazebrook KN, Ferrero A, et al. Photon-counting detector CT for musculoskeletal imaging: a clinical perspective. AJR Am J Roentgenol 2023;220(4): 551–60.
[19] Park EH, O'Donnell T, Fritz J. Dual-energy computed tomography applications in rheumatology. Radiol Clin North Am 2024;62(5):849–63.
[20] Kruk KA, Dietrich TJ, Wildermuth S, et al. Dual-energy CT in differentiating osteomyelitis from malignant bone lesions. Skelet Radiol 2022;51(5):989–97.
[21] François MA, Comby PO, Goueslard K, et al. Diagnostic performance of spectral CT in detecting bone marrow edema for vertebral fracture: a multi-reader study. Eur J Radiol 2025;182:111857.
[22] Lins CF, Salmon CEG, Nogueira-Barbosa MH. Applications of the Dixon technique in the evaluation of the musculoskeletal system. Radiol Bras 2021;54(1):33–42.
[23] Omoumi P. The Dixon method in musculoskeletal MRI: from fat-sensitive to fat-specific imaging. Skelet Radiol 2022;51(7):1365–9.
[24] Erkal Tonkaz D, Ozpar R, Tonkaz M, et al. Efficacy of fat quantification methods used in MRI to distinguish between normal, benign, and malignant bone marrow pathologies in children. Acta Radiol 2024;65(7): 841–50.
[25] Tanturi de Horatio L, Zadig PK, Von Brandis E, et al. Whole-body MRI in children and adolescents: can T2-weighted Dixon fat-only images replace standard T1-weighted images in the assessment of bone marrow? Eur J Radiol 2023;166:110968.
[26] El-Adalany MA, El-Din Eid NK, Othman S, et al. Role of diffusion-weighted MRI in evaluation of pediatric musculoskeletal soft tissue masses. Egypt J Radiol Nucl Med 2021;52:263.
[27] Chun CW, Jung JY, Baik JS, et al. Detection of soft-tissue abscess: comparison of diffusion-weighted imaging to contrast-enhanced MRI. J Magn Reson Imaging 2018; 47(1):60–8.
[28] Habre C, Botti P, Laurent M, et al. Benefits of diffusion-weighted imaging in pediatric acute osteoarticular infections. Pediatr Radiol 2022;52(6):1086–94.
[29] Kruk KA, Dietrich TJ, Wildermuth S, et al. Diffusion-weighted imaging distinguishes between osteomyelitis, bone marrow edema, and healthy bone on forefoot magnetic resonance imaging. J Magn Reson Imaging 2022; 56(5):1571–9.
[30] Barendregt AM, Mazzoli V, van Gulik EC, et al. Juvenile idiopathic arthritis: diffusion-weighted MRI in the assessment of arthritis in the knee. Radiology 2020;295(2): 373–80.
[31] Sujlana P, Skrok J, Fayad LM. Review of dynamic contrast-enhanced MRI: technical aspects and applications in the musculoskeletal system. J Magn Reson Imaging 2018;47(4):875–90.

[32] Visser JJ, Goergen SK, Klein S, et al. The value of quantitative musculoskeletal imaging. Semin Musculoskelet Radiol 2020;24(4):460–74.

[33] Inarejos Clemente EJ, Navarro OM, Navallas M, et al. Multiparametric MRI evaluation of bone sarcomas in children. Insights Imaging 2022;13(1):33.

[34] Kim EY, Kwack KS, Cho JH, et al. Usefulness of dynamic contrast-enhanced MRI in differentiating between septic arthritis and transient synovitis in the hip joint. AJR Am J Roentgenol 2012;198(2):428–33.

[35] Guimarães JB, da Cruz IAN, Ahlawat S, et al. The role of whole-body MRI in pediatric musculoskeletal oncology: current concepts and clinical applications. J Magn Reson Imaging 2024;59(6):1886–901.

[36] Zadig P, von Brandis E, Ording Müller LS, et al. Pediatric whole-body magnetic resonance imaging: comparison of STIR and T2 Dixon sequences in the detection and grading of high signal bone marrow changes. Eur Radiol 2023;33(7):5045–53.

[37] Cai W, Steinberg SM, Bredella MA, et al. Volumetric MRI analysis of plexiform neurofibromas in neurofibromatosis type 1: comparison of two methods. Acad Radiol 2018;25(2):144–52.

[38] Lu Z, Pan S, Wang B, et al. T2 mapping of the acetabular cartilage in infants and children with developmental dysplasia of the hip. Acta Radiol 2021;62(10):1418–25.

[39] Zhang N, Lv Y, Liu Y, et al. T2 mapping in the quantitative evaluation of articular cartilage changes in children with hemophilia: a pilot study. Pediatr Investig 2019; 2(4):242–7.

[40] Kim HK, Laor T, Graham TB, et al. T2 relaxation time changes in distal femoral articular cartilage in children with juvenile idiopathic arthritis: a 3-year longitudinal study. AJR Am J Roentgenol 2010;195(4):1021–5.

[41] Xia W, Zhang Y, Liu C, et al. Quantitative T2 mapping magnetic resonance imaging of articular cartilage in patients with juvenile idiopathic arthritis. Eur J Radiol 2023;160:110690.

[42] Deshmukh S, Subhawong T, Carrino JA, et al. Role of MR spectroscopy in musculoskeletal imaging. Indian J Radiol Imaging 2014;24(3):210–6.

[43] Fayad LM, Jacobs MA, Wang X, et al. Musculoskeletal tumors: how to use anatomic, functional, and metabolic MR techniques. Radiology 2012;265(2):340–56.

[44] Doganay S, Altinok T, Alkan A, et al. The role of MRS in the differentiation of benign and malignant soft tissue and bone tumors. Eur J Radiol 2011;79(2):e33–7.

[45] Subhawong TK, Wang X, Machado AJ, et al. 1H Magnetic resonance spectroscopy findings in idiopathic inflammatory myopathies at 3 T: feasibility and first results. Investig Radiol 2013;48(7):509–16.

[46] Tan EJ, Zhang S, Tirukonda P, et al. React - a novel flow-independent non-gated non-contrast MR angiography technique using magnetization-prepared 3D non-balanced dual-echo dixon method: preliminary clinical experience. Eur J Radiol Open 2020;7(7):100238.

[47] Betz LH, Dillman JR, Towbin AJ, et al. Respiratory-triggered flow-independent noncontrast non-ECG-gated MRV (REACT) versus CE-MRV for central venous evaluation in children and young adults: a six-reader study. AJR Am J Roentgenol 2023;221(2):240–8.

[48] Milks KS, Singh J, Benedict JA, et al. Fluid-attenuated inversion-recovery sequence with fat suppression as an alternative to contrast-enhanced MRI in pediatric synovitis. Pediatr Radiol 2024;54(1):96–104.

[49] Guermazi A, Omoumi P, Tordjman M, et al. How AI may transform musculoskeletal imaging. Radiology 2024; 310(1):e230764.

[50] Shelmerdine SC, White RD, Liu H, et al. Artificial intelligence for radiological paediatric fracture assessment: a systematic review. Insights Imaging 2022;13(1):94.

[51] Pape J, Rosolowski M, Pfäffle R, et al. A critical comparative study of the performance of three AI-assisted programs for bone age determination. Eur Radiol 2025; 35(3):1190–6.

[52] Lv L, Zhang Z, Zhang D, et al. Machine-learning radiomics to predict bone marrow metastasis of neuroblastoma using magnetic resonance imaging. Cancer Innov 2023;2(5):405–15.

Advances in Clinical Radiology 7 (2025) 175–186

ADVANCES IN CLINICAL RADIOLOGY

Advances in Neonatal Ultrasound Imaging

Beyond Grayscale and Color Doppler Assessment

Domen Plut, MD, PhD[a,b,*], Peter Slak, MD[a,b], Abbey J. Winant, MD[c], Edward Y. Lee, MD, MPH[c]

[a]Department of Radiology, University of Ljubljana, Vrazov Trg 2, Ljubljana 1000, Slovenia; [b]Division of Pediatric Radiology, Institute of Radiology, University Medical Centre Ljubljana, Zaloška Cesta 7, Ljubljana 1000, Slovenia; [c]Department of Radiology, Boston Children's Hospital, Harvard Medical School, 300 Longwood Avenue, Boston, MA 02215, USA

KEYWORDS

• Child • Contrast-enhanced ultrasound • Doppler imaging • Elastography • Microvascular flow imaging • Neonate • Sonography

KEY POINTS

- Improvements in ultrasound (US) technology have allowed for the development of US techniques that provide information beyond grayscale and color Doppler imaging.
- Contrast-enhanced US allows detailed evaluation of body compartments and tissue perfusion through intracavitary or intravenous application of microbubble US contrast.
- Microvascular flow imaging, an advanced Doppler imaging technique, allows visualization of very small vasculature and detection of low-velocity vascular flow without the use of contrast.
- US elastography provides diagnostic assessment of tissue stiffness.
- Clinical applications of these methods in neonatal radiology are expanding, including the evaluation of the brain, liver, kidneys, hollow organs, and vasculature.

INTRODUCTION

Ultrasound (US) is an ideal imaging tool during the neonatal period. First, it is non-invasive and safe. Unlike radiography and computed tomography (CT), US does not utilize ionizing radiation, which is particularly important for the developing organs of neonates, which are more sensitive to the deleterious effects of radiation. Unlike MRI, US generally does not require sedation in children and therefore does not expose the developing brain to the risks associated with sedation. Secondly, US is a reliable imaging tool with excellent soft tissue visualization and high diagnostic accuracy. It is particularly effective in neonates due to their smaller size, which allows imaging with higher-frequency probes to gain higher-resolution images. These high-resolution images allow detailed assessment of the organ structure and have the ability to assess blood flow with the use of the Doppler technique. In addition, the US beam can penetrate the predominantly cartilaginous growing bones of neonates allowing for sonographic assessment of structures not accessible to US in adults, such as the brain and spinal cord. Furthermore, US machines are readily portable and can be used at the bedside, even in the neonatal intensive care units. This allows for immediate evaluation without needing to move the baby, which is especially important in critically-ill

*Corresponding author. Division of Pediatric Radiology, Institute of Radiology, University Medical Centre Ljubljana, Zaloška Cesta 7, Ljubljana 1000, Slovenia. *E-mail address:* plut.domen@gmail.com

https://doi.org/10.1016/j.yacr.2025.06.003 www.advancesinclinicalradiology.com
2589-8701/25/

ABBREVIATIONS	
AKI	acute kidney injury
CEUS	contrast-enhanced ultrasound
HIE	hypoxic-ischemic encephalopathy
MV-flow	microvascular flow
MVI	microvascular imaging
NEC	necrotizing enterocolitis
US	ultrasound
VI	vascular index
VUR	vesicoureteral reflux

children with numerous support structures, such as endotracheal tubes, central lines, or extracorporeal membrane oxygenation (ECMO) cannulae. Consequently, US is an invaluable first-line imaging tool for assessment of neonates.

The use of US in medicine began during the 2nd World War, with wider dissemination following the introduction of commercially available systems from the sixties onward [1]. Rapid technologic advances in US soon led to the development of real-time grayscale moving images, which can be combined with real time color Doppler technique, which still comprise the fundamental components of US imaging technique today. More recently, further improvements in US technology have allowed for the development of US techniques that provide information beyond the grayscale and color Doppler imaging, as follows: (1) Contrast-enhanced US (CEUS) allows detailed evaluation of body compartments and tissue perfusion through intracavitary or intravenous application of microbubble contrast [2]; (2) Microvascular flow (MV-flow) imaging, an advanced Doppler imaging technique, allows visualization of very small vasculature and detection of low-velocity vascular flow without the use of contrast [3]; (3) US elastography allows evaluation of tissue stiffness [4]. In this article, we review the current and potential clinical applications of these additional sonographic methods in the field of neonatal radiology.

CONTRAST-ENHANCED ULTRASOUND

Contrast-enhanced US (CEUS) is an advanced sonographic technique that allows detailed assessment of the tissue microvasculature and perfusion following intravenous injection of contrast or assessment of hollow organs and body compartments following intracavitary injection of contrast. The advantages of CEUS are its ease of use and a high-safety profile [5]. Adverse reactions to US contrast agents are rare and usually mild in degree [6]. Because US contrast has no renal toxicity, renal function testing is not required prior to US contrast administration. In 2016, CEUS was approved for use in children by the United States Food and Drug Administration for evaluation of focal liver lesions and diagnosis of vesicoureteral reflux (VUR). US contrast is a blood pool agent, meaning that it remains confined within the blood vessels and does not diffuse into surrounding tissues or cross the blood-brain barrier. Because US contrast is distributed throughout the vascular pool after intravenous injection, additional off-label applications focused on various organs have been increasingly performed since its approval for use [5].

CEUS is performed on US systems equipped with specialized software. US contrast agents are optimized to resonate at US frequencies of 2.5 to 3.5 MHz, the center frequency of abdominal convex probes used for imaging of adults. For neonatal imaging, higher-frequency convex or linear transducers are more commonly used, which require an increased dose of US contrast to achieve the same contrast-enhanced image quality [7]. CEUS is performed using either a single-screen contrast-only display or more commonly, on a dual-screen display, with the grayscale reference and contrast-only images shown side-by-side. During a CEUS study, several still images at different phases of enhancement are typically recorded. For quantification studies based on time-intensity curves (TICs), 2- to 3-minute videos are recorded. Perfusion kinetics parameters (i.e., time to peak, wash-in slope, peak intensity, wash-in and wash-out area under the curve, and the wash-out slope) can be determined from TICs [8].

Neuroimaging Applications

The open anterior fontanelle allows assessment of the infant's brain by US, therefore also CEUS. US serves a primary role in the evaluation of many clinically important intracranial disorders in infants, while CEUS has a growing role in the assessment of disorders that affect vascular patency and cerebral perfusion.

Ischemic stroke

Neonatal ischemic stroke occurs in 1 in 2500 full-term infants and even more commonly in premature infants [9]. Infants with stroke often present with seizures, lethargy, hypotonia, feeding difficulties, apnea, or localized neurologic impairment. The majority of neonatal ischemic stroke occurs within the brain area supplied by the middle cerebral artery [10].

Cranial US can be used to detect perinatal stroke, but infarcts located peripherally and small infarcts are not easily identified by grayscale US. In general, MRI is the preferred imaging method for diagnosing neonatal stroke. However, MRI can be difficult to perform in critically-ill newborns and CEUS may be a helpful alternative imaging modality in infants who are unable to undergo MRI. [11]. CEUS can show varying levels of enhancement in ischemic brain tissue depending on the time elapsed since the onset of stroke and the time of evaluation, ranging from non-enhancement to hyper-enhancement. A study evaluating brain CEUS in comparison to MRI (as the reference standard) for the detection of neonatal stroke showed that CEUS had a sensitivity of 87.5% for acute/subacute ischemia and 100% for chronic ischemia [12].

Intracranial hemorrhage

Epidural, subdural, subarachnoid, intraventricular, and intraparenchymal hemorrhage are uncommon in term neonates but occur more frequently in preterm and low birth-weight infants [13]. Intracranial hemorrhage may be asymptomatic or present with nonspecific signs, such as altered consciousness, hypotonia, reduced movement, seizures, dilated pupils, or a bulging fontanelle due to increased intracranial pressure.

Cranial US is the first-line diagnostic tool, while MRI with susceptibility-weighted imaging serves as the gold standard. CEUS can also identify intracranial hemorrhage, appearing as either a region of heterogeneous hypoperfusion or a completely avascular area (Fig. 1). In a study comparing head CEUS to MRI, CEUS showed a sensitivity of 75% and specificity of 86.4% for detecting germinal matrix hemorrhage, and a sensitivity of 50.0% and specificity of 100.0% for intraparenchymal hemorrhage [12].

Brain tumors

The incidence of neonatal brain tumors is low. Neonates with brain tumors may present with large head circumference, symptoms of elevated intracranial pressure, bulging fontanelle, irritability, drowsiness, vomiting, failure to thrive, neurologic deficits, or seizures. MRI remains the mainstay of diagnosis for neonatal brain tumors. In comparison to grayscale US, CEUS can improve the visualization of brain tumors and identify highly-perfused zones within the tumor that are most suitable for tissue sampling [14]. CEUS can also depict the major feeding arteries, which is important for operative planning [11].

Intracranial vascular anomalies

The most common vascular malformation in neonates is the vein of Galen malformation. It typically presents dramatically with features of high-output cardiac failure. Treatment of choice is endovascular occlusion of pathologic vessels [15]. CEUS of the brain can serve as a valuable supplement to MRI in establishing the diagnosis, providing anatomic information about feeding arteries, draining veins, and nidus configuration, and assessing residual flow after endovascular treatment (Fig. 2) [16].

Hypoxic-ischemic encephalopathy

Hypoxic-ischemic encephalopathy (HIE) develops in newborns who experience brain hypoxia or ischemia in the perinatal period. HIE can result in death or severe neurologic impairment and is one of the most common causes of cerebral palsy [17]. MRI is the standard imaging method for evaluating the severity of brain

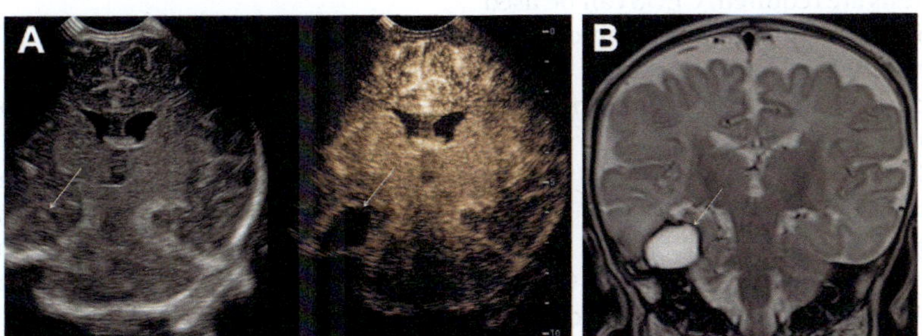

FIG. 1 2-week-old girl (gestational age 38 weeks) with brain hemorrhage following surgery for congenital diaphragmatic hernia repair. **(A)** Dual display coronal contrast-enhanced US (left display, grayscale reference image; right display, contrast-enhanced image). Grayscale image shows an ovoid heterogeneously hypoechoic lesion within the right temporal area of the brain (*arrow*). The lesion is better visualized as a hypoechoic non-enhanced area in the contrast enhanced image (*arrow*). **(B)** Coronal T2-weighted MR image performed at age 6-week-old shows hyperintense right temporal lesion (*arrow*), in keeping with encephalomalacia after hemorrhage.

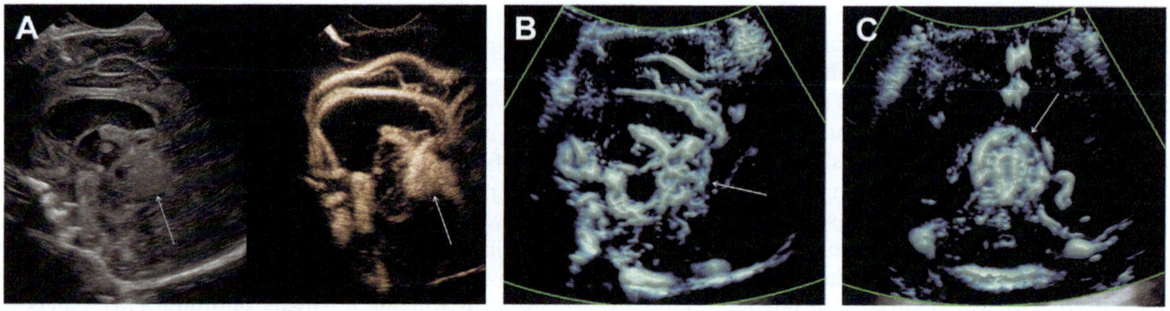

FIG. 2 Newborn boy (gestational age 33 weeks) presenting with heart failure due to vein of Galen malformation. (**A**) Dual display sagittal contrast-enhanced US (left display, grayscale reference image; right display, contrast-enhanced image). Grayscale image shows a hyperechoic lesion posterior to the 3rd ventricle (*arrow*). Contrast-enhanced image shows that the lesion is composed of convoluted vasculature (*arrow*). (**B**, **C**) Microvascular flow imaging in sagittal (**B**) and coronal (**C**) plane demonstrates the convoluted vessels of this complex vascular malformation (*arrow*).

injury in neonates with HIE. MRI is typically performed several days after the hypoxic event, after completion of therapeutic hypothermia. CEUS can be performed in the neonatal intensive care unit, even after initiation of therapeutic hypothermia, and may be helpful in earlier establishment of diagnosis. Studies involving small patient groups suggest that quantitative assessment of brain perfusion with CEUS can help differentiate less affected infants from those with severe HIE [18–20].

Brain death

Brain death is defined as the complete and irreversible loss of brain functions, defined by the cessation of cortical and brainstem activities [21]. It is diagnosed based on the presence of coma, a positive apnea test, and the absence of brainstem reflexes. In some clinical situations ancillary tests are required. CEUS can be used as an ancillary test for confirming brain death or near-brain death. In the setting of brain death, an almost complete absence of perfusion of the intracranial vessels can be demonstrated by CEUS [22,23].

Abdominopelvic Imaging Applications

Focal liver lesion

Evaluation of focal hepatic lesions was one of the first indications for CEUS in children. There is a broad differential diagnosis for hepatic lesions in children. Common benign solid hepatic lesions in neonates are congenital and infantile hemangioma, whereas focal nodular hyperplasia, mesenchymal hamartoma, and other benign tumors are infrequent [24]. The most common primary hepatic malignant tumor in children is hepatoblastoma, although it is not common in the neonatal period [25]. When multiple focal liver lesions are encountered in a neonate, metastatic neuroblastoma should be considered [26]. CEUS can help better characterize focal hepatic lesions in children based on patterns of US contrast enhancement. The dual blood supply of the liver from the hepatic artery and portal vein enables lesion differentiation, because different lesions have different patterns of contrast enhancement in the arterial, portal venous, and delayed phases, which may obviate the need for additional imaging or biopsy [27,28]. Benign hepatic lesions, such as focal nodular hypreplasia (FNH), typically demonstrate contrast retention in the portal venous and delayed phases of enhancement (Fig. 3), while malignant lesions, such as hepatoblastoma, are suspected when the early wash-out of contrast from the lesion is observed [28,29].

Necrotizing enterocolitis

Necrotizing enterocolitis (NEC) is among the most common gastrointestinal emergencies in neonates. It typically affects preterm and low-birthweight newborns or term infants with congenital heart disease [30]. In addition to abdominal radiograph and grayscale/Doppler US, which are standardly used for NEC evaluation, CEUS can be used as a supplementary tool for assessing bowel wall viability in NEC [5]. CEUS provides clear characterization of bowel wall vascularization without the interference of motion artifacts that often interfere with Doppler imaging. In the early phases of NEC, CEUS reveals thickened, well-perfused bowel walls. As NEC progresses, bowel dilation occurs, the bowel walls become thinner, and contrast enhancement diminishes. In cases of severe ischemia from NEC, a

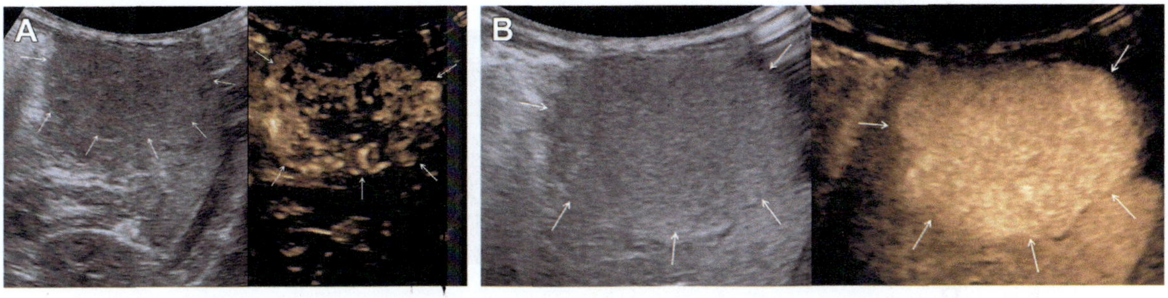

FIG. 3 5-month-old boy with a congenital liver hemangioma in the left lobe. (**A**, **B**) Dual display transverse contrast-enhanced US image (left display, grayscale reference image; right display, contrast-enhanced image) at 7 seconds (**A**) and 2 minutes (**B**) after contrast application. Grayscale images show a homogenous lesion within the left liver lobe (*arrows*). Contrast-enhanced images show centripetal enhancement of the lesion with contrast retention in the delayed phase.

non-viable bowel loop will appear fixed and dilated, with no mural enhancement on CEUS (Fig. 4) [31].

Acute kidney injury

Acute kidney injury (AKI) is a sudden impairment of renal function characterized by decreased glomerular filtration rate. Development of AKI is common in hospitalized critically-ill children, with reported rates up to 27% [32]. Neonates are especially susceptible to developing AKI due to immature kidney function. Early diagnosis of AKI is important, because it can guide therapeutic interventions, which may improve patient outcomes and long-term prognosis [33]. CEUS provides a comprehensive assessment and quantification of renal blood flow through the analysis of TICs (Fig. 5). A meta-analysis examining CEUS in adults with AKI found a marked decrease in renal perfusion compared to individuals without AKI [34]. Research on the predictive value of CEUS perfusion parameters for the development of AKI in pediatric patients is still lacking [35].

Genitosonography and distal colostosonography

Urogenital sinus abnormalities are commonly seen in neonates with ambiguous genitalia and require imaging evaluation to delineate the precise urogenital anatomy. CEUS (i.e., contrast-enhanced genitosonography) has been shown to be useful in evaluation of children with urogenital anomalies [36,37]. For example, CEUS

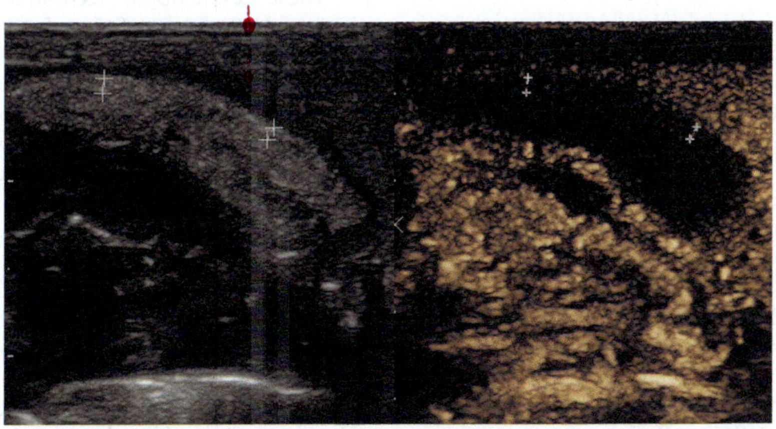

FIG. 4 6-week-old premature girl (gestational age 26 weeks) with necrotizing enterocolitis. Dual display longitudinal contrast-enhanced US (left display, grayscale reference image; right display, contrast-enhanced image). Grayscale image shows a pathologic bowel segment with a thick hyperechoic wall (cursors indicate the bowel wall) filled with hyperechoic content. Contrast-enhanced image shows non-opacification of the bowel wall. At surgery, this bowel segment was found to be necrotic.

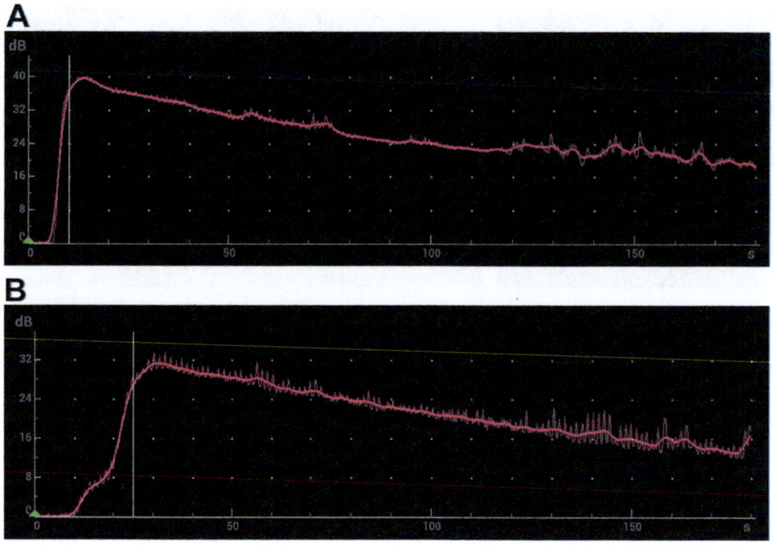

FIG. 5 Time-intensity curve (TIC) analysis of contrast-enhanced US of the kidney. (**A**, **B**) The TIC in a child with acute kidney injury (**B**) demonstrates lower "peak intensity" and prolonged "time-to-peak" in comparison to the TIC in a child with normal kidney function (**A**).

(e.g. US contrast-enhanced distal colostosonography) can be used in neonates with anorectal malformation without perineal fistula to demonstrate a frequently occurring fistula between the distal colon and the urinary/genital tract. [38,39]. These CEUS examinations can be performed after intracavitary instillation of US contrast, either through the perineal orifices for genitosonography or the distal stoma for colostosonography.

MICROVASCULAR FLOW IMAGING

Historically, color and power Doppler US imaging have been the primary sonographic tools for evaluating blood flow, using Doppler shifts to construct images with directional information for color Doppler and magnitude-based data for power Doppler [3]. CEUS allows a more detailed evaluation of small vasculature, beyond the ability of color and power Doppler imaging, utilizing intravenous US contrast. In recent years, several new sonographic techniques have been developed to assess smaller blood vessels with slow-flow dynamics without the need for intravenous contrast agents. These methods selectively filter out random motion while maintaining the ability to detect directional movement of blood flow, offering greater sensitivity and higher resolution compared to color and power Doppler imaging (Fig. 6). Similar to power Doppler, these US techniques generate a flow map overlaid on a grayscale image; however, they lack directional flow information. Because these techniques still rely on Doppler shifts, they are subject to limitations, such as angle and depth dependency, and motion sensitivity. Quantification of tissue vascularity is possible with MV-flow imaging through the use of the Vascular Index (VI) calculation (Fig. 7). VI denotes the ratio between the pixels within the designated area of the image with flow signal present and all the pixels in the designated area.

These new Doppler techniques are integrated into high-end US systems of several manufacturers. Although the proprietary algorithms behind these methods vary on the manufacturer, all incorporate strategies to minimize noise and enhance sensitivity to slow flow signals. These advancements include motion suppression, artifact reduction techniques, and adaptive filtering approaches like singular value decomposition to eliminate clutter. Display modes resemble color or power Doppler imaging, presenting flow information as an overlay on grayscale images with different color hues. These techniques are branded under different names, depending on the manufacturer: Superb Microvascular Imaging from Canon Medical Systems, Slow Flow from Siemens Healthineers, Microvascular Imaging (MVI) from GE Healthcare, MicroFlow Imaging from Philips, MV-flow from Samsung Medison, and Ultra-Microangiography from Mindray.

The ability of MV-flow imaging to depict small vessels without intravenous contrast makes it a tool of

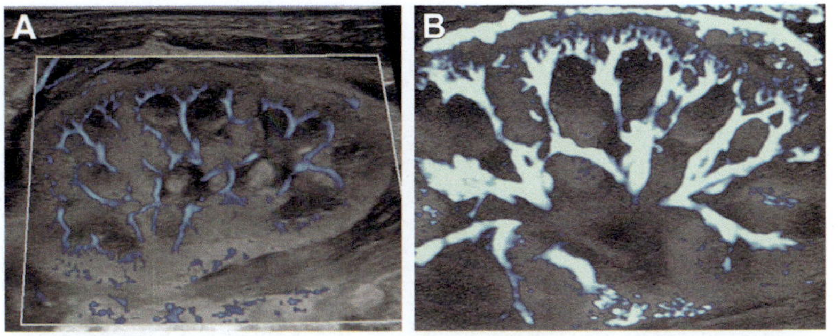

FIG. 6 Newborn premature girl (gestational age 32 weeks). Microvascular flow imaging of the kidney performed with a 15 MHz (**A**) and 20 MHz (**B**) linear array demonstrates detailed kidney vasculature.

great interest in pediatric imaging. It has been applied in various pediatric settings, proving useful in mapping the microvascular anatomy of the neonatal brain (see Figs. 2 and 8) [40] and other organs [41], assessing vascular flow in undescended testes [42], assessing ovarian vasculature in the setting of non-ovarian pathology [43], detecting increased vascularity in thyroiditis [44], assessing vascular changes in various hepato-gastrointestinal disorders [45], evaluating the kidney perfusion in the setting of AKI in critically-ill children [35], identifying areas of reduced blood flow in acute pyelonephritis [41], and follow-up of traumatic solid organ injuries for detection of arterial pseudoaneurysms [3].

In addition, MV-flow imaging has shown potential in the evaluation of the distal ureters for the presence of VUR, allowing for non-invasive detection of high-grade VUR (with reported sensitivity up to 75%), which could reduce the need for catheter-based procedures [46].

In adults, the use of MV-flow imaging for evaluating focal liver lesions has already been documented and may be similarly applied in children. The characteristic "spoke wheel" vascular pattern of focal nodular hyperplasia, including its feeding vessel and central vascular nidus, can be demonstrated. In addition, MVI can help differentiate between benign hepatic lesions, such as hemangiomas, which typically show peripheral globular vascularity, and malignant liver tumors, such as hepatoblastomas, which are characterized by a disorganized vascular pattern due to abnormal blood vessel growth [47]. However, pediatric studies confirming these findings in children should be performed.

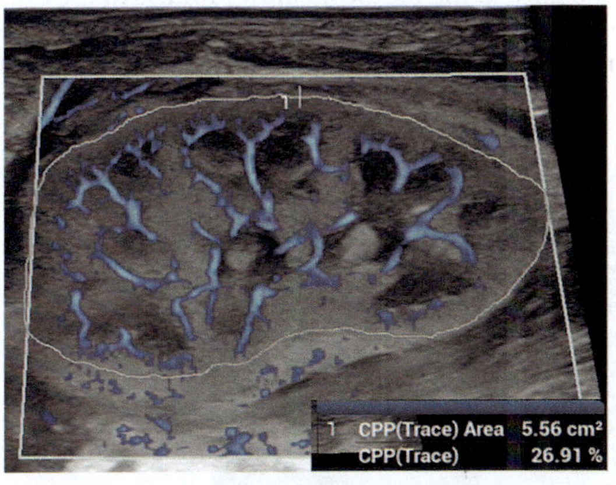

FIG. 7 The measurement of the vascular index for microvascular flow imaging. Vascular index denotes the ratio between the pixels with flow signal present (blue) and all the pixels in the designated area (white outline of the kidney).

ULTRASOUND ELASTOGRAPHY

Many disease processes, such as tumor, inflammation, and fibrosis, result in changes in tissue stiffness. Consequently, quantitative assessment of parenchymal tissue stiffness is a clinically useful diagnostic parameter. US elastography is a technique with expanding clinical applications that uses US waves to assess the elasticity of tissues. Elasticity is the tendency of the tissue to resist deformation with an applied force, or to resume its original shape after removal of the force. Deformation can be perpendicular to surface, tangential to surface, or result in volume loss. These deformations can be measured by various US elastography techniques. Different US elastography techniques measure different physical quantities (i.e. strain imaging and shear wave imaging) and cannot be interchangeably compared [4]. For example, US strain elastography quantifies the amount of lesion deformation by applying stress through repeated manual compression of the transducer.

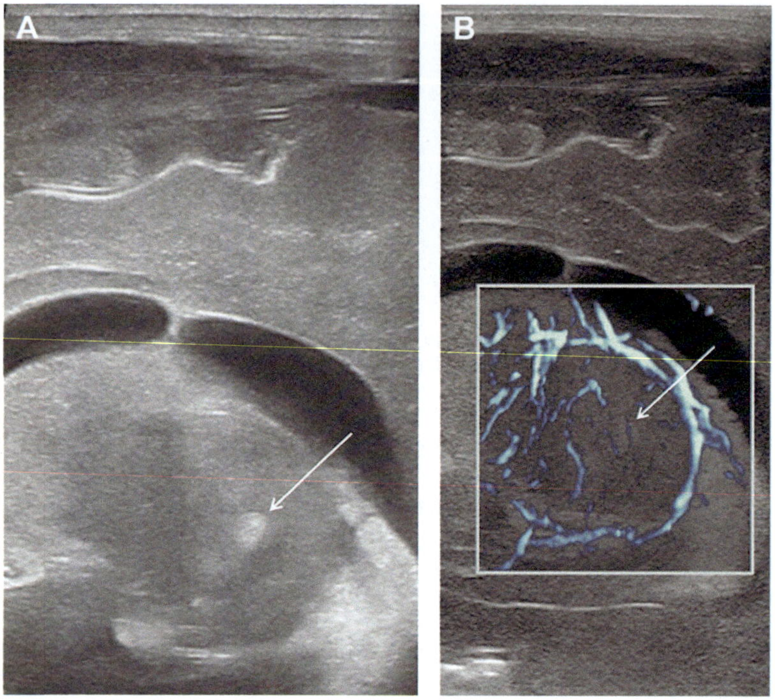

FIG. 8 6-week-old premature girl (gestational age 26 weeks) with a hyperechoic lesion within the right thalamus following surgery for necrotizing enterocolitis. (**A**) Grayscale US image shows a hyperechoic lesion within the right thalamus (*arrow*). (**B**) Microvascular flow imaging shows small vessels within the hyperechoic lesion, in keeping with an ischemic lesion.

Quantitative evaluation is not feasible with this technique [20]. In shear-wave elastography, an acoustic radiation force is sent from the transducer into the tissue toward the region of interest to quantify tissue stiffness. Shear-wave elastography has been reported to be highly reproducible with low-interobserver variability [20]. Nonetheless, shear-wave elastography is subject to artifacts caused by reflection and refraction due to the variations in shear wave velocity. Standardization and strict adherence to the protocols show promise in the evaluation of liver in adult patients, but it is still in the preliminary stages of clinical use for pediatric indications. The

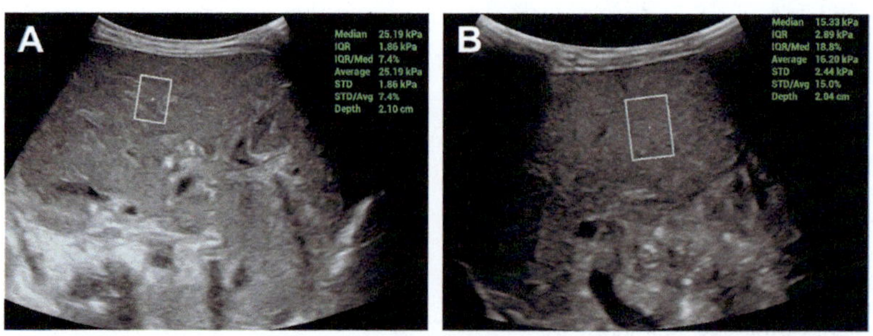

FIG. 9 Shear-wave elastography measurements of liver stiffness in a 2-month-old girl with biliary atresia prior to surgery (**A**) and 3 weeks following the Kasai procedure (**B**). The elastography measurements demonstrate a decrease in liver stiffness, as evidenced by the decreased median elastography measurements in kPA, following the procedure.

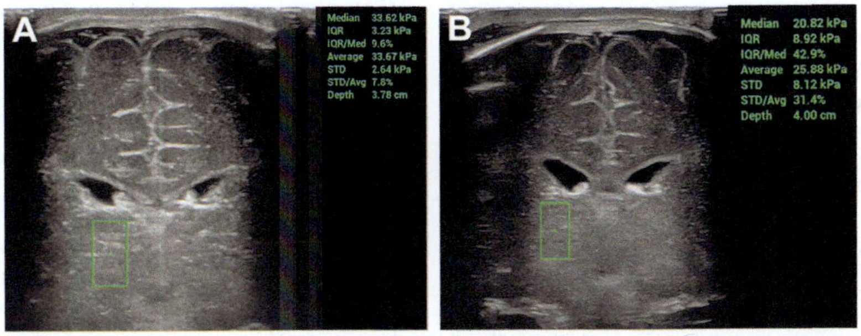

FIG. 10 Shear-wave elastography measurements of brain stiffness in a newborn girl with hypoxic-ischemic encephalopathy on day 1 (**A**) and following completion of therapeutic hypothermia on day 5 (**B**). The elastography measurements demonstrate a decrease in brain stiffness following the treatment, denoting a decrease of intracranial pressure due to resolution of brain edema.

inadequate standardization of the method and therefore its high variability of measurement and lack of normative standard values are a great limitation.

The most commonly researched application of US elastography in children is in the evaluation of the liver. A meta-analysis of 27 studies demonstrated that US elastography is able to diagnose cirrhosis, distinguish healthy from fibrotic liver tissue, and show consistent liver stiffness values in children without liver disease across studies [48]. US elastography also shows potential in the follow-up of patients with chronic liver disease (e.g. cystic fibrosis-associated liver disease, metabolic liver diseases, Gaucher's disease, Wilson's disease, α1-antitrypsin deficiency, glycogen storage disease, biliary disease, steatohepatitis, corrective surgery of congenital heart diseases, short bowel syndrome, etc.) to be used as a non-invasive alternative to repeated liver biopsies for monitoring disease progression (Fig. 9) [49].

Spleen stiffness measured by US elastography was found to be useful in children with portal hypertension for detecting venous complications [50–52]. The degree of spleen stiffness was also valuable in monitoring the severity of portal hypertension in patients with biliary atresia after the Kasai procedure [53] and after liver transplantation [50].

Several applications of US elastography of the brain in neonates have been studied. One study evaluating neonatal brain elasticity at different gestational ages found that term neonates brain parenchyma demonstrated higher stiffness in comparison to preterm neonates [54]. Future larger studies would be useful to determine normative values of elasticity for the developing brain. Another study reported that neonates with brain edema following perinatal hypoxia exhibited increased stiffness of the brain (Fig. 10) [20]. Similarly, a study that compared neonates with hydrocephalus to healthy children discovered increased stiffness of the brain in children with hydrocephalus [55]. These studies show potential for US elastography to be useful in non-invasive monitoring of these patients and monitoring their response to treatment.

SUMMARY

In recent years, contrast-enhanced US, MV-flow imaging, and US elastography have emerged as valuable imaging techniques with practical applicability in the diagnosis and management of various neonatal disorders. These techniques are safe and easy to perform at the bedside and may obviate the need for contrast-enhanced CT, MRI, or biopsy. Further research and clinical experience with these techniques will strengthen our knowledge and diagnostic confidence with their current applications and inform additional future applications.

CLINICS CARE POINTS

- Novel sonographic techniques like CEUS, MV-flow imaging, and elastography, provide a safe and effective imaging tool in neonates, reducing the need for more invasive or higher-risk procedures like MRI, CT, or biopsies.
- US is portable and can be used at the bedside, which is especially useful in neonatal intensive care units, allowing immediate evaluation without moving critically-ill infants.
- CEUS is useful in characterization of focal liver lesions, diagnosing ischemic strokes and intracranial hemorrhages, assessing bowel wall viability in

necrotizing enterocolitis, and evaluating perfusion of brain and kidneys in the setting of acute injury.

- MV-flow imaging provides enhanced visualization of small vasculature and slow blood flow without intravenous contrast and can be helpful in assessing conditions like AKI, brain lesions, liver tumors, and VUR.
- US elastography is useful in initial evaluation and follow-up of neonates with liver diseases, such as fibrosis, cirrhosis, and portal hypertension, and in neonatal brain imaging, particularly in conditions like hypoxia and hydrocephalus.

DISCLOSURES

The authors have no relevant commercial or financial conflicts of interest to disclose. The article received no funding.

REFERENCES

[1] Rajamani A, Arun Bharadwaj P, Hariharan S, et al. A historical timeline of the development and evolution of medical diagnostic ultrasonography. J Clin Ultrasound 2024;52(9):1419–37.
[2] Wilson SR, Greenbaum LD, Goldberg BB. Contrast-enhanced ultrasound: what is the evidence and what are the obstacles? Am J Roentgenol 2009;193(1):55–60.
[3] Aziz MU, Eisenbrey JR, Deganello A, et al. Microvascular flow imaging: a state-of-the-art review of clinical use and promise. Radiology 2022;305(2):250–64.
[4] Sigrist RMS, Liau J, Kaffas AE, et al. Ultrasound elastography: review of techniques and clinical applications. Theranostics 2017;7(5):1303–29.
[5] Plut D, Slak P, Williams-Weekes T, et al. Contrast-enhanced ultrasound in children: current and new applications. Adv Clin Radiol 2023;5(1):75–89.
[6] Ntoulia A, Anupindi SA, Back SJ, et al. Contrast-enhanced ultrasound: a comprehensive review of safety in children. Pediatr Radiol 2021;51(12):2161–80.
[7] Piscaglia F, Nolsøe C, Dietrich CF, et al. The EFSUMB guidelines and recommendations on the clinical practice of contrast enhanced ultrasound (CEUS): update 2011 on non-hepatic applications. Ultraschall Med 2012;33(1):33–59.
[8] Tranquart F, Mercier L, Frinking P, et al. Perfusion quantification in contrast-enhanced ultrasound (CEUS)–ready for research projects and routine clinical use. Ultraschall Med 2012;33(Suppl 1):S31–8.
[9] Munoz D, Hidalgo MJ, Balut F, et al. Risk factors for perinatal arterial ischemic stroke: a case-control study. Cell Med 2018;10:2155179018785341. https://doi.org/10.1177/2155179018785341.
[10] Govaert P, Ramenghi L, Taal R, et al. Diagnosis of perinatal stroke I: definitions, differential diagnosis and registration. Acta Paediatr 2009;98(10):1556–67.
[11] Plut D, Prutki M, Slak P. The use of contrast-enhanced ultrasound (CEUS) in the evaluation of the neonatal brain. Children (Basel) 2023;10(8). https://doi.org/10.3390/children10081303.
[12] Squires JH, Beluk NH, Lee VK, et al. Feasibility and safety of contrast-enhanced ultrasound of the neonatal brain: a prospective study using MRI as the reference standard. AJR Am J Roentgenol 2022;218(1):152–61.
[13] Yeo KT, Thomas R, Chow SS, et al. Improving incidence trends of severe intraventricular haemorrhages in preterm infants <32 weeks gestation: a cohort study. Arch Dis Child Fetal Neonatal Ed 2020;105(2):145–50.
[14] Prada F, Perin A, Martegani A, et al. Intraoperative contrast-enhanced ultrasound for brain tumor surgery. Neurosurgery 2014;74(5):542–52 [discussion: 552].
[15] Spazzapan P, Milosevic Z, Velnar T. Vein of Galen aneurismal malformations - clinical characteristics, treatment and presentation: three cases report. World J Clin Cases 2019;7(7):855–62.
[16] Hwang M, Barnewolt CE, Jüngert J, et al. Contrast-enhanced ultrasound of the pediatric brain. Pediatr Radiol 2021;51(12):2270–83.
[17] Shankaran S, Pappas A, McDonald SA, et al. Childhood outcomes after hypothermia for neonatal encephalopathy. N Engl J Med 2012;366(22):2085–92.
[18] Hwang M, Sridharan A, Darge K, et al. Novel quantitative contrast-enhanced ultrasound detection of hypoxic ischemic injury in neonates and infants: pilot study 1. J Ultrasound Med 2019;38(8):2025–38.
[19] Sridharan A, Riggs B, Darge K, et al. The wash-out of contrast-enhanced ultrasound for evaluation of hypoxic ischemic injury in neonates and infants: preliminary findings. Ultrasound Q 2021;38(1):36–42.
[20] Hwang M, Riggs BJ, Katz J, et al. Advanced pediatric neurosonography techniques: contrast-enhanced ultrasonography, elastography, and beyond. J Neuroimaging 2018;28(2):150–7.
[21] Nakagawa TA, Ashwal S, Mathur M, et al, Society of Critical Care Medicine, Section on Critical Care and Section on Neurology of American Academy of Pediatrics, Child Neurology Society. Clinical report—guidelines for the determination of brain death in infants and children: an update of the 1987 task force recommendations. Pediatrics 2011;128(3):e720–40.
[22] Hwang M, Riggs BJ, Saade-Lemus S, et al. Bedside contrast-enhanced ultrasound diagnosing cessation of cerebral circulation in a neonate: a novel bedside diagnostic tool. NeuroRadiol J 2018;31(6):578–80.
[23] Slak P, Pušnik L, Plut D. Contrast-enhanced ultrasound (CEUS) as an ancillary imaging test for confirmation of brain death in an infant: a case report.

Children (Basel) 2022;9(10). https://doi.org/10.3390/children9101525.

[24] Chung EM, Cube R, Lewis RB, et al. Pediatric liver masses: radiologic-pathologic correlation part 1. Benign tumors. Radiographics 2010;30(3):801–26.

[25] Chattopadhyay S, Mukherjee S, Boler A, et al. Hepatoblastoma in the neonatal period: an unusual presentation. J Cytol 2012;29(4):252–4.

[26] Fernandez-Pineda I, Sandoval JA, Davidoff AM. Hepatic metastatic disease in pediatric and adolescent solid tumors. World J Hepatol 2015;7(14):1807–17.

[27] Burrowes DP, Medellin A, Harris AC, et al. Contrast-enhanced US approach to the diagnosis of focal liver masses. Radiographics 2017;37(5):1388–400.

[28] Jacob J, Deganello A, Sellars ME, et al. Contrast enhanced ultrasound (CEUS) characterization of grey-scale sonographic indeterminate focal liver lesions in pediatric practice. Ultraschall Med 2013;34(6):529–40.

[29] Durot I, Wilson SR, Willmann JK. Contrast-enhanced ultrasound of malignant liver lesions. Abdom Radiol (NY) 2018;43(4):819–47.

[30] Holman RC, Stoll BJ, Curns AT, et al. Necrotising enterocolitis hospitalisations among neonates in the United States. Paediatr Perinat Epidemiol 2006;20(6):498–506.

[31] Benjamin JL, Dennis R, White S Jr, et al. Improved diagnostic sensitivity of bowel disease of prematurity on contrast-enhanced ultrasound. J Ultrasound Med 2020;39(5):1031–6.

[32] Meena J, Mathew G, Kumar J, et al. Incidence of acute kidney injury in hospitalized children: a meta-analysis. Pediatrics 2023;151(2). https://doi.org/10.1542/peds.2022-058823.

[33] Hanna M, Brophy PD, Giannone PJ, et al. Early urinary biomarkers of acute kidney injury in preterm infants. Pediatr Res 2016;80(2):218–23.

[34] Wang XY, Pang YP, Jiang T, et al. Value of early diagnosis of sepsis complicated with acute kidney injury by renal contrast-enhanced ultrasound. World J Clin Cases 2019;7(23):3934–44.

[35] Ogorevc N, Slak P, Nikšić S, et al. Contrast-enhanced ultrasound (CEUS) and ultra-microangiography (UMA) in critically ill children with acute kidney injury. Children 2024;11(10):1205.

[36] Seranio N, Darge K, Canning DA, et al. Contrast enhanced genitosonography (CEGS) of urogenital sinus: a case of improved conspicuity with image inversion. Radiol Case Rep 2018;13(3):652–4.

[37] Chow JS, Paltiel HJ, Padua HM, et al. Case series: comparison of contrast-enhanced genitosonography (ceGS) to fluoroscopy and cone-beam computed tomography in patients with urogenital sinus and the cloacal malformation. Clin Imag 2020;60(2):204–8.

[38] Chow JS, Paltiel HJ, Padua HM, et al. Contrast-enhanced colosonography for the evaluation of children with an imperforate anus. J Ultrasound Med 2019;38(10):2777–83.

[39] Tirrell TF, Demehri FR, McNamara ER, et al. Contrast enhanced colostography: new applications in preoperative evaluation of anorectal malformations. J Pediatr Surg 2021;56(1):192–5.

[40] Goeral K, Hojreh A, Kasprian G, et al. Microvessel ultrasound of neonatal brain parenchyma: feasibility, reproducibility, and normal imaging features by superb microvascular imaging (SMI). Eur Radiol 2019;29(4):2127–36.

[41] Yoo J, Je BK, Choo JY. Ultrasonographic demonstration of the tissue microvasculature in children: microvascular ultrasonography versus conventional color Doppler ultrasonography. Korean J Radiol 2020;21(2):146–58.

[42] Lee YS, Kim MJ, Han SW, et al. Superb microvascular imaging for the detection of parenchymal perfusion in normal and undescended testes in young children. Eur J Radiol 2016;85(3):649–56.

[43] Ayaz E, Aslan A, İnan İ, et al. Evaluation of ovarian vascularity in children by using the "superb microvascular imaging" ultrasound technique in comparison with conventional Doppler ultrasound techniques. J Ultrasound Med 2019;38(10):2751–60.

[44] Bayramoglu Z, Kandemirli SG, Caliskan E, et al. Assessment of paediatric Hashimoto's thyroiditis using superb microvascular imaging. Clin Radiol 2018;73(12):1059.e9-e15.

[45] Ohno Y, Fujimoto T, Shibata Y. A new era in diagnostic ultrasound, superb microvascular imaging: preliminary results in pediatric hepato-gastrointestinal disorders. Eur J Pediatr Surg 2017;27(1):20–5.

[46] Kim HK, O'Hara S, Je BK, et al. Feasibility of superb microvascular imaging to detect high-grade vesicoureteral reflux in children with urinary tract infection. Eur Radiol 2018;28(1):66–73.

[47] He MN, Lv K, Jiang YX, et al. Application of superb microvascular imaging in focal liver lesions. World J Gastroenterol 2017;23(43):7765–75.

[48] Andersen SB, Ewertsen C, Carlsen JF, et al. Ultrasound elastography is useful for evaluation of liver fibrosis in children-a systematic review. J Pediatr Gastroenterol Nutr 2016;63(4):389–99.

[49] Sönmez S, Boşat M, Yurtseven N, et al. The role of elastography in the assessment of chronic liver disease in children. Afr Health Sci 2019;19(3):2806–11.

[50] Goldschmidt I, Brauch C, Poynard T, et al. Spleen stiffness measurement by transient elastography to diagnose portal hypertension in children. J Pediatr Gastroenterol Nutr 2014;59(2):197–203.

[51] Sutton H, Fitzpatrick E, Davenport M, et al. Transient elastography measurements of spleen stiffness as a predictor of clinically significant varices in children. J Pediatr Gastroenterol Nutr 2018;67(4):446–51.

[52] Tomita H, Fuchimoto Y, Ohkuma K, et al. Spleen stiffness measurements by acoustic radiation force impulse imaging after living donor liver transplantation in children: a potential quantitative index for

venous complications. Pediatr Radiol 2015;45(5): 658–66.
[53] Uchida H, Sakamoto S, Kobayashi M, et al. The degree of spleen stiffness measured on acoustic radiation force impulse elastography predicts the severity of portal hypertension in patients with biliary atresia after portoenterostomy. J Pediatr Surg 2015;50(4): 559–64.
[54] Su Y, Ma J, Du L, et al. Application of acoustic radiation force impulse imaging (ARFI) in quantitative evaluation of neonatal brain development. Clin Exp Obstet Gynecol 2015;42(6):797–800.
[55] Dirrichs T, Meiser N, Panek A, et al. Transcranial shear wave elastography of neonatal and infant brains for quantitative evaluation of increased intracranial pressure. Investig Radiol 2019;54(11):719–27.

Advances in Clinical Radiology 7 (2025) 187–198
ADVANCES IN CLINICAL RADIOLOGY

An Overview of the Different Intrinsic Muscular Abnormalities of the Head and Neck

Irene Dixe de Oliveira Santo, MD, CIIP[a], Bindu N. Setty, MD[b,*]
[a]Department of Radiology, Yale University, New Haven, CT, USA; [b]Department of Radiology, Boston University, Boston, MA, USA

KEYWORDS
• Head and neck muscles • Muscle neoplasms • Muscle inflammation • Muscle infection

KEY POINTS
- Disease processes affecting the intrinsic muscles of the head and neck region can result in great functional impairment and psychological distress.
- Abnormalities in the muscle may be a manifestation of an occult systemic disease and its recognition is important for timely therapy.
- Plethora of muscle related entities exist with few unique to the head and neck such as fibromatosis colli and longus colli tendinitis.

INTRODUCTION

Muscles of the head and neck can be divided into muscles of the eye, ear, mastication, facial expression, and suprahyoid and infrahyoid regions with extraocular muscles being a distinctive subset. Disorders of head and neck musculature can be varied in etiologies and include congenital, reactive or use-related, traumatic, inflammatory, infectious, neoplastic, or systemic processes. These can lead to physical and psychological consequences due to their prime locational and functional value. Most entities of the head and neck musculature such as infection, neoplasms, use-related, and posttraumatic changes are similar to that seen elsewhere in the body. Fibromatosis colli and calcific tendinitis of the longus colli muscle are unique entities to the neck musculature. Lastly, disorders like orbital myositis and tuberculous myositis in the neck may unmask the presence of a systemic disease process.

CONGENITAL

Fibromatosis colli

Fibromatosis colli is an uncommon cause of neck mass in infants, usually noted around 2 weeks after birth. Associated neck movement restriction and a history of birth trauma may be present [1]. Ultrasound may be requested to confirm the suspected diagnosis or to rule out soft tissue mass or lymphadenopathy. It is key to identify the fusiform enlargement of the sternocleidomastoid muscle in its long axis and discontinuity of the expected parallel fibers displaced by a fibroma of

*Corresponding author. Department of Radiology, Boston Medical Center, 840 Harrison Avenue 1st Floor, Boston, MA 02118. *E-mail address:* Bindu.setty@bmc.org

https://doi.org/10.1016/j.yacr.2025.06.004
www.advancesinclinicalradiology.com
2589-8701/25/

ABBREVIATIONS	
CN	cranial nerve
CT	computed tomography
EOM	extraocular muscle
ICA	internal carotid artery
IgG4	immunoglobulin G4
IOIS	idiopathic orbital inflammatory syndrome
SCM	sternocleidomastoid
TB	tuberculosis

variable echogenicity [2–4]. Occasionally small calcifications may be seen [2] (Fig. 1). While this condition is generally self-limited managed with passive stretching and physiotherapy [5], it may lead to congenital muscular torticollis and positional plagiocephaly [6].

REACTIVE (USE-RELATED)

Masticatory muscle hypertrophy

Masticatory muscle hypertrophy is an uncommon condition, with a slight male predominance, usually bilateral and may affect the masseter and/or temporalis muscles. Common presentations include facial squaring, trismus, and bruxism [7,8]. Factors such as temporomandibular disorder, malocclusion, and emotional stress may be associated [9]. Ultrasound may confirm uniform increased muscle mass with preserved muscle echotexture. Increased muscle bulk with preserved density or signal intensity may be seen on computed tomography (CT) [10] (Fig. 2) and magnetic

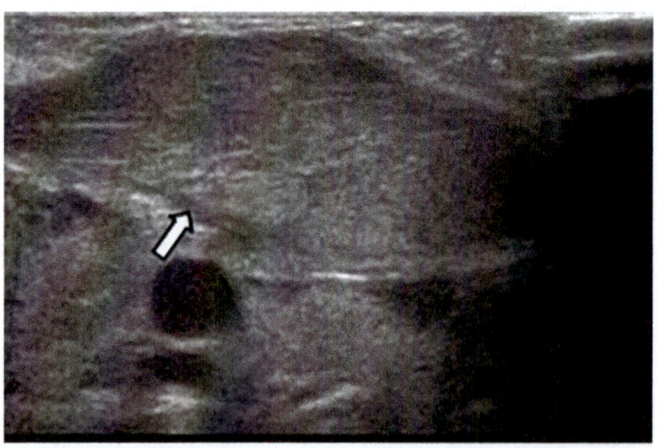

FIG. 1 Fibromatosis coli. Ultrasound of the right neck of a 4 week old female patient presenting with torticollis shows a fusiform mass like right sternocleidomastoid muscle (*arrow*) with increased echogenicity. Normal adjacent soft tissues.

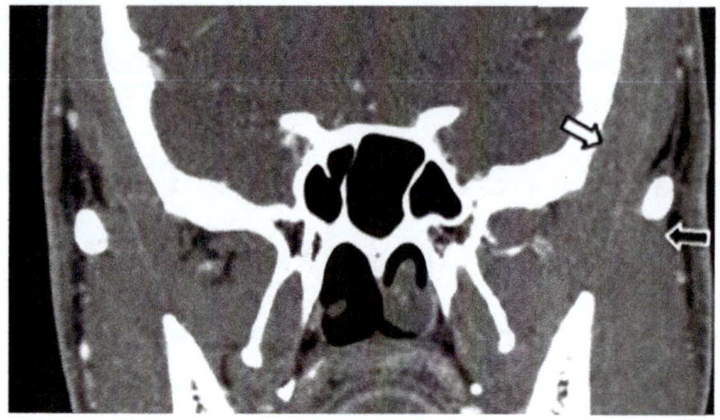

FIG. 2 Masseter hypertrophy. Coronal CT of the face in a 30 year old male patient with slowly progressive soft tissue swelling over the left temple shows asymmetric thickening of the left masseter (*black arrow*) and temporalis (*white arrow*) muscles compared to those on the right.

resonance imaging (MRI), respectively. These modalities are also useful to rule out other pathologies [11]. Management includes physical therapy, mouth guards, medications, botulinum toxin A injection, or surgery [12].

Denervation atrophy

Deafferentation of skeletal muscle leads to denervation atrophy. Precise knowledge of the cranial nerve anatomy and muscle innervation is essential (Table 1) for identifying the etiology (Fig. 3). Denervation is typically classified in 3 sequential phases: acute, subacute, and chronic. The length of each phase is variable, differing between individuals, affected nerves, or type of injury [13]. Clinical manifestations vary depending on the affected muscle/s (Figs. 4 and 5). In the acute phase (<1 month), following the initial insult, there is shift of fluid in the affected muscle, to the extracellular compartments. These changes may cause increased muscle volume and hyperintensity on T2-weighted/STIR images secondary to edema with increased intramuscular blood flow. Confinement of edema to the muscle and lack of surrounding inflammatory changes or fascial edema should help differentiate this from other entities such as inflammation or infection [13]. Edema may be less conspicuous on CT images. During the subacute phase (range 12–20 months), the increased blood volume and extracellular fluid decrease and the muscular size normalizes. T2/STIR hyperintensity and mild contrast enhancement may be present , and increased T1 signal intensity from fatty replacement may be more evident. The chronic phase (>1 year) is characterized by muscle atrophy with fatty infiltration, which is reflected by muscle hypodensity on CT, and hyperintensity on T1-weighted images reflecting increased fat content [14]

TABLE 1
Innervation of the various muscles of head and neck region[a]

Cranial Nerves	Muscles	Function	Foramen	Examples
Oculomotor (III)	Superior rectus, medial rectus, inferior rectus, inferior oblique, and levator palpebrae	Eye movement	Superior orbital fissure	Fig. 3
Trochlear (IV)	Superior oblique	Eye movement	Superior orbital fissure	Fig. 3
Trigeminal (V)	Masticator muscles (masseter, temporalis, lateral pterygoid, and medial pterygoid) and tensor tympani	Mastication and dampens sound	Superior orbital, fissure, foramen rotundum, and foramen ovale	Fig. 3
Abducens (VI)	Lateral rectus	Eye movement	Superior orbital fissure	Fig. 3
Facial (VII)	Muscles of facial expression and stapedius	Facial expression and dampens sound	Internal auditory meatus	—
Glossopharyngeal (IX)	Stylopharyngeus	Elevates pharynx and speech + swallow	Jugular foramen	—
Vagus (X)	Cricothyroid, levator veli palatini, palatoglossus, palatopharyngeus, pharyngeal constrictors, and larynx	Speech and swallowing	Jugular foramen	Fig. 4
Accessory (XI)	Sternocleidomastoid and trapezius	Move head and neck	Jugular foramen	Fig. 5
Hypoglossal (XII)	Tongue	Tongue movement	Hypoglossal canal	Fig. 6

[a] To the exception of cranial nerves I, II, and VIII, all other cranial nerves have motor functions, supplying muscles in the head and neck. Insults to these nerves can be recognized by denervation.

(Fig. 6). Compensatory hypertrophy of other muscle groups may be seen.

TRAUMATIC

The main types of traumatic muscle injury include strain, lacerations, contusions, hematomas, compartment syndrome, and myositis ossificans. These can generally be classified according to mechanism of injury (ie, direct or indirect) and presentation (ie, acute, subacute/delayed, and chronic).

Rhabdomyolysis

Rhabdomyolysis results from muscle fiber breakdown and leakage of contents into circulation and can be either due to traumatic or nontraumatic causes. Local symptoms include tenderness, swelling and weakness, and systemic manifestations are tea-colored urine or anuria, fever, malaise, and confusion. Products of the skeletal muscle breakdown released into the serum result in laboratory abnormalities, being serum creatinine kinase, the gold standard for laboratory diagnosis (>1000 UI/L) [15]. Muscles of the legs and back are the most common sites affected but can also occur in the head and neck [16–19]. Two types of CT and MR imaging findings have been described. Type 1 presents as enlargement of the involved muscles, which appear hypodense on CT due to edema (Fig. 7) and isointense to hyperintense on T1-WI (from blood

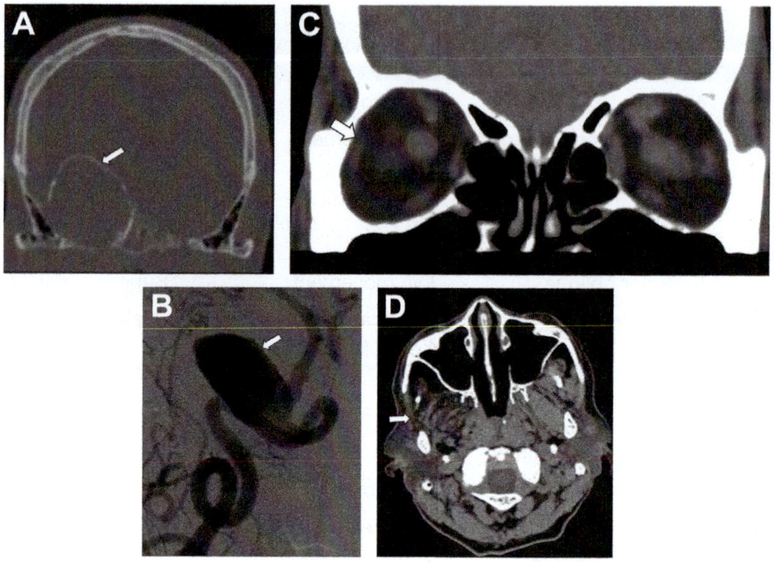

FIG. 3 (*A*) Denervation atrophy. Coronal non enhanced CT (NECT) (bone window) of the brain in a 60 year old female patient demonstrates a large lesion with peripheral rim of calcification in the right paracavernous/sellar region (*arrow*) suspicious for a giant right cavernous internal carotid artery (ICA) aneurysm. (*B*) Denervation atrophy. Digital subtraction angiogram in a 60 year old female patient confirms the giant aneurysm arising from the cavernous portion of the ICA (*arrow*). (*C*) Denervation atrophy. Coronal CT of the orbits in a 60 year old female patient shows atrophic extraocular muscles on the right as compared to the left (*arrow*), and decreased muscle density representing fatty replacement, consistent with involvement of cranial nerve (CN) III, IV, and VI, all of which travel through the cavernous sinus. (*D*) Denervation atrophy. Axial CT of the infratemporal fossa in a 60 year old female patient shows atrophic muscles of mastication with fatty replacement on the right (*arrow*) compared to the left, consistent with CN V involvement.

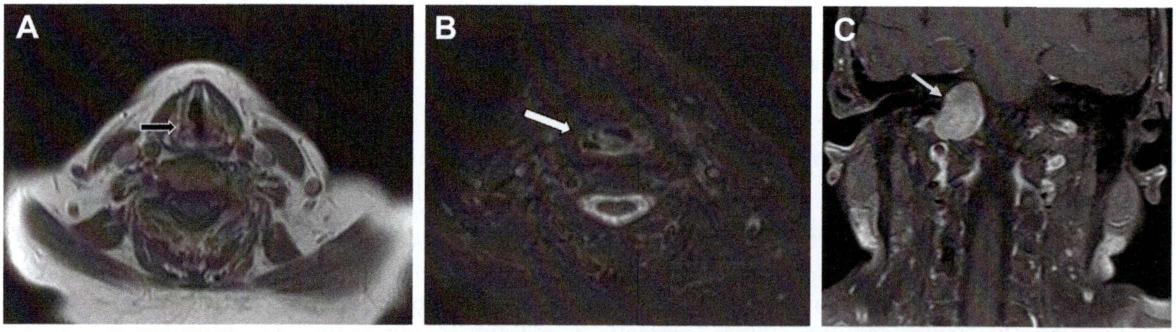

FIG. 4 (*A*) Denervation atrophy: Axial T1 MRI in a 70 year old female patient shows ipsilateral vocal cord palsy with medial rotation of the right arytenoid cartilage demonstrated by medialization of the vocal cord (*arrow*) presenting with recurrent hoarseness resulting from compression of the right X cranial nerve due to a jugular schwannoma. (*B*) Denervation atrophy: Axial STIR MRI in a 70 year old female patient showing ipsilateral vocal cord palsy demonstrated by dilatation of the right pyriform sinus (*arrow*) presenting with recurrent hoarseness resulting from compression of the right X cranial nerve due to a jugular schwannoma. (*C*) Denervation atrophy: Coronal postcontrast MRI in a 70 year old female patient demonstrates an enhancing lesion in the right jugular foramen, where the vagus nerve exits the skull (*arrow*) presenting with recurrent hoarseness resulting from compression of the right X cranial nerve due to a jugular schwannoma.

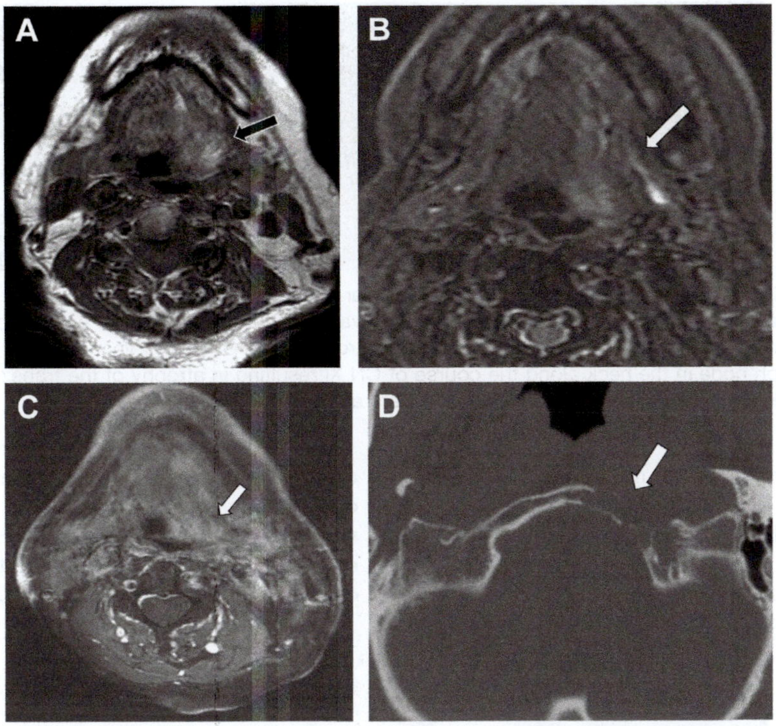

FIG. 5 (*A*) Denervation atrophy. Axial T1 precontrast MRI in a 70 year old female patient shows fatty replacement of the left tongue, which is visibly atrophic as compared to the right and prolapses posteriorly to efface the vallecula (*arrow*) secondary to subacute denervation of the left side of the tongue secondary to a metastasis to the left occipital condyle affecting the hypoglossal (XII) cranial nerve. (*B*) Denervation atrophy. Axial STIR MRI in a 70 year old female patient shows signal abnormality in the left tongue consistent with edema, which should not be confused with a mass (*arrow*) secondary to subacute denervation of the left side of the tongue secondary to a metastasis to the left occipital condyle affecting the hypoglossal (XII) cranial nerve. (*C*) Denervation atrophy. Axial T1 postcontrast MRI in a 70 year old female patient shows enhancement in the left tongue secondary to denervation, which should not be confused with a mass (*arrow*) secondary to subacute denervation of the left side of the tongue secondary to a metastasis to the left occipital condyle affecting the hypoglossal (XII) cranial nerve. (*D*) Denervation atrophy. Axial cervical spine CT in a 70 year old female patient shows a lytic lesion in the left occipital condyle with involvement of the hypoglossal canal resulting in CN XII palsy (*arrow*).

products and debris) and diffusely hyperintense on T2-WI with homogenous enhancement. In type 2 (which is more common) [15], muscles are heterogeneously hypodense on CT, variably hyperintense on T1-weighted images and heterogeneously hyperintense on T2-weighted images with rim-enhancement after contrast. The "stipple sign," which is a dot-like or linear streaky enhancement, may be seen and thought to be residual viable muscle fibers or inflamed vessels within necrotic infarcted muscle [15,16,20]. Ultrasound may demonstrate loss of normal striated echotexture of the affected muscles [15]. Treatment is supportive.

Extraocular muscle entrapment and herniation

Blowout fractures of the orbital floor in adults are usually of "open door" type, characterized by bone displacement and herniation of the orbital contents into the adjacent sinus [21]. In children, after herniation, the bone recoils back into its original position leading to extraocular muscle (EOM) entrapment with the presence of a nondisplaced, or minimally displaced fracture line, a phenomenon known as "trapdoor" fracture [22]. Adults may present with periorbital edema, pain, and limited EOM mobility

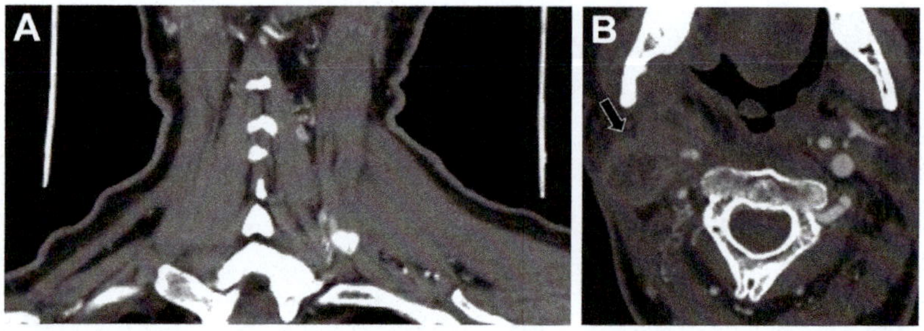

FIG. 6 (*A*) Denervation atrophy. Coronal CT in a 71 year old male patient shows atrophy of the right trapezius muscle (*arrow*), consistent with chronic denervation of the right trapezius with history of multiple head and neck cancers and surgeries. (*B*) Denervation atrophy. Axial CT in a 71 year old male patient shows necrotic lymph node in the neck along the course of CN XI resulting in atrophy of the trapezius muscle (*arrow*) with history of multiple head and neck cancers and surgeries.

[22], and in children, diplopia may be present without periorbital swelling or evidence of trauma ("white-eyed blowout fracture") [22]. Careful ophthalmologic examination is essential for diagnosis (Fig. 8). While there may be imaging findings raising concern for entrapment, such a frank herniation of the EOMs through the osseous defect, this is a clinical diagnosis and cannot be diagnosed with imaging alone [23]. Trapdoor fractures are considered a surgical emergency, which require surgical repair. Less commonly, blow out fractures of the medial orbital wall can lead to entrapment of the medial rectus [24].

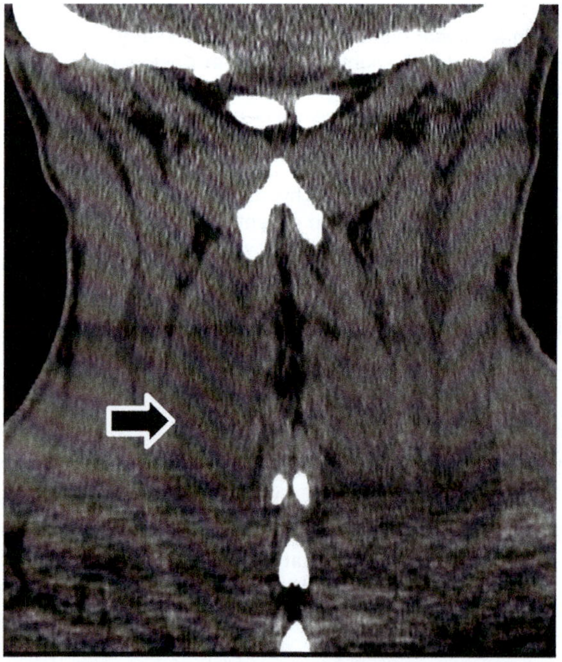

FIG. 7 Rhabdomyolysis. Coronal neck CT 29 year old male patient shows hypodensity and enlargement of the paraspinal muscles (*arrow*), worse on the right found after 10 to 14 hours of prolonged immobility secondary to narcotic use.

INFLAMMATION

Calcific tendinitis of the longus colli muscle

Calcific tendinitis of the longus colli muscle is an uncommon, inflammatory response to calcium hydroxyapatite crystal deposition in the tendons of the longus colli muscle. Patients may present with neck pain or stiffness, odynophagia, and low-grade fever [25]. Imaging findings may help differentiate this condition from other processes such retropharyngeal abscess, which is crucial to prevent unnecessary medical or surgical interventions [25,26]. Contrast-enhanced CT is the

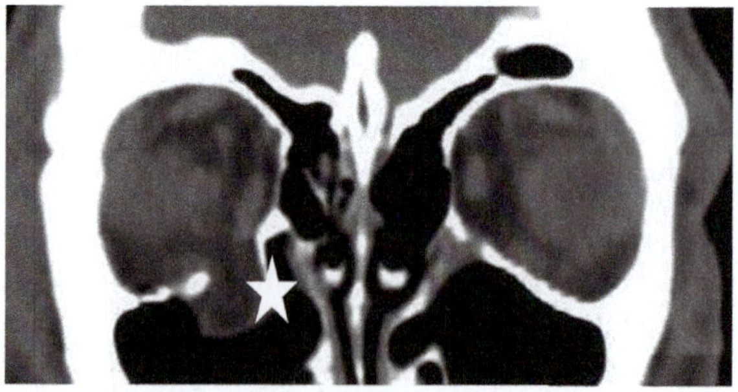

FIG. 8 EOM herniation due to "open door" fracture. Coronal CT of the orbits in a 22 year old male patient shows a blowout orbital floor fracture with herniation of the right inferior rectus and orbital fat into the maxillary sinus who presents with diplopia and restricted gaze after being punched in the right eye. The orbital floor fracture fragment projects inferiorly (*asterisk*).

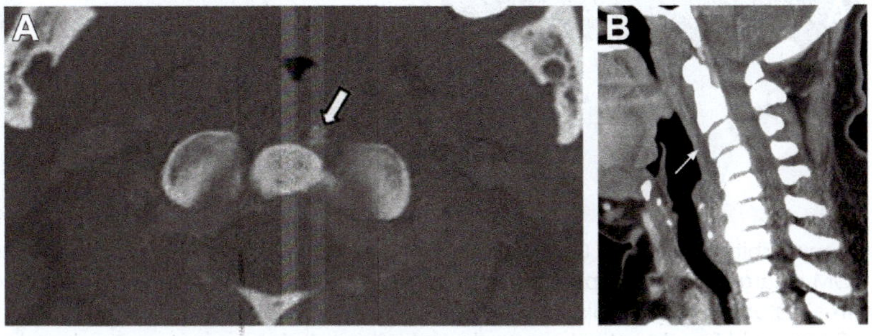

FIG. 9 (*A*) Calcific tendinitis of the longus colli muscle. Axial CT scan (bone window) in a 55 year old male patient at the level of the dens shows an amorphous calcific density (*arrow*) at the area of the superior longus colli muscle. (*B*) Calcific tendinitis of the longus colli muscle. Sagittal CT neck with contrast in a 55 year old male patient shows a tapering effusion (*arrow*) from the level of C1 to C5. There is no surrounding enhancement or bony destruction to suggest abscess.

modality of choice [27], and it reveals amorphous calcifications in the superior fibers of the longus colli muscle tendons at the C1 to C2 level [26] (Fig. 9) and may demonstrate hypoattenuation of the muscles due to edema. MR is excellent in detecting edema in the muscle and prevertebral soft tissues and effusions, but not as sensitive as CT in the evaluation of calcification [27]. MR may also reveal marrow edema in the adjacent vertebrae [27]. The condition is self-limited and responds to nonsteroidal anti-inflammatory drugs.

Orbital myopathies

Extraocular muscles are unique in their cytoarchitecture with higher blood flow compared with skeletal muscle, which facilitates easier circulation of the inflammatory cells and likely lead to distinctive subset of diseases that affect these muscles [28].

Thyroid-associated myopathy

Thyroid-associated ophthalmopathy is the most frequent extrathyroidal manifestation of Graves' disease and is the most common orbitopathy. Lid retraction, proptosis, ophthalmoplegia, conjunctivitis, chemosis, and, rarely, dysthyroid optic neuropathy may be present [29]. Although most patients present with concurrent systemic hyperthyroid clinical manifestations, in 10% to 20% of cases, ophthalmopathy may precede thyrotoxicosis, and in 10% to 15%, it may present with current or previous hypothyroidism [29]. The disease has a self-limited active phase that usually lasts 18 to 24 months and abates slowly, followed by an inactive (static) phase [30]. Although diagnosis usually relies on the clinical features, imaging may play a role in assessing the extent and severity of the disease and to follow up changes after treatment [30]. EOM enlargement occurs in a classic spindle-shaped morphology with sparing of the tendinous insertions (Fig. 10) may be observed on CT or MR images. The inferior, medial, superior, and lateral rectus muscles (listed in order of decreasing frequency of involvement) may be affected. It is usually bilateral but can be unilateral [31]. Additional imaging findings include increased orbital fat, lacrimal gland enlargement, eyelid edema, exophthalmos, stretching of the optic nerve, and tenting of the posterior globe. Management includes control of thyroid disease, corticosteroids, and other medication (such as monoclonal antibodies) or orbital decompression [32].

Idiopathic orbital inflammatory syndrome-orbital myositis

Idiopathic orbital inflammatory syndrome (IOIS) is a benign inflammatory condition characterized by orbital inflammation of unknown etiology and may be classified into subgroups according to the location [33,34]. EOM involvement of the inflammatory process is known as orbital myositis. Symptoms include unilateral painful proptosis and diplopia [34]. Imaging reveals EOM thickening, with involvement of the muscle myotendinous junction, resulting in tubular morphology (Fig. 11). The most frequently affected muscle is the medial rectus, followed by the superior rectus and lateral rectus and is most often unilateral [34,35]. Affected muscles reveal marked enhancement [35]. In addition to asymmetric enlargement of muscles, there may be ill-defined infiltrates throughout the orbital fat [35]. Sparing of the myotendinous junction may be a clue to thyroid-associated orbitopathy, although this finding alone does not exclude IOIS [36]. Contrast-enhanced T1 MR images with fat suppression best visualize the inflammation of the muscles, tendons, and surrounding fat [36]. Diagnosis is based on the medical history, clinical course, laboratory findings, and response to steroids [31]. Steroids

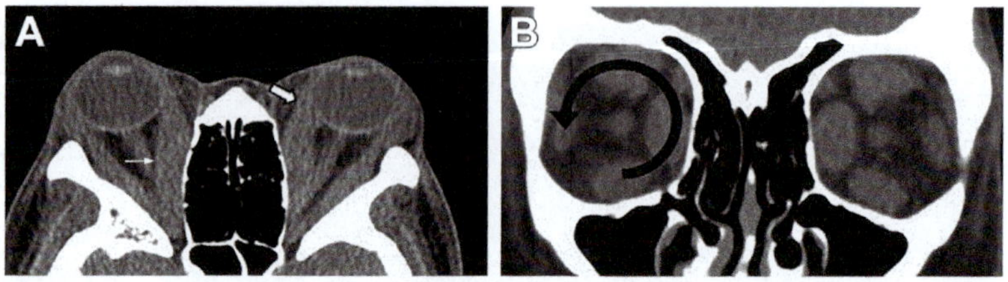

FIG. 10 (*A*) Thyroid orbitopathy. Axial CT through the orbits in a 33 year old female patient shows proptosis and bilateral EOM enlargement with sparing of the myotendinous junctions (*arrow*), giving the "Coca-Cola bottle" sign with a history of Grave's disease presents with exophthalmos. (*B*) Thyroid orbitopathy. Coronal CT shows in a 33 year old female patient shows the enlargement of the inferior, medial, and superior rectus muscles bilaterally (*arrow* depicting the right side in the image). The Mnemonic "I'M SLOw" reflects the involvement of the extraocular muscle in decreasing order of frequency: inferior, medial, superior, and lateral rectus followed by the oblique muscles.

classically results in rapid improvement [31]. Additional treatment may include immunosuppressant drugs, radiation therapy, or surgery [33].

Orbital cellulitis, lymphoproliferative disease, immunoglobulin G4 (IgG4)-related disease, metastases, and sarcoidosis should be ruled out before labeling a patient with IOIS [36–38]. Distinguishing features of lymphoma may be the absence of pain and increased intensity on diffusion-weighted images [31]. Sarcoid-related orbital myopathy mainly affects the superior rectus/levator complex and lateral rectus, possibly due to associated dacryoadenitis, and up to 80% of patients may have systemic manifestations [39] and is typically painless [37]. Affected muscles are isodense on CT and hyperintense on T2-WI and enlarged with diffuse homogenous enhancement (Fig. 12). IgG4-related myopathy is another differential to consider where there is predominantly lateral rectus involvement with tendinous sparing [40]. The muscles may have relatively low signal intensity on T2-WI due to increased cellularity and amount of fibrosis [38].

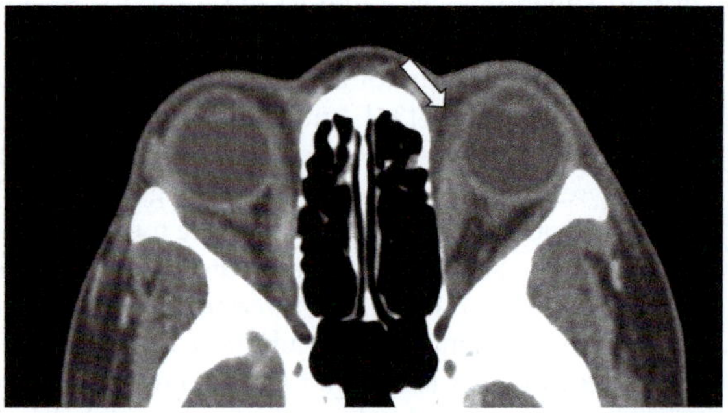

FIG. 11 Idiopathic orbital inflammatory syndrome. Axial CT with contrast through the orbits in a 48 year old female patient shows diffuse enlargement of the right lateral rectus muscle as well as the bilateral medial recti with the involvement of the myotendinous junctions, a ragged, fluffy border of the involved muscles, and inward bowing of the muscle belly posterior to the globe (*arrow*) presenting with eye pain and diplopia.

INFECTION

Infectious myositis can be either viral, bacterial, fungal, or parasitic in etiology.

Pyomyositis and pyogenic abscess

Pyomyositis is a rare purulent infection of skeletal muscle, most commonly due to hematogenous spread [41]. It usually affects the extremities, lower back, but may seldom be seen in the neck [42,43]. *Staphylococcus aureus* is responsible for 75% to 95% of cases, and

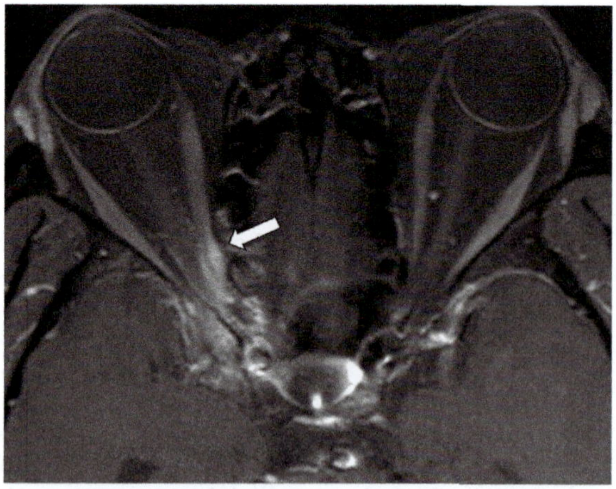

FIG. 12 Sarcoidosis. Axial T1 fat-saturated image with contrast in a 51 year old gentleman demonstrates an enhancement along the right orbital apex with secondary involvement of the right medial rectus (*arrow*) who presented with right eye vision changes. This was a biopsy proven case of orbital sarcoid with pathology showing chronic granulomatous inflammation with giant cell reaction.

risk factors include immunodeficiency, trauma, and intravenous drug use. [41]. Ultrasound demonstrates an enlarged muscle due to edema, and, if present, an abscess may be seen. CT demonstrates enlarged hypodense muscle, stranding of the surrounding fat and, as the infection evolves, an abscess may be seen as an area of fluid density with peripheral enhancement (Fig. 13). MR imaging reveals diffuse muscle enlargement and T2/STIR hyperintensity. The signal intensity of an abscess may vary and depend on its age and content, but usually may appear as T2/STIR hyperintense fluid collections, with rim-enhancement after contrast administration [41,44]. Management is with antibiotic therapy and drainage if an abscess is present.

Tuberculous myositis and abscess

Extrapulmonary manifestations are estimated to occur in approximately 20% of the patients with tuberculosis (TB). Tuberculous myositis is a rare form of extrapulmonary TB, as striated muscle is one of the most resistant tissues to mycobacterial infection [45]. It can affect virtually any muscle, including the head and neck region [43]. MR imaging is the modality of choice and is similar to pyomyositis. Abscess formation manifests as a peripherally enhancing T2 hyperintense fluid collection. The walls of the abscess may demonstrate subtle T1 hyperintensity possibly related to oxygen free radical and iron within macrophages [45] (Fig. 14). Management is with a prolonged, multiagent antimycobacterial regimen [45].

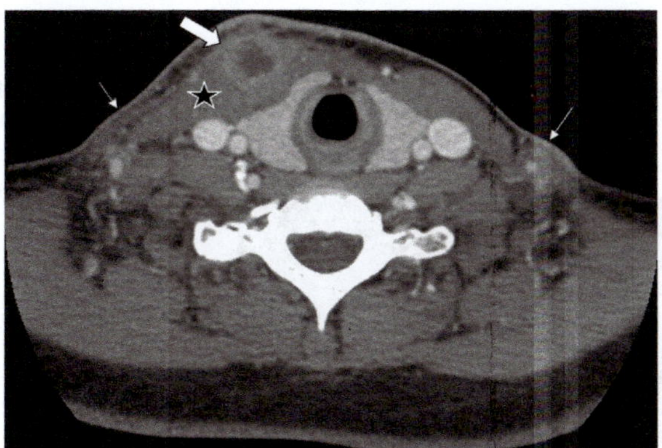

FIG. 13 Pyogenic abscess. Axial postcontrast images of the neck of a 40 year old male intravenous drug user show a small abscess within the right sternocleidomastoid (SCM; *thick white arrow*). Also seen is associated thickening of the muscle (black *asterisk*) with surrounding inflammatory changes within the subcutaneous fat. Additionally, skin thickening and subcutaneous fat stranding bilaterally at the base of the neck over both external jugular veins (*thin white arrows*) consistent with the clinical history of bilateral neck injections who presents with redness and swelling of the right neck.

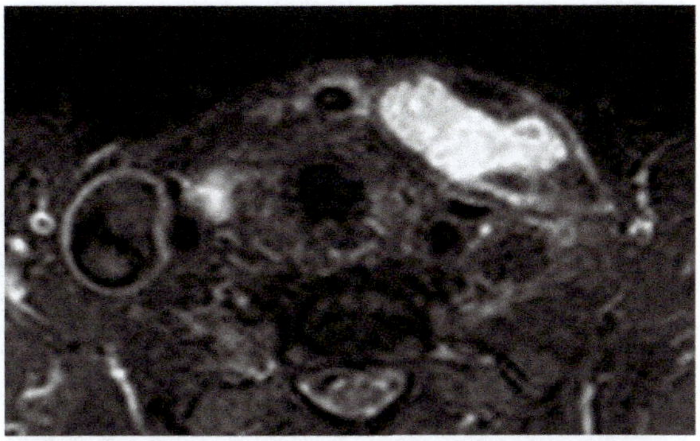

FIG. 14 Tuberculous abscess. Axial T2W MR image of the neck in a 30 year old male patient shows a fluid collection with central hyperintensity located within the inferior left sternocleidomastoid muscle (*arrow*) that resolved after prolonged, multiagent, antimycobacterial regimen.

NEOPLASTIC

Muscle-related neoplasms of the head and neck may be due to a primary muscle tumor or systemic disease.

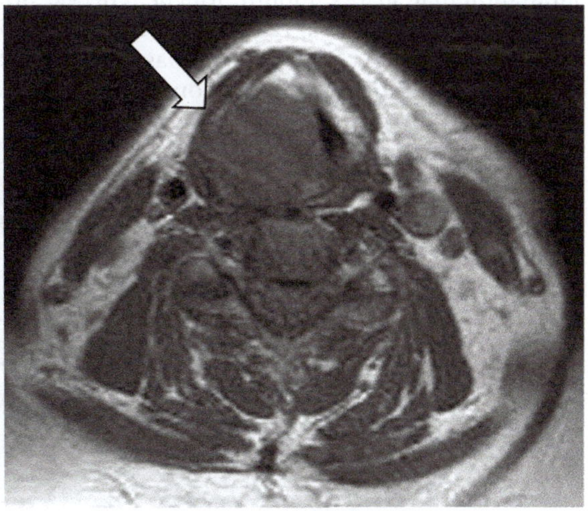

FIG. 15 Rhabdomyoma. Axial T1W MR image of the neck in a 58 year old male patient shows a large laryngeal mass (*arrow*) that is isointense to the surrounding muscle, with smooth medial contours that suggest submucosal origin who presents with hoarseness. Pathology was consistent with a rhabdomyoma.

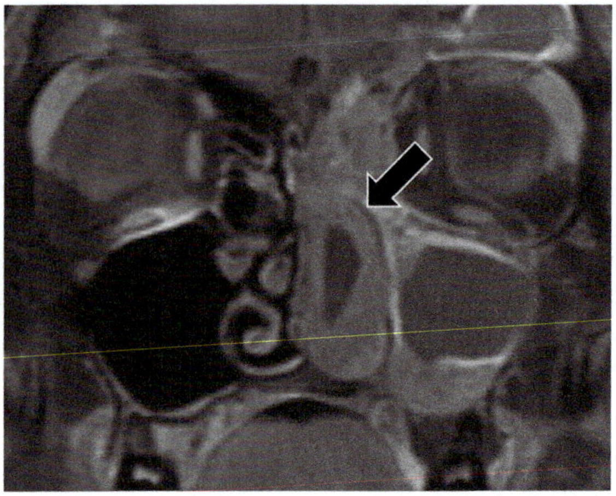

FIG. 16 Rhabdomyosarcoma: Coronal CE T1-weighted image with fat saturation in a 37 year old patient shows a left nasal cavity mass (*arrow*) with central sparing suggestive of necrosis and resultant obstruction to the drainage of the left maxillary sinus.

Rhabdomyoma

Rhabdomyoma is a benign tumor of striated muscle. While cardiac rhabdomyomas may occur in infants, extracardiac rhabdomyomas often affect male individuals aged over 40 years, with a predilection for the head and neck [46,47], including the larynx, pharynx, sternocleidomastoid, parapharyngeal and submandibular spaces, mouth, tongue, cheeks, lips, and eyelids [47]. Clinical findings depend on localization and size. Rhabdomyomas are well-circumscribed, homogenous lesions isointense to the muscle on T1-weighted and T2-weighted MR images (Fig. 15), and isodense on CT to the adjacent musculature, with homogenous enhancement after contrast administration [46,48]. Definitive diagnosis through fine needle aspiration (FNA) cytology is important to prevent unnecessarily aggressive management. Surgical excision is recommended for symptomatic or cosmetically disturbing lesions [46].

Rhabdomyosarcoma

Rhabdomyosarcoma is a malignant tumor of striated muscle and the most common soft tissue sarcoma in children but may also affect adults [48]. Approximately 40% involve the head and neck and can be classified according to location into parameningeal (50%), non-parameningeal (25%), and orbital (25%) [49]. Parameningeal tumors, which include the paranasal sinuses, nasopharynx, middle ear, mastoid, and infratemporal fossa, portend a worst prognosis. Rhabdomyosarcomas are large soft tissue masses often accompanied by lytic bone destruction [48]. Signal intensities are variable, from low to intermediate on T1 and heterogeneously low to high signal on T2-weighted images (Fig. 16) usually with restricted diffusion [50]. Enhancement after contrast administration is also variable on both CT and MR images [48]. Management may include surgery, chemotherapy, radiation, or hormonal therapy.

Leiomyosarcoma

Leiomyosarcoma is a rare, malignant neoplasm arising from smooth muscle or from undifferentiated mesenchymal cells that may affect middle-aged to older

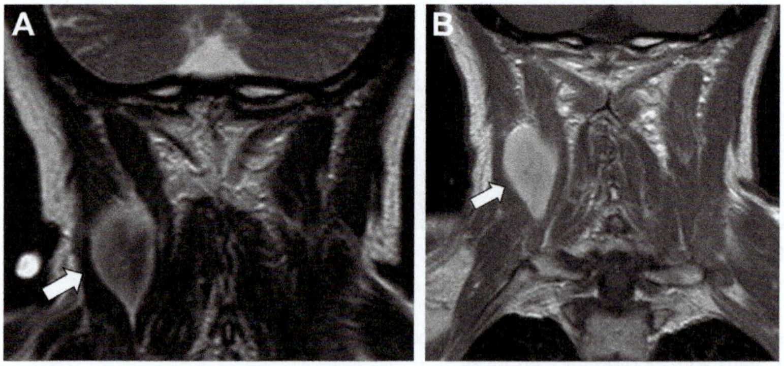

FIG. 17 (*A*) Leiomyosarcoma. Coronal T2 MRI of the neck in a 69 year old female patient shows a T2 hyperintense lesion in the right posterior paraspinal muscles (*arrow*) with a history of metastatic leiomyosarcoma of unknown primary site who presents with right posterior neck mass. (*B*) Leiomyosarcoma. Coronal CE- MRI in a 69 year old female patient of the neck shows an avidly enhancing lesion in the right posterior paraspinal muscles (*arrow*) with a history of metastatic leiomyosarcoma of unknown primary site who presents with right posterior neck mass.

adults [48]. Between 3% and 10% of leiomyosarcomas occur in the head and neck [48], primarily in the nasal cavity and paranasal sinuses. Possible contributing factors include prior radiation, human immunodeficiency virus infection and acquired immunodeficiency syndrome, and chemotherapy [48,49]. Leiomyosarcoma presents as a rapidly enlarging mass, with varied symptoms depending on location [49] and a low incidence of nodal metastasis [51]. Recurrence is estimated in 34% [52]. On CT, they appear as bulky masses with little enhancement and remodeling of the adjacent osseous structures. On MR imaging, they are isointense to hypointense to muscle on T1 with variable signal on T2-weighted images and prominent enhancement (Fig. 17) [48] demonstrating lower diffusion coefficients in comparison with benign tumors [50]. Diffusion-weighted images may be also useful on delineating the margins of the tumor [50]. Malignant tumors may show early arterial enhancement and higher peak contrast enhancement on dynamic contrast-enhanced MR imaging in comparison with benign tumors [50]. Treatment is surgical.

SUMMARY

This pictorial essay illustrates the important clues for the recognition of intrinsic muscle disorders in the head and neck. Correlation of clinical presentation and imaging findings is the mantra of the radiologist to achieve a correct diagnosis.

CLINICS CARE POINTS

- Disease processes affecting the intrinsic muscles of the head and neck region can result in great functional impairment and psychological distress and accurate diagnosis, management and counseling is important.
- Abnormalities in the muscle may be a manifestation of an occult systemic disease and its recognition is important for timely therapy.

DISCLOSURE

The authors have nothing to disclose.

REFERENCES

[1] Kulkarni AR, Tinmaswala MA, Shetkar SV. Fibromatosis colli in neonates: an ultrasound study of four cases. J Clin Neonatol 2016;5(4):271–3.

[2] Chauvin NA, Khwaja A. Musculoskeletal imaging in neonates: use of ultrasound. Pediatr Radiol 2022;52(4): 765–76, Epub 2021 Sep 7. PMID: 34490498.

[3] Caprio MG, Di Serafino M, Pontillo G, et al. Paediatric neck ultrasonography: a pictorial essay. J Ultrasound 2019;22(2):215–26 [published correction appears in J Ultrasound. 2018 Oct 31].

[4] Ludwig BJ, Foster BR, Saito N, et al. Diagnostic imaging in nontraumatic pediatric head and neck emergencies. Radiographics 2010;30(3):781–99.

[5] Oliveira JC, Abreu MS, Gomes FM. Sternocleidomastoid tumour in neonate: fibromatosis colli. BMJ Case Rep 2018;2018:bcr2017223543.

[6] Rousslang LK, Rooks EA, Smith AC, et al. Fibromatosis colli leading to positional plagiocephaly with gross anatomical and sonographic correlation. BMJ Case Rep 2021;14(1):e239236. https://doi.org/10.1136/bcr-2020-239236:PMID: 33431471; PMCID: PMC7802680.

[7] Graziano P, Dell'Aversana Orabona G, Astarita F, et al. Bilateral hypertrophy of masseteric and temporalis muscles, our fifteen patients and review of literature. Eur Rev Med Pharmacol Sci 2016;20(1):7–11.

[8] Kebede B, Megersa S. Idiopathic masseter muscle hypertrophy. Ethiop J Health Sci 2011;21(3):209–12.

[9] Braun IF, Torres WE, Landman JA, et al. Computed tomography of benign masseteric hypertrophy. J Comput Assist Tomogr 1985;9(1):167–70.

[10] Shetty N, Malaviya RK, Gupta MK. Management of unilateral masseter hypertrophy and hypertrophic scar - a case report. Case Rep Dent 2012;2012:521427.

[11] Sonar PR, Panchbhai AS. Case Report: masseter hypertrophy: a case and review. F1000Res 2024;12:1263, PMID: 39036345; PMCID: PMC11258545.0.1136/bcr.07.2011.4557. PMID: 22679271; PMCID: PMC3185404.

[12] Ranasinghe JC, Wickramasinghe C, Rodrigo G. Isolated unilateral temporalis muscle hypertrophy in a child: a case report with literature review. BMC Pediatr 2018; 18(1):71, PMID: 29458353; PMCID: PMC5817789.

[13] Saks R, Shatzkes D, Gillespie J. Pictorial review of cranial nerve denervation in the head and neck. Radiographics 2024;44(10):e240023. https://doi.org/10.1148/rg.240023: PMID: 39298352.

[14] Borges A. Imaging of denervation in the head and neck. Eur J Radiol 2010;74(2):378–90.

[15] Rixey AB, Glazebrook KN, Powell GM, et al. Rhabdomyolysis: a review of imaging features across modalities. Skelet Radiol 2024;53(1):19–27, Epub 2023 Jun 15. PMID: 37318587.

[16] Mian AZ, Saito N, Sakai O. Rhabdomyolysis of the head and neck: computed tomography and magnetic resonance imaging findings. Dentomaxillofac Radiol 2011;40(6):390–2.

[17] Jain V, Ellingson AN, Smoker WR. Lateral pterygoid muscle rhabdomyolysis. AJNR Am J Neuroradiol 2007; 28(10):1876–7.

[18] Shah HV, Irvine GH, Bradley M. Rhabdomyolysis of the masseter muscle: case report. Br J Oral Maxillofac Surg 2008;46(2):138–40.

[19] Lin SP, Sung CS, Chan KH. Compartment syndrome and rhabdomyolysis as a positioning complication following retrosigmoid craniotomy. Acta Anaesthesiol Taiwan 2013;51(4):184–6.
[20] Lu CH, Tsang YM, Yu CW, et al. Rhabdomyolysis: magnetic resonance imaging and computed tomography findings. J Comput Assist Tomogr 2007;31(3):368–74.
[21] Merali FI, Grant MP, Mahoney NR. Orbital floor fracture with atypical extraocular muscle entrapment pattern and intraoperative asystole in an adult. Craniomaxillofac Trauma Reconstr 2015;8(4):370–4.
[22] Barh A, Swaminathan M, Mukherjee B. Orbital fractures in children: clinical features and management outcomes. J aapos 2018;22(6):415.e1–7.
[23] Thatcher J, Chang YM, Chapman MN, et al. Clinical-radiologic correlation of extraocular eye movement disorders: seeing beneath the surface. Radiographics 2016; 36(7):2123–39.
[24] Thiagarajah C, Kersten RC. Medial wall fracture: an update. Craniomaxillofac Trauma Reconstr 2009;2(3):135–9.
[25] Abdelbaki A, Abdelbaki S, Bhatt N, et al. Acute calcific tendinitis of the longus colli muscle: report of two cases and review of the literature. Cureus 2017;9(8):e1597.
[26] Kim YJ, Park JY, Choi KY, et al. Case reports about an overlooked cause of neck pain: calcific tendinitis of the longus colli: case reports. Medicine (Baltim) 2017; 96(46):e8343.
[27] Qureshi PAAA, Bollason G, Ágústsson KL. Acute calcific tendinitis of the longus colli muscles: an entity that should Be known by emergency radiologists. Cureus 2022;14(5):e25518.
[28] Yu Wai Man CY, Chinnery PF, Griffiths PG. Extraocular muscles have fundamentally distinct properties that make them selectively vulnerable to certain disorders. Neuromuscul Disord 2005;15(1):17–23.
[29] Perros P, Neoh C, Dickinson J. Thyroid eye disease. BMJ 2009;338:b560.
[30] Gonçalves ACP, Gebrim E, Monteiro MLR. Imaging studies for diagnosing Graves' orbitopathy and dysthyroid optic neuropathy. Clinics (Sao Paulo) 2012;67-(11):1327–34.
[31] LeBedis CA, Sakai O. Nontraumatic orbital conditions: diagnosis with CT and MR imaging in the emergent setting. Radiographics 2008;28(6):1741–53.
[32] Hoang TD, Stocker DJ, Chou EL, et al. 2022 update on clinical management of Graves disease and thyroid eye disease. Endocrinol Metab Clin North Am 2022;51(2): 287–304, Epub 2022 May 11. PMID: 35662442; PMCID: PMC9174594.
[33] Ferreira TA, Saraiva P, Genders SW, et al. CT and MR imaging of orbital inflammation. Neuroradiology 2018; 60(12):1253–66.
[34] Yeşiltaş YS, Gündüz AK. Idiopathic orbital inflammation: review of literature and new advances. Middle East Afr J Ophthalmol 2018;25(2):71–80.
[35] Ding ZX, Lip G, Chong V. Idiopathic orbital pseudotumour. Clin Radiol 2011;66:886–92.
[36] Pakdaman MN, Sepahdari AR, Elkhamary SM. Orbital inflammatory disease: pictorial review and differential diagnosis. World J Radiol 2014;6(4):106–15.
[37] Chapman MN, Fujita A, Sung EK, et al. Sarcoidosis in the head and neck: an Illustrative review of clinical presentations and imaging findings. Am J Roentgenol 2017; 208(1):66–75.
[38] Fujita A, Sakai O, Chapman MN, et al. IgG4-related disease of the head and neck: CT and MR imaging manifestations. Radiographics 2012;32(7):1945–58.
[39] Vahdani K, Rose GE. Sarcoid orbital myopathy: clinical presentation and outcomes. Ophthalmic Plast Reconstr Surg 2020;36(1):61–6.
[40] Tiegs-Heiden CA, Eckel LJ, Hunt CH, et al. Immunoglobulin G4-related disease of the orbit: imaging features in 27 patients. AJNR Am J Neuroradiol 2014;35(7):1393–7.
[41] Hayeri MR, Ziai P, Shehata ML, et al. Soft-tissue infections and their imaging mimics: from cellulitis to necrotizing fasciitis. Radiographics 2016;36(6):1888–910.
[42] Tucciarone M, Taliente S, Gómez-Blasi Camacho R, et al. Extensive pyomyositis of prevertebral muscles after acupuncture: case report. Turk J Emerg Med 2019;19(3):113–4.
[43] Gosnell EJ, Anwar B, Varadarajan V, et al. Sternocleidomastoid pyomyositis. Eur Ann Otorhinolaryngol Head Neck Dis 2016;133(4):273–5, Epub 2016 Feb 12. PMID: 26879580.
[44] Perez M, MEDINA E, Noriega M, Arango MC, Swelling and pain: pyomyositis of the neck. European Congress of Radiology-ECR, 2017.
[45] Vanhoenacker FM, Sanghvi DA, De Backer AI. Imaging features of extraaxial musculoskeletal tuberculosis. Indian J Radiol Imaging 2009;19(3):176–86.
[46] de Trey LA, Schmid S, Huber GF. Multifocal adult rhabdomyoma of the head and neck manifestation in 7 locations and review of the literature. Case Reports in Otolaryngology 2013;2013:758416.
[47] Brys AK, Sakai O, DeRosa J, et al. Rhabdomyoma of the larynx: case report and clinical and pathologic review. Ear Nose Throat J 2005;84(7):437–40.
[48] Razek AA, Huang BY. Soft tissue tumors of the head and neck: imaging-based review of the WHO classification. Radiographics 2011;31(7):1923–54.
[49] Scelsi CL, Wang A, Garvin CM, et al. Head and neck sarcomas: a review of clinical and imaging findings based on the 2013 world health organization classification. Am J Roentgenol 2018;212(3):644–54.
[50] Rodriguez JD, Selleck AM, Abdel Razek AAK, et al. Update on MR imaging of soft tissue tumors of head and neck. Magn Reson Imaging Clin N Am 2022;30(1): 151–98, PMID: 34802577.
[51] Yadav J, Bakshi J, Chouhan M, et al. Head and neck leiomyosarcoma. Indian J Otolaryngol Head Neck Surg 2013;65(Suppl 1):1–5.
[52] Jafarian M, Azizi S. Leiomyosarcoma of the maxilla: a case report and literature review. J Dent (Shiraz) 2022; 23(1 Suppl):244–50, PMID: 36380835; PMCID: PMC 9652062.

Advances in Clinical Radiology 7 (2025) 199–214
ADVANCES IN CLINICAL RADIOLOGY

Dual-energy Computed Tomography Applications of Pediatric Disorders

Practical Imaging Approach to Diagnosis

Maude S. Tabigue, MD[a,*], Nathan David P. Concepcion, MD[a,b], Bernard F. Laya, MD, MHM, DO[a,b,c], Edward Y. Lee, MD, MPH[d]

[a]Section of Pediatric Radiology, Institute of Radiology, St. Luke's Medical Center - Quezon City, 279 E. Rodriguez Sr. Avenue, Quezon City 1112, Philippines; [b]Section of Pediatric Radiology, Institute of Radiology, St. Luke's Medical Center - Global City, Rizal Dr. cor. 32nd Street and 5th Avenue, Taguig City 1634, Philippines; [c]St. Luke's Medical Center College of Medicine - William H. Quasha Memorial, Sta. Ignaciana Street, Cathedral Heights, Quezon City 1112, Philippines; [d]Department of Radiology, Boston Children's Hospital and Harvard Medical School, 300 Longwood Avenue, Boston, MA 02115, USA

KEYWORDS

• Dual-energy computed tomography • Multienergy computed tomography • Spectral computed tomography • Dual-source • Single-source • Virtual non-contrast • Virtual monoenergetic

KEY POINTS

- Reduction in the radiation dose and volume of iodinated-contrast material required are particularly helpful for the thoracoabdominal imaging in children.
- The 2 post-processing techniques that best exploit the advantages of dual-energy computed tomography (DECT) in children are material-decomposition images and virtual monoenergetic (or monochromatic) images.
- Virtual non-contrast images can be generated without added radiation dose eliminating the need to obtain an actual pre-contrast unenhanced image.
- Virtual monoenergetic images result to increased attenuation for structures containing iodine (at low-keV setting) and reduces beam hardening and metal artifact (at high-keV setting).
- High-iodine concentrations on DECT may indicate residual or viable tumors, but decreased intralesional iodine content may signify successful treatment.

INTRODUCTION

Dual-energy computed tomography (DECT), also called multienergy or spectral CT, utilizes 2 different radiograph energy spectra (e.g., 80 and 140 kVp) during simultaneous image acquisition. This technique takes advantage of the innate properties and attenuation differences of body tissues and materials (e.g., contrast material, metallic stents, and prostheses) [1–3].

Radiograph photons primarily interact with matter through the photoelectric effect and Compton scatter [4,5]. DECT applications rely on generating photoelectric and Compton scatter components from obtained data to create spectral and multiple virtual reconstructed images that highlight the pathology or anatomy in question, depending on the clinical need [5,6].

*Corresponding author. Section of Pediatric Radiology, Institute of Radiology, St. Luke's Medical Center - Quezon City, 279 E. Rodriguez Sr. Avenue, Quezon City 1112, Philippines. *E-mail address:* dramaude27@gmail.com

https://doi.org/10.1016/j.yacr.2025.06.005 www.advancesinclinicalradiology.com
2589-8701/25/

ABBREVIATIONS

BPS	bronchopulmonary sequestration
CHD	congenital heart disease
CLDP	chronic lung disease of prematurity
CPAM	congenital pulmonary airway malformation
CT	computed tomography
DECT	dual-energy computed tomography
DS	dual-source
SECT	single-energy computed tomography
SS	single-source
VMI	virtual monoenergetic image
VNC	virtual non-contrast

An increased attenuation is observed when the photons' incoming energy surpasses the binding energy of the K-shell electrons (K-edge). Knowledge of this property is crucial to understanding DECT applications. The differences in K-edges of the different elements, such as calcium and iodine, and soft tissues, with the former being higher in K-shell binding energies are also important. This distinctiveness allows for the effective differentiation of these elements from soft tissues. For instance, iodine, which is a component of contrast agents, attenuates at lower energies (i.e., 40 – 50 keV) because these energies are close to its K-edge (33.2 keV) [5].

There are different DECT technologies used in clinical settings and these vary in their approaches to data acquisition, post-processing, and display algorithms. These are dual-source (DS) using 2 x-ray tubes and the single-source (SS) or single-tube systems where the latter include rapid kilovoltage switching, dual-layer detector, and split-filter with twin-beam systems, [1,7] as well as a sequential dual-scan system [6,8].

The differences in specifications, advantages, and disadvantages of each of the aforementioned DECT acquisition systems are not within the scope of this article. This article provides practical information regarding the advantages of DECT over single-energy CT (SECT) and its commonly used and emerging clinical applications in pediatric chest and abdomen.

DUAL-ENERGY COMPUTED TOMOGRAPHY POST-PROCESSING TECHNIQUES

The 2 post-processing techniques that best utilize the advantages of DECT in children are material-decomposition images and virtual monoenergetic (or monochromatic) images [1].

Material Decomposition (or Material-specific) Images

Depending on the DECT acquisition system, 2-material or 3-material decomposition algorithms are used. SS systems apply a 2-material decomposition algorithm in the projection space before image reconstruction, while DS systems utilize a 3-material decomposition algorithm in the image space domain following the reconstruction of the images [1].

Virtual non-contrast (VNC) images can be generated eliminating the need to obtain an actual pre-contrast unenhanced image, which is particularly beneficial in pediatric imaging as a potential means of substantially reducing radiation exposure (Fig. 1) [7]. It has been reported that split-bolus DECT urography reduced radiation dose by 56.4% by omitting the pre-contrast scan [9]. VNC images can also help differentiate contrast enhancement from calcification within thoracic or abdominal masses in a single-phase contrast-enhanced examination [6]. However, calcifications may appear smaller on the VNC images when compared to the actual non-enhanced scan [8].

Material decomposition images that utilize various materials, such as iodine, contrast, calcification, or acute hemorrhage, are also valuable for accurately differentiating among materials [7]. Hyperdense lesions on contrast-enhanced DECT that remain attenuated on VNC likely indicate proteinaceous content or hematoma and do not represent true contrast enhancement [5,7,10].

Iodine content appears as either color-coded iodine maps that exclusively show iodine content or as iodine overlay images that superimpose iodine content on virtual-unenhanced images (Fig. 2) [11]. Quantitative analysis is possible by placing a reference region of interest in an area of concern on a contrast-enhanced iodine map or the overlay images [1].

Bone-subtraction algorithms can also aid in optimally evaluating vessels in angiographic studies [12,13], although this can also be done in SECT depending on the vendor software applications available.

Virtual Monoenergetic (or Monochromatic) Images

Dual-energy CT analyzes and differentiates tissues and materials in the body. Materials, such as iodine, calcium, uric acid, soft tissue, and water interact, uniquely with photons of varying energies, enabling differentiation [14,15].

Virtual monoenergetic images (VMIs) are gray-scale virtually reconstructed images at a chosen keV ranging

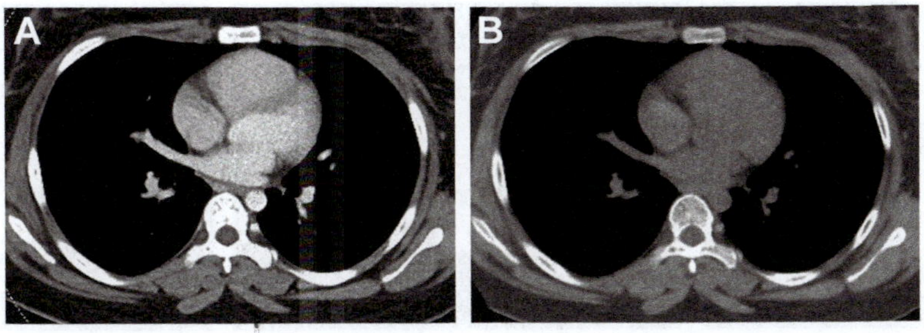

FIG. 1 Material-decomposition image in a healthy 15-y-old girl. Contrast-enhanced axial computed tomography image in soft tissue setting is shown at the level of the heart (*A*). After post-processing the same cut with removal of the iodine-containing materials, a virtual non-contrast image (*B*) is generated. The acquisition of an actual unenhanced image is no longer required.

from 40 to 200 keV (depending on the vendor) that depict the expected appearance of an image that would otherwise be achieved using a true single-energy x-ray source without additional radiation or contrast administration [16]. These are generated by breaking down 2 basis materials, one with low density (e.g., water) and the other with high density (e.g., bone). The bone and water density maps are reconstructed in the projection domain, and then linearly merging the low-kVp and high-kVp mass density maps [8,17].

Low keV setting: increased attenuation or enhancement

Low-energy photons (e.g., near 40 kVp to 60 kVp) are near the K-edge of iodine (33.2 keV) [16]. Thus, VMI at low keV results to increased attenuation or enhancement for vessels, or tissues containing iodine (Fig. 3) [7,16]. However, image noise can increase [7,18]. Energy levels can be optimized with respect to resolution and noise between 40 and 60 keV [16] (between 40 – 70 keV in another study) [19]. An energy level of 50 keV is considered the most suitable to optimize contrast as it offers a reasonable combination of increased density and image sharpness [16]. Smoothing or iterative reconstruction can also minimize noise [18].

Applications for low-keV VMI include improved delineation of abnormalities (e.g., iodine-containing or enhancing lesions), analysis of vessels, salvage of poor contrast studies, reduction of iodine load, and optimization of image quality [16].

High keV setting: beam hardening and metal artifact reduction

Metal implants cause artifacts from beam hardening and photon-starvation effects, which appear as bright and dark streaks that can degrade image quality and obscure visualization of adjacent structures and pathologic processes [1].

High-energy photons (e.g. near 120 – 140 kVp) have less attenuation by materials in the body [16]. High keV VMI simulates increased radiograph beam penetration and helps reduce blooming and metallic artifacts [7]. Metal artifacts can be diminished between 95 keV and 150 keV, although contrast enhancement is reduced (Fig. 4) [17]. An energy level of 120 keV has been suggested to be optimal for minimizing beam-hardening artifacts during the initial assessment [16].

High keV monoenergetic images can also reduce beam hardening artifacts from injected contrast material in the subclavian veins, axillary veins (Fig. 5), or superior vena cava during chest computed tomography (CT) scans. In addition, VMI also enhances image quality, with optimal evaluations best achieved between 100 keV and 130 keV [20].

In pelvic CT scans of patients with hip implants, VMI at 200 keV are preferred for evaluating bone. At the same time, the dedicated metal artifact reduction algorithm is deemed more effective for assessing soft tissue [16,21].

The combination of metal artifact reduction software with high-keV VMI optimizes artifact reduction in patients with orthopedic foreign bodies in the spine [22]. Spinal fusion for scoliosis and repair of developmental hip dysplasia are clinical scenarios where metal implants may degrade the quality of CT images [1]. Beam hardening and metallic streak artifacts can be reduced using high-energy VMIs between 110 keV and 150 keV, preferentially removing the low-energy photons contributing to artifact degradation [1,10]. Optimal keV setting provides the lowest artifacts and highest diagnostic value is at 105 keV for routine high-energy reconstruction [23].

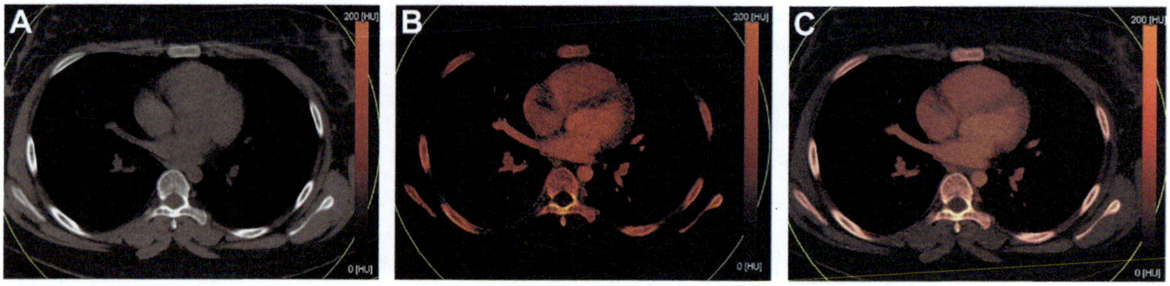

FIG. 2 Post-processing technique using material decomposition iodine-specific images in an axial computed tomography (CT) study of the chest of a healthy 12-y-old girl. (*A*) Virtual non-contrast CT image after subtraction of iodine content. (*B*) Iodine map image shows pure iodine content. (*C*) Iodine overlay image after superimposition of B on A.

This application can also assist in evaluating stent placement or stent-graft procedures [16,24].

ADVANTAGES OF THE DUAL-ENERGY COMPUTED TOMOGRAPHY POST-PROCESSING TECHNIQUES

Due to the material decomposition and VMIs generated by DECT, there is a reduction in the radiation dose and volume of iodinated-contrast material required, which is particularly helpful for the imaging of children [25].

Radiation-dose Reduction

Radiation-induced pediatric malignancies pose a constant concern because children are more vulnerable to radiation effects than adults. As they are still maturing, their cells are still rapidly dividing, making them vulnerable to mutations, and their smaller stature inadvertently exposes the adjacent organs beyond the imaging region of interest. Since they have a longer lifespan at the time of radiation exposure, there is extended latency period for developing long-term radiation-induced effects [26].

Radiation dose can vary depending on the manufacturer and the dual-energy systems used, and it may be reduced by substituting actual unenhanced images with virtual unenhanced images [1,5]. A study that compared weight-matched and region-matched SECT and DS-DECT of the chest and abdomen in children and young adults (mean age of 11 ± 6 y) concluded that DS-DECT resulted in a substantial reduction in radiation dose and contrast volume [27]. There have been many publications that show radiation level exposure from DECT is equivalent to or even lower than the comparable SECT examinations. This is attributed to better iterative reconstruction techniques, improved detector efficiency, and the addition of spectral filtration that attenuates photons at higher-energy tubes [1,2,28–31].

Contrast-enhanced abdominopelvic DECT studies for children, regardless of effective diameter, can be performed with a similar or lower dose and similar image quality compared with SECT examinations. DECT size-specific dose estimates were lower across all effective patient diameters compared with SECT (mean: 8.5 ± 1.8 mGy vs 9.3 ± 2.0 mGy, respectively, $P \leq .001$). Dual-energy CT dose index-volume ($CTDI_{vol}$) was lower compared to SECT (mean: 5.6 ± 2.4 mGy vs 6.1 ± 2.7 mGy, respectively, $P \leq .001$) except in the smallest diameter group (<15 cm) where it was comparable to SECT ($P = .065$) [32].

DECT, particularly the DS system, uses an ultra-high pitch mode, which can perform a CT procedure in less than a second. It is currently the fastest and lowest-dose scanner, providing the least motion degradation and optimizing image quality. Due to the inherent risk of radiation dose and anesthesia, notwithstanding the cost, fast acquisition, and non-sedate options can be opted for [33]. The DS-DECT also has tin filter in front of the high-kilovolt peak radiograph tube. The tin filter attenuates the lower-energy photons, thereby decreasing radiation exposure and increasing spectral separation [2].

Contrast Volume and Injection Rate Reduction

VMIs generated in DECT were also beneficial in imaging children with compromised renal functions or those who can only receive a small amount of contrast medium (infants, neonates, and very small children) or

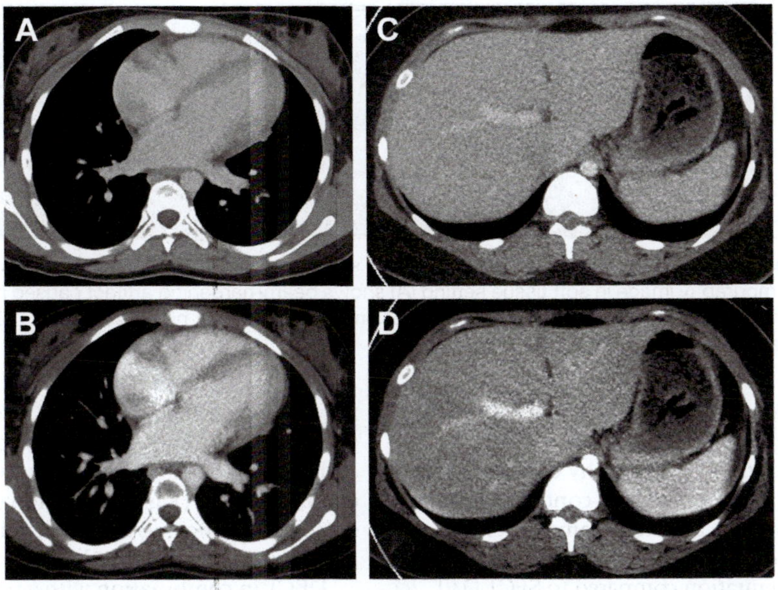

FIG. 3 Contrast-enhanced axial computed tomography images of the chest at the level of the heart (*A*) and abdomen at the level of the portal vein (*C*) in soft tissue window at 80 keV setting show faint enhancement of the cardiac chambers, aorta, portal vein, spleen, and other vessels. Post-processing technique using virtual monoenergetic images at 40 keV (*B* and *D*) demonstrates increased enhancement of these structures without added radiation exposure.

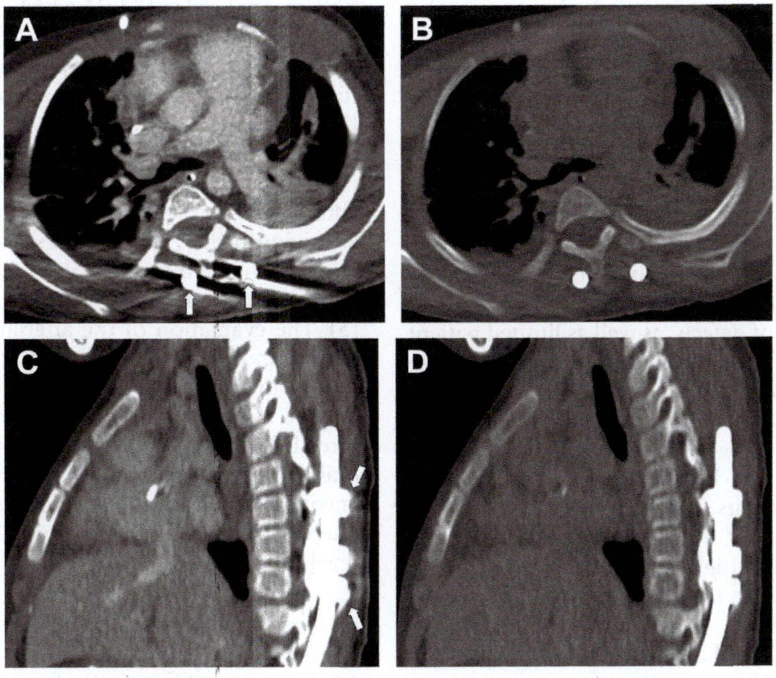

FIG. 4 Virtual monoenergetic image in a 6-y-old boy diagnosed to have congenital scoliosis, status-post spinal fusion. The spinal orthopedic devices (*arrows*) cause severe metal artifact in axial (*A*) and sagittal reformatted (*C*) images. Post-processing using a high keV setting (150 keV) decreases the artifact (*B* and *D*).

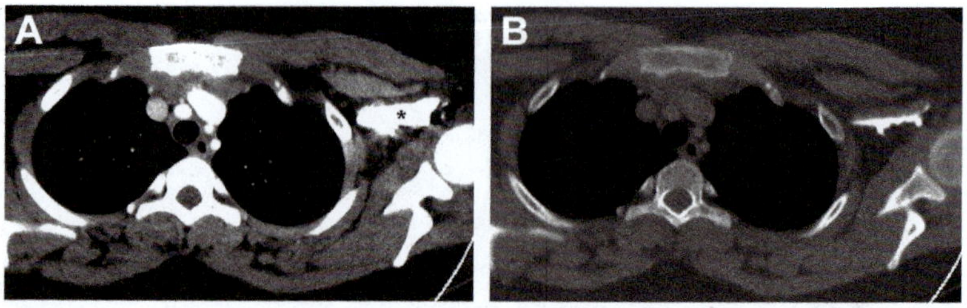

FIG. 5 Virtual monoenergetic image in 14/M who was suspected of pulmonary tuberculosis. Axial computed tomography image in soft tissue setting (*A*) shows beam-hardening artifact caused by intravenous contrast in the left axillary vein (*asterisk*). Post-processing image (*B*) with high keV setting (120 keV) shows significant decrease in the artifact.

slower contrast-medium injection rate (small-caliber intravenous [IV] catheter) [6,27]. Moreover, iodine-specific images used in CT angiography enhance vessel contrast and may allow a reduced-contrast medium dose [7]. This technique also maintains or enhances the contrast-to-noise ratio, and deliver better subjective vascular contrast attenuation compared to SECT [16].

CLINICAL APPLICATIONS OF DUAL-ENERGY COMPUTED TOMOGRAPHY IN PEDIATRIC IMAGING

DECT applications are used in vascular imaging, evaluating pulmonary parenchymal perfusion and pulmonary vasculature, characterizing solid organ lesions and bowel pathology, determining renal calculi composition, and assessing tumor viability and response to treatment [1].

Thoracic Applications

Congenital cardiac disease and vascular imaging

Imaging of pediatric congenital heart disease (CHD) is challenging due to the broad spectrum of diseases and the complex nature of defects, as well as limited patient cooperation, higher heart rate, and the need to minimize for radiation dose. Third-generation DS-DECT scanners are characterized by high-pitch, extended-anatomic coverage, and a more flexible electrocardiogram-synchronized scan, which allows procedures even for non-cooperative patients with minimal sedation, free breathing, and without administration of β-blockers for the heart rate. The high-temporal resolution minimizes motion artifacts. Dual-energy applications provide additional clinical information about vascular structures and myocardial and lung perfusion, allowing artifact reduction [12].

VMIs at lower energies can enhance the attenuation of vessels, thereby improving vascular imaging, as these lower energies are closer to the K-edge of iodine (33.2 keV) [5]. There is a better contrast-to-noise ratio and enhanced-image quality at low-keV VMI levels of 60 keV or lower (Fig. 6). Additionally, at 40 keV, the accuracy of diagnosing acute arterial bleeding and endoleaks is improved [34–37].

DECT in combination with a prospective (instead of retrospective) electrocardiogram (ECG)-gating during cardiac CT angiography reduces radiation dose by 64% and iodine doses by 40% in pediatric patients with CHD. Moreover, neither the quality of the images nor its diagnostic accuracy is compromised. The optimal VMI energy level is 45 keV, which demonstrated similar or higher luminal CT values, signal-to-noise and contrast-to-noise ratios compared to conventional scanning. Contrast-agent-related artifacts are also reduced [38].

Although uncommon in the pediatric age group, mural vascular calcifications may be observed in the chronic stage of arteritis (i.e., Kawasaki disease). Characterizing heavily calcified vessels in this clinical scenario using subtraction algorithms in DECT scans may eliminate the need for actual unenhanced images [5]. The evaluation of the arterial system also utilizes bone removal software in DECT angiography, which results in images that show only contrast-enhanced vessels, facilitating optimal evaluation of the vasculature [13]. This application is beneficial for the optimal evaluation of congenital and acquired conditions encountered in children, such as aortic coarctation, arteritis, and non-inflammatory aortitis, to mention a few [1,13].

Pulmonary perfusion and lung vessel evaluation

DECT scan is widely utilized in evaluating pulmonary vasculature [39–42]. Clinical indications for pulmonary CT angiography in children encompass the evaluation of vascular anatomy and parenchymal morphology in patients with pulmonary embolism, pulmonary atresia, and pulmonary hypertension. The advantage of DECT over conventional CT angiography lies in the additional information it provides regarding pulmonary perfusion and the evaluation of vessels and parenchyma without added radiation in one acquisition [1].

Iodine maps illustrate the distribution of iodine or the volume of perfused-lung parenchyma, enabling the visualization and quantification of perfusion defects. Increased perfusion may be expected in the dependent areas of the lung [1,43]. Otherwise, there is uniform blood flow in normal lung parenchyma (Fig. 7). Perfusion defects associated with occlusive pulmonary embolism appear as peripheral wedge-shaped areas with decreased or absent iodine content beyond the occluded, non-visualized segmental, or subsegmental vessel (Figs. 8 and 9) [1,44]. In contrast, non-occlusive emboli show variable amounts of lung perfusion. DECT perfusion findings in cases of pulmonary embolism correlate with scintigraphy and single-photon emission CT [1,45,46].

The DECT findings in chronic thromboembolic pulmonary hypertension and non-embolic pulmonary hypertension show peripheral triangular defects in the former and smaller non-segmental defects with a mottled pattern in the latter (Fig. 10) [1,47].

Neonates and infants with chronic lung disease of prematurity (CLDP, previously known as bronchopulmonary dysplasia) undergo CT angiography with DECT perfusion to evaluate for pulmonary hypertension. A finding of a heterogenous perfusion abnormalities seen throughout the lungs may reflect severe CLDP. However, the dense nature of the infant lung and limited ability of commercial software to accurately record and tabulate perfusion in these regions make the diagnosis challenging. Various abnormal perfusion patterns might have prognostic value. Patients with poorer perfusion are likely to have a higher risk for long-term ventilation dependence. Thus, further research is needed in this area [44].

Lung vessel iodine images reflect the distribution of iodine in the vasculature, allowing for the evaluation

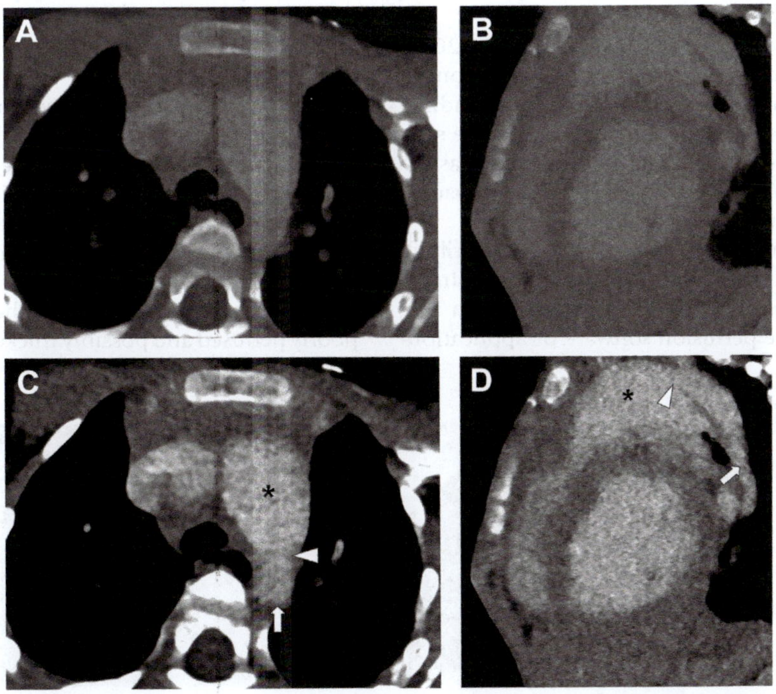

FIG. 6 Virtual monoenergetic post-processing technique in a 3-y-old girl diagnosed to have a complex congenital heart disease with patent ductus arteriosus (PDA). Contrast-enhanced axial (*A*) and sagittal reformatted (*B*) images in soft tissue window show suboptimal enhancement of the cardiac chambers and major vessels due to improper bolus timing. Using a low-keV (40 keV) setting (*C* and *D*), there is better delineation of the PDA (*arrowheads*) from the roof of the pulmonary artery (*asterisks*) to the descending thoracic aorta (*arrows*).

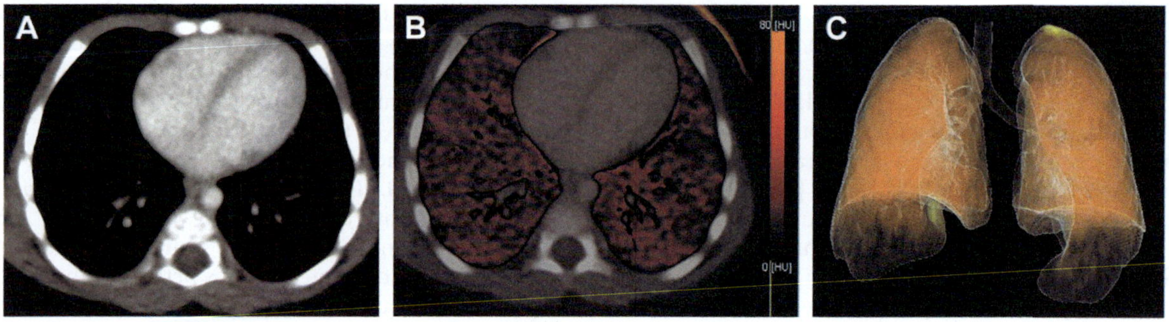

FIG. 7 Axial computed tomography image in soft tissue setting without (*A*) and with lung perfusion analysis showing normal uniform and homogenous blood flow bilaterally in 2-dimensional imaging (*B*) and 3-D (*C*) reconstruction.

of both enhancing and non-enhancing vessels. This technique may also be applied in assessing patients suspected of having an absent or hypoplastic pulmonary artery [1]. In cases of suboptimal CT pulmonary angiography scans caused by technical issues or incorrect contrast bolus timing, low-keV VMIs can effectively improve vessel visibility, thus eliminating the need for an additional scan or repeat examination [48].

Pulmonary infections (i.e., coronavirus disease 2019 [COVID-19] pneumonia) show increased perfusion or iodine distribution in the parenchyma surrounding the opacity or consolidation. This finding may be secondary to vascular dilation, contributing to increased-perfused blood volume. However, the lung opacity showed reduced perfusion on iodine maps [10].

Perfusion to pulmonary nodules has been described in adults. Pediatric lung lesions, like bronchopulmonary foregut malformations, can be evaluated in the similar manner. The perfusion software or application can determine the degree of enhancement, which may help differentiate a congenital pulmonary airway malformation (CPAM) from a bronchopulmonary sequestration (BPS). CPAM shows decreased perfusion compared to the normal lung (Fig. 11), while BPS can demonstrate increased perfusion because of the presence of a systemic arterial supply [33].

Abdominal Applications

Bowel evaluation

Non-ischemic bowel disease in children includes infectious colitis and inflammatory bowel disease, such as Crohn disease and ulcerative colitis. DECT findings of inflammatory-infectious bowel diseases show bowel wall thickening with associated hyperemia and increased iodine content on iodine overlay images (Fig. 12) [1].

Ischemic bowel diseases, on the other hand, exhibit poorly perfused and possibly thickened bowel segments

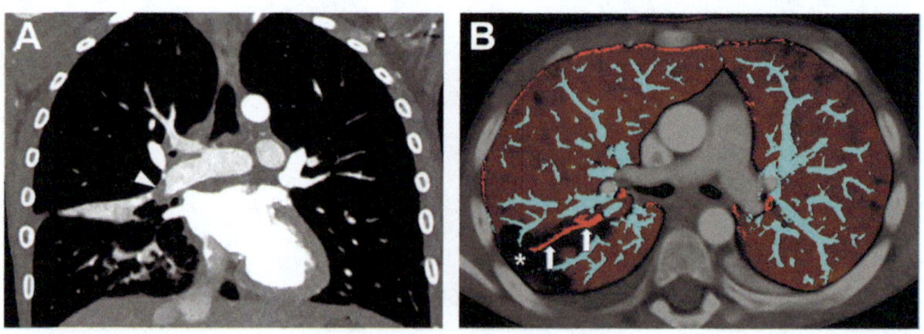

FIG. 8 Lung perfusion and vessel algorithm in pulmonary embolism. Contrast-enhanced coronal reformatted computed tomography image (*A*) shows a filling defect in the lower lobe branch (*arrowhead*) of the right pulmonary artery. Axial lung vessel image (*B*) better illustrates the vasculature demonstrating good flow (*in light blue*) and no flow (*in red, arrows*) with a corresponding wedge-shaped perfusion defect (*asterisk*). (*Courtesy of* Prof. M. Siegel, MD of the Edward Mallinckrodt Institute of Radiology, Washington University School of Medicine, St. Louis, Missouri.)

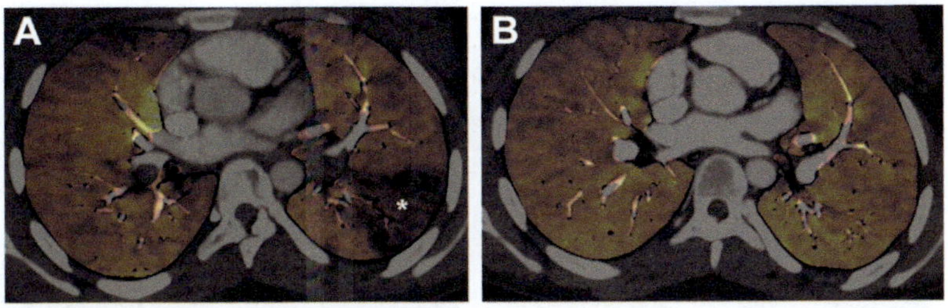

FIG. 9 Pulmonary embolism in an 18-y-old female. Axial computed tomography lung perfusion image at the time of diagnosis (*A*) shows a wedge-shaped defect in the left lower lobe (*asterisk*). Follow-up study (*B*) after treatment no longer demonstrates the perfusion defect.

with decreased or absent wall iodine content. This can occur in CHD, bowel obstruction due to intussusception, midgut volvulus or incarcerated hernia, hemolytic uremic syndrome, and necrotizing colitis [1,49].

In inflammatory-infectious and ischemic bowel diseases, the differences in enhancement between the hyperperfused, hypoperfused, and adjacent normally-perfused segments are highlighted using low-keV virtual-monoenergetic and iodine-specific images, which can maximize iodine contrast while minimizing the impact of noise [1]. Recent studies have shown that iodine overlay and virtual-monoenergetic imaging at lower energy levels (40 keV) can detect and differentiate mural hypoperfused segments from the normally perfused bowel wall [50]. Furthermore, the 40 keV VMI increases the conspicuity of wall vascularization in inflammatory intestinal lesions in Crohn disease [49,51] and acute bowel ischemia when combined with iodine maps [49,50]. Similarly in patients with small bowel obstruction, enhancement of the bowel wall can be appreciated with increasing confidence on 70 keV images compared with linearly blended images [49,52].

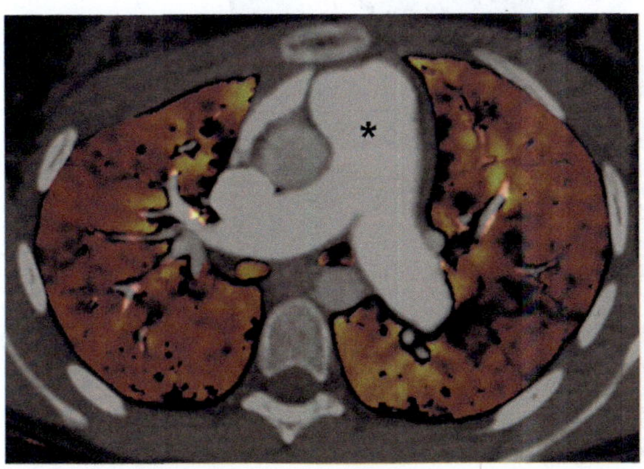

FIG. 10 Pulmonary arterial hypertension in an 11-y-old girl. Axial lung perfusion image shows dilated pulmonary arteries (*asterisk*) with the typical mottled pattern of perfusion in both lungs.

In the trauma setting, iodine map images can also increase the visibility of the iodine content in the bowel walls and VNC images, thus increasing diagnostic confidence in visualizing intramural hemorrhage [53].

Appendicitis

In early acute and uncomplicated appendicitis, there is increased conspicuity of appendiceal wall hyperemia on low-keV VMIs and increased transmural iodine content on iodine overlay images (Fig. 13) [1]. There is a statistically significant overall increased attenuation (average ratio of 1.7; $P<.05$), signal-to-noise-ratio ($P<.001$), and contrast-to-noise-ratio ($P<.001$) in the inflamed-appendiceal wall for the monoenergetic images (mean 107.1 $\pm$ 40 HU) compared to conventional ones (mean 62.9 $\pm$ 20.4 HU) ($P<.001$). Improved detection and increased conspicuity of subtle enhancement are observed compared to conventional CT, using low-monoenergetic images [54]. VMI reconstructions at 80 kVp with 70 keV yielded the best diagnostic performance ($P<.001$) in diagnosing acute appendicitis [55].

In non-perforated appendicitis with signs of necrosis or gangrene, focal or diffuse loss of transmural enhancement is seen on low-keV VMI with a corresponding transmural absence of iodine content on iodine overlay images. This additional information provides clinical value, as the presence of gangrene indicates impending perforation and necessitates prompt surgical intervention [1]. Similar principles can also be applied in cases of cholecystitis [10].

Renal stone

A non-enhanced CT scan confirms and evaluates renal stones suspected on sonography in patients with flank

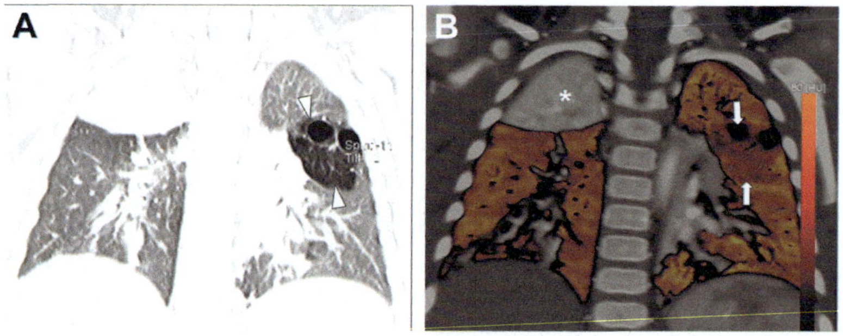

FIG. 11 Lung perfusion study in a 23-mo-old girl with congenital pulmonary airway malformation (CPAM). Coronal reformatted computed tomography image in lung window setting (*A*) shows confluent air-filled cystic structures (*arrowheads*) in the left upper lobe. Coronal lung perfusion image (*B*) demonstrates decreased perfusion (*arrows*) more so in the larger cysts superiorly. There is also note of a right upper lobe atelectasis (*asterisk*).

pain. In children, although uncommon, the most frequent stones are calcium oxalate, calcium phosphate, struvite, cystine, and uric acid in decreasing frequency. Differentiating uric from non-uric acid stones is clinically significant, as the composition may affect treatment strategies. Uric acid stones are treated with urine alkalinization, while calcium, struvite, and cystine stones may require mechanical removal or fragmentation depending on their size [1,5].

SECT is limited by partial volume averaging effects, precluding optimal stone composition analysis [5]. DECT can be used to analyze the differences in density or atomic number of the predominant materials within stones, with increased accuracy when larger than 3 to 5 mm in diameter (Fig. 14) [1,56]. Further characterization of non-uric acid stones to other subtypes (cystine, struvite, calcium oxalate, and hydroxyapatite) is also possible by applying additional tin filtration to the high-energy spectrum [1,57–60].

Using virtual non-enhanced images through the iodine-subtraction method, it is possible in DECT to help identify stones in contrast-opacified collecting

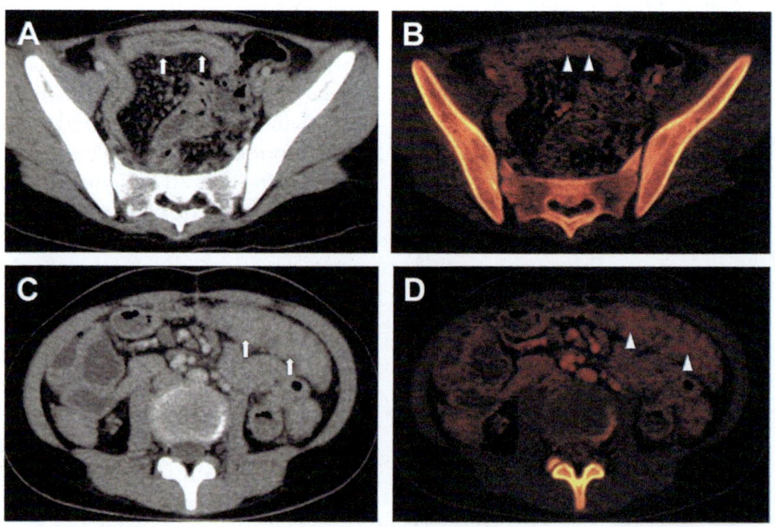

FIG. 12 Material-decomposition image in an 11-y-old girl diagnosed with Crohn disease. Contrast-enhanced axial computed tomography images in soft tissue setting show bowel wall thickening (*arrows*) in an ileal segment (*A*) and in the distal transverse colon (*C*). Post-processing with iodine overlay images (*B* and *D*) shows more conspicuous mucosal enhancement (*arrowheads*).

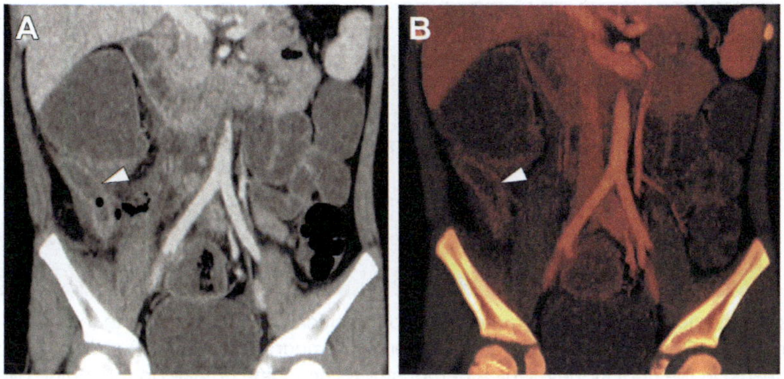

FIG. 13 Material-decomposition image in a 5-y-old boy with appendicitis. Contrast-enhanced coronal computed tomography reformatted image (*A*) shows a fluid-filled dilated appendix (*arrowheads*) with increased conspicuity of the transmural enhancement on the iodine overlay image (*B*).

systems enabling the detection of urinary calculi that may otherwise remain hidden. This technique is, however, limited by stones less than 3 mm, but these tiny calculi may not be clinically significant, as they can be passed spontaneously [1,5,61].

Solid organ evaluation

DECT can be helpful in further evaluation of solid organ lesions, like in the liver and pancreas, using the material-decomposition and VMIs. The conspicuity of hyperattenuating and hypervascular liver lesions

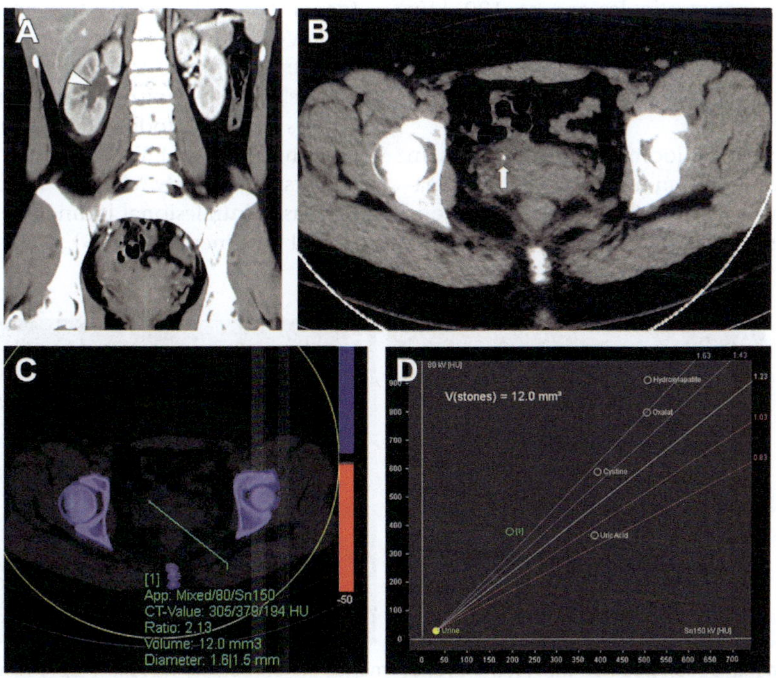

FIG. 14 Renal stone composition analysis in an 18-y-old girl with right flank pain. Contrast-enhanced coronal computed tomography (CT) image (*A*) shows mild dilation of the right renal pelvis (*arrowhead*). Axial CT image (*B*) reveals a tiny calcific focus (*arrow*) along the course of the right distal ureter. Renal stone algorithm auto-detects the ureterolithiasis with corresponding values (*C*) and its predominant non-uric acid composition (*D*).

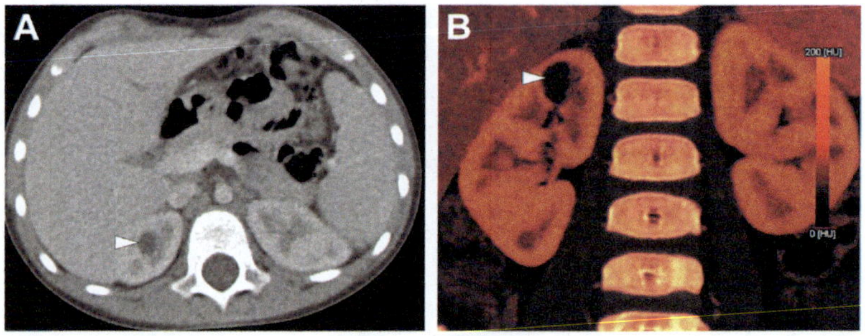

FIG. 15 Lesion characterization using material decomposition post-processing technique in a 4-y-old boy with abdominal pain. Contrast-enhanced axial computed tomography image (*A*) shows a hypodense ovoid focus (*arrowheads*) in the right kidney, which demonstrates no iodine uptake on the iodine overlay image (*B*) indicating a simple cyst. (*Courtesy of* Prof. M. Siegel, MD of the Edward Mallinckrodt Institute of Radiology, Washington University School of Medicine, St. Louis, Missouri.)

is increased at low-keV VMI (i.e., 80 keV) compared to conventional SECT scanners, and there is increased detection when obtained at the late arterial phase of enhancement [5,62]. For the pancreas, the attenuation differences between normal pancreatic parenchyma and pancreatic lesions were also more pronounced at lower energy levels of 80 kVp, enhancing the visibility of undetectable pancreatic lesions at 120 kVp [5,63].

Chest and abdominal masses and mass-like lesion evaluation

The increased visibility of iodine and differences in contrast enhancement between tumors and normal parenchyma aid in tumor staging [1,11,64,65]. There is also improved vessel conspicuity with low-energy VMIs (suggested at 50 keV to 55 keV) to achieve optimal image contrast, improving the definition of vessel-tumor margins and vessel enhancement, which has significant implications in tumor staging and surgical planning [11,64]. There is also improved detection of hypovascular lesions by improved differentiation with the normal parenchyma. The suggested VMI levels for soft tissue characterization are between 60 keV and 77 keV (Fig. 15) [64].

The response to treatment and tumor viability can also be assessed using qualitative and quantitative iodine images [1,2,66]. Iodine enhancement or high-iodine concentrations on DECT may indicate residual or viable tumors. Conversely, changes in tumor perfusion with decreased intralesional iodine content may signify successful treatment (Fig. 16) [1,2,11]. Areas of fibrosis

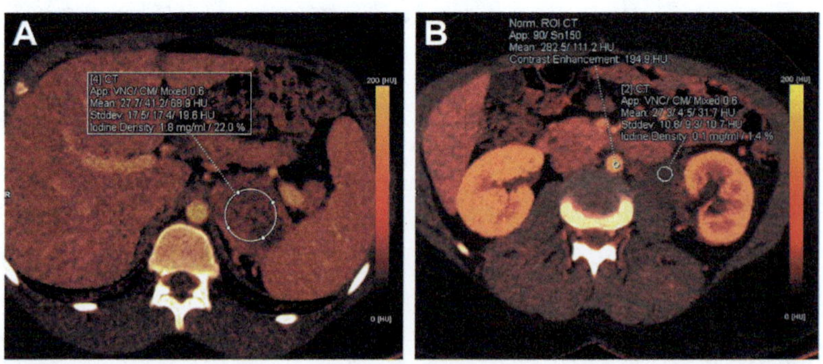

FIG. 16 Material decomposition with iodine overlay images in neuroblastoma follow-up. Pre-chemotherapy study (*A*) shows a left suprarenal tumor with baseline iodine concentration of 1.8 mg/mL. Post-chemotherapy study (*B*) shows a residual soft tissue structure with no iodine uptake reflective of complete treatment response. This was subsequently confirmed on scintigraphy using metaiodobenzylguanidine (MIBG) tracer. (*Courtesy of* Prof. M. Siegel, MD, Edward Mallinckrodt Institute of Radiology, Washington University School of Medicine, St. Louis, Missouri.)

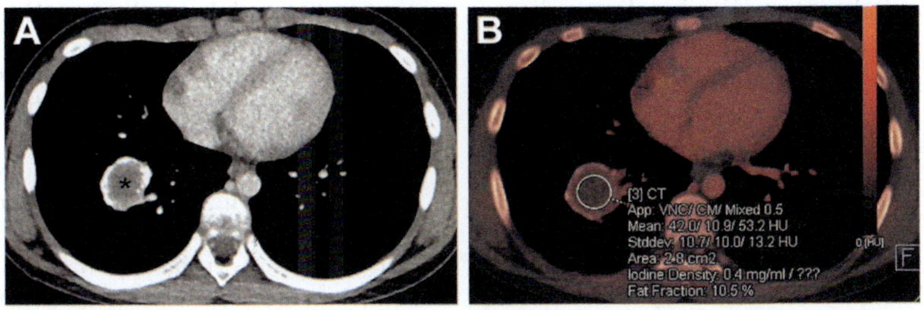

FIG. 17 Iodine concentration quantification in a 12-y-old boy previously treated for pulmonary tuberculosis (TB). Axial computed tomography (CT) image in soft tissue setting (*A*) shows a peripherally calcified, solid homogenous mass in the right lung (*asterisk*). Dual-energy CT iodine mapping (*B*) demonstrates a low iodine concentration (0.4 mg/mL) more in keeping with a benign or granulomatous disease like that of the known TB of the patient.

that can be seen in fibrosing mediastinitis or due to post-treatment changes in tumors like neuroblastoma or lymphoma show diminished iodine content relative to vessels on iodine-specific images [1,2].

Chest mass evaluation. Common thoracic masses in children include lymphoma, teratoma, neurogenic tumors (e.g., neuroblastoma), and bronchopulmonary foregut cysts. Cysts are non-enhancing and well-marginated lesions that are relatively homogeneous and of near water attenuation. They may occasionally be hyperattenuating due to proteinaceous or hemorrhagic content. In a single-phase contrast-enhanced DECT examination, VNC, and iodine-specific images may be generated to differentiate enhancing and non-enhancing tissues, and to reduce radiation exposure by eliminating actual non-enhanced studies. In VNC images, a hyperdense cyst that does not display iodine content supports a diagnosis of a complex cyst [1].

Iodine-specific images increase the conspicuity of the presence of iodine within a hyperattenuating mediastinal mass or pulmonary nodule, which raise concern for malignancy. Quantification of iodine content measured in mg/ml may differentiate malignant from benign tumors. Iodine concentration is greater than or equal to 1 mg/mL in malignant tumors (Fig. 17) [1,2].

Lymphadenopathy is commonly caused by lymphoma, metastases, and granulomatous disease. However, the nodal location, size, and attenuation values are non-specific to distinguish benign from malignant lymph nodes. Using DECT iodine-enhanced images and iodine concentration measurements may aid in the differentiation. The iodine content of malignant nodes is also higher when compared to that in granulomatous or inflammatory nodes [2].

Abdominal mass evaluation. Similar to chest masses, DECT with virtual monoenergetic and material decomposition techniques, such as VNC images and iodine mapping with quantification, are helpful in the setting of a pediatric abdominal mass [1,11] where a single-phase contrast-enhanced study is preferred also to reduce the radiation dose by eliminating actual non-contrast studies. VNC images help detect or confirm the presence of tumoral calcification and hemorrhage on a contrast-enhanced DECT examination. A potential pitfall, however, is that faint or small calcifications are sometimes not apparent, similar to tiny renal calculi discussed previously [11].

SUMMARY

Pediatric clinical applications of DECT encompass congenital cardiac and vascular imaging, pulmonary perfusion and vessel assessment, evaluation of solid and hollow organ pathology, determination of renal calculi composition, assessment of masses and mass-like lesions, tumor viability and treatment response, and reduction of metal and beam hardening artifacts.

Among various benefits of DECT, 2 post-processing techniques of DECT that best leverage its advantages in pediatric imaging are material-decomposition images and VMIs (or monochromatic). Radiation dose is optimized and reduced by eliminating the need for actual non-enhanced images in keeping with the 'As Low As Reasonably Achievable' principle. Improved visibility of lesions, even in suboptimal scans, is also achieved through multiple post-processing techniques that aid in characterizing the anatomy or pathology of concern, without the need for additional radiation exposure or increased contrast volume and injection rate.

A clear understanding of the technical aspects and characteristic imaging appearance of DECT applications in a variety of congenital and acquired pediatric disorders is a key to its optimal utilization and maximum benefit for managing pediatric patients in a daily clinical setting.

CLINICS CARE POINTS

- DECT is one of the newer innovations in CT technology that has many clinical applications in various organ systems.
- As long as the study was scanned using DECT, its applications and tools can be performed anytime without the physical presence of the patient and without prolonging the procedure time.
- DECT is not only in black, white, and gray, but can now be color-coded to provide functional information or disease activity qualitatively and quantitatively.
- DECT can increase the conspicuity of the lesions by virtually increasing the enhancement and lessening the artifacts without additional radiation exposure.

DISCLOSURE

The authors have nothing to disclose.

REFERENCES

[1] Siegel MJ, Ramirez-Giraldo JC. Dual-energy CT in children: imaging algorithms and clinical applications. Radiology 2019;291(2):286–97.

[2] Siegel MJ, Bhalla S, Cullinane M. Dual-energy CT material decomposition in pediatric thoracic oncology. Radiol Imaging Cancer 2021;3(1):e200097.

[3] Johnson TRC. Dual-energy CT: general principles. AJR Am J Roentgenol 2012;199:S3–8.

[4] Rassouli N, Etesami M, Dhanantwari A, et al. Detector-based spectral CT with a novel dual-layer technology: principles and applications. Insights Imaging 2017;8(6):589–98.

[5] Coursey CA, Nelson RC, Boll DT, et al. Dual-energy multidetector CT: how does it work, what can it tell us, and when can we use it in abdominopelvic imaging? Radiographics 2010;30(4):1037–55.

[6] Gottumukkala RV, Kalra MK, Tabari A, et al. Advanced CT techniques for decreasing radiation dose, reducing sedation requirements, and optimizing image quality in children. Radiographics 2019;39(3):709–26.

[7] Goo HW, Goo JM. Dual-energy CT: new horizon in medical imaging. Korean J Radiol 2017;18(4):555–69.

[8] Machida H, Tanaka I, Fukui R, et al. Dual-energy spectral CT: various clinical vascular applications. Radiographics 2016;36(4):1215–32.

[9] Chen CY, Hsu JS, Jaw TS, et al. Split bolus portal venous phase dual energy CT urography: protocol design, image quality, and dose reduction. AJR Am J Roentgenol 2015;205:W492–501.

[10] Hamid S, Nasir MU, So A, et al. Clinical applications of dual-energy CT. Korean J Radiol 2021;22(6):970–82.

[11] Kamps SE, Otjen JP, Stanescu AL, et al. Dual-energy CT of pediatric abdominal oncology imaging: private tour of new applications of CT technology. AJR Am J Roentgenol 2020;214(5):967–75.

[12] Schicchi N, Fogante M, Esposto Pirani P, et al. Third-generation dual-source dual-energy CT in pediatric congenital heart disease patients: state-of-the-Art. Radiol Med 2019;124(12):1238–52.

[13] Schulz B, Kuehling K, Kromen W, et al. Automatic bone removal technique in whole-body dual-energy CT angiography: performance and image quality. AJR Am J Roentgenol 2012;199(5):W646–50.

[14] Kalender W, Bautz W, Felsenberg D, et al. Material-selective imaging and density measurement using the dual-energy method. I. Principles and methodology [in German]. Digitale Bilddiagn 1987;7(2):66–72.

[15] Patino M, Prochowski A, Agrawal MD, et al. Material separation using dual- energy CT: current and emerging applications. Radiographics 2016;36(4):1087–105.

[16] Albrecht MH, Vogl TJ, Martin SS, et al. Review of clinical applications for virtual monoenergetic dual-energy CT. Radiology 2019;293(2):260–71.

[17] Yu L, Leng S, McCollough CH. Dual-energy CT-based monochromatic imaging. AJR Am J Roentgenol 2012;199(5 Suppl):S9–15.

[18] Geyer LL, Schoepf UJ, Meinel FG, et al. State of the art: iterative CT reconstruction techniques. Radiology 2015;276(2):339–57.

[19] McCollough CH, Leng S, Yu L, et al. Dual- and multi-energy CT: principles, technical approaches, and clinical applications. Radiology 2015;276:637–53.

[20] Kim C, Kim D, Lee KY, et al. The optimal energy level of virtual monochromatic images from spectral CT for reducing beam-hardening artifacts due to contrast media in the thorax. AJR Am J Roentgenol 2018;211(3):557–63.

[21] Laukamp KR, Lennartz S, Neuhaus VF, et al. CT metal artifacts in patients with total hip replacements:for artifact reduction monoenergetic reconstructions and post-processing algorithms are both efficient but not similar. Eur Radiol 2018;28(11):4524–33.

[22] Große Hokamp N, Neuhaus V, Abdullayev N, et al. Reduction of artifacts caused by orthopedic hardware in the spine in spectral detector CT examinations using virtual monoenergetic image reconstructions and metal-artifact-reduction algorithms. Skelet Radiol 2018;47:195–201.

[23] Bamberg F, Dierks A, Nikolaou K, et al. Metal artifact reduction by dual energy computed tomography using monoenergetic extrapolation. Eur Radiol 2011;21(7):1424–9.

[24] Mangold S, Cannaó PM, Schoepf UJ, et al. Impact of an advanced image-based monoenergetic reconstruction algorithm on coronary stent visualization using third

generation dual-source dual-energy CT: a phantom study. Eur Radiol 2016;26(6):1871–8.
[25] Yu T, Gao J, Liu ZM, et al. Contrast dose and radiation dose reduction in abdominal enhanced computerized tomography scans with single-phase dual-energy spectral computerized tomography mode for children with solid tumors. Chin Med J 2017;130:823–31.
[26] Tabari A, Patino M, Westra SJ, et al. Initial clinical experience with high-pitch dual-source CT as a rapid technique for thoraco-abdominal evaluation in awake infants and young children. Clin Radiol 2019;74(12): 977.e9-e15.
[27] Tabari A, Gee MS, Singh R, et al. Reducing radiation dose and contrast medium volume with application of dual-energy CT in children and young adults. AJR Am J Roentgenol 2020;214(6):1199–205.
[28] Goo HW. Initial experience of dual-energy lung perfusion CT using a dual-source CT system in children. Pediatr Radiol 2010;40(9):1536–44.
[29] Siegel MJ, Curtis WA, Ramirez-Giraldo JC. Effects of dual-energy technique on radiation exposure and image quality in pediatric body CT. AJR Am J Roentgenol 2016; 207(4):826–35.
[30] Siegel MJ, Street T, Ramirez-Giraldo JC. Pediatric diagnostic reference ranges for dual-energy dual-source abdominopelvic CT. In: abstract Archives of the Radiological Society of North America. 2018. Available at: https://archive.rsna.org/2018/18023128.html.
[31] Weinman JP, Mirksy DV, Jensen AM, et al. Dual energy head CT to maintain image quality while reducing dose in pediatric patients. Clin Imaging 2019;93:83–6.
[32] Siegel MJ, Mhlanga JC, Salter A, et al. Comparison of radiation dose and image quality between contrast-enhanced single- and dual-energy abdominopelvic computed tomography in children as a function of patient size. Pediatr Radiol 2021;51(11):2000–8.
[33] Rapp JB, Ho-Fung VM, Ramirez KI, et al. Dual-source computed tomography protocols for the pediatric chest - scan optimization techniques. Pediatr Radiol 2023; 53(7):1248–59.
[34] Albrecht MH, Trommer J, Wichmann JL, et al. Comprehensive comparison of virtual monoenergetic and linearly blended reconstruction techniques in third-generation dual-source dual-energy computed tomography angiography of the thorax and abdomen. Investig Radiol 2016;51:582–90.
[35] Albrecht MH, Scholtz JE, Hüsers K, et al. Advanced image-based virtual monoenergetic dual-energy CT angiography of the abdomen: optimization of kiloelectron volt settings to improve image contrast. Eur Radiol 2016;26:1863–70.
[36] Martin SS, Wichmann JL, Scholtz JE, et al. Noise-optimized virtual monoenergetic dual-energy CT improves diagnostic accuracy for the detection of active arterial bleeding of the abdomen. J Vasc Interv Radiol 2017;28:1257–66.
[37] Martin SS, Wichmann JL, Weyer H, et al. Endoleaks after endovascular aortic aneurysm repair: improved detection with noise- optimized virtual monoenergetic dual-energy CT. Eur J Radiol 2017;94:125–32.
[38] Xie M, Wang H, Tang S, et al. Application of dual-energy CT with prospective ECG-gating in cardiac CT angiography for children: radiation and contrast agent dose. Eur J Radiol 2024;170:111229.
[39] Alis J, Latson LA Jr, Haramati LB, et al. Navigating the pulmonary perfusion map: dual-energy computed tomography in acute pulmonary embolism. J Comput Assist Tomogr 2018;42(6):840–9.
[40] Goo HW. Dual-energy lung perfusion and ventilation CT in children. Pediatr Radiol 2013;43(3):298–307.
[41] Hwang HJ, Hoffman EA, Lee CH, et al. The role of dual-energy computed tomography in the assessment of pulmonary function. Eur J Radiol 2017;86:320–34.
[42] Ikeda Y, Yoshimura N, Hori Y, et al. Analysis of decrease in lung perfusion blood volume with occlusive and non-occlusive pulmonary embolisms. Eur J Radiol 2014;83-(12):2260–7.
[43] Lu GM, Zhao Y, Zhang LJ, et al. Dual-energy CT of the lung. AJR Am J Roentgenol 2012;199(5 Suppl):S40–53.
[44] Rapp JB, Biko DM, Barrera CA, et al. Current and future applications of thoracic dual-energy CT in children: pearls and pitfalls of technique and interpretation. Semin Ultrasound CT MR 2020;41(5):433–41.
[45] Thieme SF, Becker CR, Hacker M, et al. Dual energy CT for the assessment of lung perfusion: correlation to scintigraphy. Eur J Radiol 2008;68(3):369–74.
[46] Thieme SF, Graute V, Nikolaou K, et al. Dual energy CT lung perfusion imaging: correlation with SPECT/CT. Eur J Radiol 2012;81(2):360–5.
[47] Ameli-Renani S, Rahman F, Nair A, et al. Dual-energy CT for imaging of pulmonary hypertension: challenges and opportunities. Radiographics 2014;34(7):1769–90.
[48] Leithner D, Wichmann JL, Vogl TJ, et al. Virtual monoenergetic imaging and iodine perfusion maps improve diagnostic accuracy of dual- energy computed tomography pulmonary angiography with suboptimal contrast attenuation. Investig Radiol 2017;52:659–65.
[49] Çağlar Ö, Cesur E, Sade R, et al. Dual energy CT in necrotizing enterocolitis; a novel diagnostic approach. Turk J Med Sci 2021;51:2575–83.
[50] Lourenco PDM, Rawski R, Mohammed MF, et al. Dual-energy CT iodine mapping and 40-keV monoenergetic applications in the diagnosis of acute bowel ischemia. AJR Am J Roentgenol 2018;211:564–70.
[51] Lee SM, Kim SH, Ahn SJ, et al. Virtual monoenergetic dual-layer, dual-energy CT enterography: optimization of keV settings and its added value for Crohn's disease. Eur Radiol 2018;28:2525–34.
[52] Darras KE, McLaughlin PD, Kang H, et al. Virtual monoenergetic reconstruction of contrast-enhanced dual energy CT at 70keV maximizes mural enhancement in acute small bowel obstruction. Eur J Radiol 2016; 85(5):950–6.
[53] Potretzke TA, Brace CL, Lubner MG, et al. Early small-bowel ischemia: dual-energy CT improves conspicuity

compared with conventional CT in a swine model. Radiology 2015;25:119–26.

[54] Lev-Cohain N, Sosna J, Meir Y, et al. Dual energy CT in acute appendicitis: value of low mono-energy. Clin Imaging 2021;77:213–8.

[55] Topel Ç, Onur MR, Akpınar E, et al. Low tube voltage increases the diagnostic performance of dual-energy computed tomography in patients with acute appendicitis. Diagn Interv Radiol 2019;25(4):257–64.

[56] Kaza RK, Ananthakrishnan L, Kambadakone A, et al. Update of dual- energy CT applications in the genitourinary tract. AJR Am J Roentgenol 2017;208(6): 1185–92.

[57] Ascenti G, Siragusa C, Racchiusa S, et al. Stone-targeted dual-energy CT: a new diagnostic approach to urinary calculosis. AJR Am J Roentgenol 2010;195(4):953–8.

[58] Hidas G, Eliahou R, Duvdevani M, et al. Determination of renal stone composition with dual-energy CT: in vivo analysis and comparison with x-ray diffraction. Radiology 2010;257(2):394–401.

[59] Leng S, Huang A, Cardona JM, et al. Dual-energy CT for quantification of urinary stone composition in mixed stones: a phantom study. AJR Am J Roentgenol 2016; 207(2):321–9.

[60] Mansouri M, Aran S, Singh A, et al. Dual-energy computed tomography characterization of urinary calculi: basic principles, applications and concerns. Curr Probl Diagn Radiol 2015;44(6):496–500.

[61] Mangold S, Thomas C, Fenchel M, et al. Virtual nonenhanced dual-energy CT urography with tin-filter technology: determinants of detection of urinary calculi in the renal collecting system. Radiology 2012;264(1): 119–25.

[62] Marin D, Nelson RC, Samei E, et al. Hypervascular liver tumors: low tube voltage, high tube current multidetector CT during late hepatic arterial phase for detection - initial clinical experience. Radiology 2009; 251(3):771–9.

[63] Macari M, Spieler BM, Godoy MCB, et al. Dual source dual energy MDCT: comparison of 80 kVp and weighted average kVp data on pancreatic lesion conspicuity. In: abstract archives of the radiological society of north America. 2008. Available at: https://archive.rsna.org/2008/6009358.html.

[64] Agrawal MD, Pinho DF, Kulkarni NM, et al. Oncologic applications of dual-energy CT in the abdomen. Radiographics 2014;34(3):589–612.

[65] De Cecco CN, Darnell A, Rengo M, et al. Dual-energy CT: oncologic applications. AJR Am J Roentgenol 2012;199(5 Suppl):S98–105.

[66] Lee SH, Lee JM, Kim KW, et al. Dual-energy computed tomography to assess tumor response to hepatic radiofrequency ablation: potential diagnostic value of virtual non-contrast images and iodine maps. Investig Radiol 2011;46(2):77–84.

9780443413438